"Classical Chinese medicine emphasizes the concept of ShangGongZhiShen 上工治神, which states that the most highly skilled physicians treat their patients on the spiritual level (and not just the physical body). In this book, CT Holman shares very effective tools for practitioners who seek to heal every aspect of their patients—physical, emotional, and spiritual. May this book help countless people feel whole again."

—*Master Zhongxian Wu, lifelong Daoist practitioner and author of 12 books on Chinese wisdom traditions*

"Like a river approaching the sea, Chinese medicine textbooks published in the West have increased, not only in sheer volume, but also in their depth and breadth. There has been an ever-increasing literary focus on specialist areas of treatment. This book is an excellent example of this trend. Holman combines solid theory with practical hands-on approaches to the treatment of trauma. This very readable, yet also erudite text will be a welcome addition to any acupuncturist's bookshelf."

—*Nigel Ching, author of* The Fundamentals of Acupuncture *and* The Art and Practice of Diagnosis in Chinese Medicine

"This comprehensive guide to working with emotional trauma is an invaluable and timely addition to the field of Chinese medicine. While never minimizing the gravity of the impact of trauma on personal as well as collective levels, Holman consistently stands for the possibility of profound healing and transformation through our work with these wounds. This eminently optimistic book offers a wealth of information that is both practical and inspiring."

—*Lorie Eve Dechar, author of* Five Spirits: Alchemical Acupuncture for Psychological and Spiritual Healing

"As a patient, friend, and colleague of CT Holman, I can vouch for the powerful efficacy of his trauma treatment methods. This book represents a wonderful balance between solid traditional Chinese medicine and CT's own personal take on an important subject with immense clinical potential. You can see CT's courage, passionate enthusiasm, and inquisitive spirit sparkle in these pages!"

—*Sabine Wilms, Ph.D., www.happygoatproductions.com*

"I found this a stimulating and useful book, wide-ranging in its sources, unswervingly practical in its aim, backed by numerous research studies and trials, drawing on the author's experience of a multi-faceted approach to the diagnosis and treatment of emotional trauma, amply illustrated by examples and case studies. A valuable addition to an over-looked subject."

—*Peter Firebrace, international lecturer, writer, and practitioner*

"This book is the result of years of work integrating many of the seemingly disparate threads of Chinese medicine into a clinical tapestry. I have watched CT at work and can attest to the seriousness of his pursuit, his dedication to bringing the work of many teachers into a new vision and his compassion for his patients. This text represents a significant step in the treatment of trauma as it adds much-needed precision to diagnosis with well-described methodology. It takes aspects of channel palpation and diagnosis into new frontiers while providing an excellent example of how Chinese medicine can evolve in the face of the new challenges. I look forward to using these techniques in my own clinic."

—*Jason Robertson, L.Ac., Seattle, USA*

Treating Emotional Trauma with Chinese Medicine

*of related interest*

**Neuropuncture**
**A Clinical Handbook of Neuroscience**
**Acupuncture, Second Edition**
*Michael D. Corradino*
ISBN 978 1 84819 331 4
eISBN 978 0 85701 287 6

**Heavenly Stems and Earthly Branches—TianGan DiZhi**
**The Heart of Chinese Wisdom Traditions**
*Master Zhongxian Wu and Dr Karin Taylor Wu*
*Foreword by Fei BingXun*
HB ISBN 978 1 84819 151 8
PB ISBN 978 1 84819 208 9
eISBN 978 0 85701 158 9

**Psycho-Emotional Pain and**
**the Eight Extraordinary Vessels**
*Yvonne R. Farrell, DAOM, L.Ac.*
ISBN 978 1 84819 292 8
eISBN 978 0 85701 239 5

**The Art and Practice of**
**Diagnosis in Chinese Medicine**
*Nigel Ching*
ISBN 978 1 84819 314 7
eISBN 978 0 85701 267 8

# Treating Emotional Trauma with Chinese Medicine

## Integrated Diagnostic and Treatment Strategies

CT HOLMAN, M.S., L.AC.

Foreword by Lillian Bridges

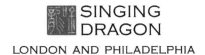
SINGING DRAGON

LONDON AND PHILADELPHIA

First published in 2018
by Singing Dragon
an imprint of Jessica Kingsley Publishers
73 Collier Street
London N1 9BE, UK
and
400 Market Street, Suite 400
Philadelphia, PA 19106, USA

*www.singingdragon.com*

**Library of Congress Cataloging in Publication Data**
Names: Holman, CT, author.
Title: Treating emotional trauma with Chinese medicine : integrated
   diagnostic and treatment strategies / CT Holman.
Description: London ; Philadelphia : Jessica Kingsley Publishers, 2017. |
   Includes bibliographical references.
Identifiers: LCCN 2017022522 (print) | LCCN 2017023136 (ebook) | ISBN
   9780857012715 () | ISBN 9781848193185 (alk. paper)
Subjects: | MESH: Psychological Trauma--therapy | Psychological
   Trauma--diagnosis | Medicine, Chinese Traditional--methods | Integrative
   Medicine | Case Reports
Classification: LCC RC552.T7 (ebook) | LCC RC552.T7 (print) | NLM WM 172.4 |
   DDC 616.85/21--dc23

**British Library Cataloguing in Publication Data**
A CIP catalogue record for this book is available from the British Library

ISBN 978 1 84819 318 5
eISBN 978 0 85701 271 5
Printed and bound by CPI Group (UK) Ltd, Croydon, CR0 4YY

For Dean and Julian,
the two gems continuing to shine light on my path

# Contents

# Foreword

Trauma is an unfortunate side-effect of living and when it occurs, as it does in everyone's life, there are emotional, psychological, and physical repercussions. Trauma can range from very mild to extremely debilitating, whether caused by a natural disaster, a war, a bad accident, or a personal tragedy. While many techniques have been developed for treating the intense manifestations of what is now called post-traumatic stress disorder or PTSD, the focus has been primarily on alleviating the physical symptoms that inhibit normal functioning. However, emotional trauma has insidious effects on health that have been less recognized and emotional trauma has often been undertreated.

Recent studies have proven that the body stores memories and trauma. Even inherited or epigenetic traumas manifest in a variety of physiological and psychological symptoms that often seem far removed from the original traumatic event. This is where Chinese medicine and other holistic treatments can be of great value in working with trauma. Chinese medicine has never differentiated between the mind, the emotions, and the body and teaches that what affects one affects all.

Chinese medicine also offers a variety of specific techniques for diagnosing dysfunction sometimes seen in the subtlest of signs. These diagnostic techniques include five element analysis, facial diagnosis, pulse diagnosis, channel palpation, tongue diagnosis, and more. Combining diagnostic methods allows Chinese medicine practitioners to get a clear picture of the blockages, whatever the cause, and also offers numerous methods for releasing and treating those blockages that have inhibited optimal functioning.

CT Holman spent many years intensely studying various diagnostic techniques with me and other eminent teachers. He was a dedicated student of facial diagnosis and was most interested in the application of these teachings in his clinic. He became one of the few advanced students with whom I conducted clinic visits. These visits involved a slightly longer intake, which included using facial diagnosis as a way to pinpoint and uncover traumas from the Facial Map of Life Experience, along with several other diagnostic techniques. A treatment plan was then developed from the signs on the face utilizing the map of emotions and the coloration of the face indicating particular organ involvement. At the end of the treatment, patients were evaluated for changes based on the facial signs and these changes were validated by before and after photos.

The results of CT Holman's treatments were phenomenal and manifested in obvious changes on the face including healthier coloration, an increase in Shen, and distinct changes in emotional affect. The most startling response to the treatments was the disappearance of some deep markings, including wrinkles! Ultimately, the treatments to release emotional trauma manifested in some profound health changes. My relationship with CT evolved to the point where he now co-teaches with me at conferences about clinical applications of facial diagnosis, where he presents and shares the protocols he has developed. I am so pleased to see facial diagnosis applied in the clinic in such a worthy way.

CT was and continues to be a skillful Chinese medicine practitioner dedicated to uncovering emotional trauma, treating it with the result of alleviating the suffering of his patients. I feel privileged to have been able to watch his evolution into a specialist in this field, which has culminated in this book.

CT Holman has given readers a thorough overview of the causes and the physiological manifestations of emotional trauma, in both Western and Eastern medical terms. There is a detailed discussion of five element diagnosis and facial diagnosis, both of which provide an understanding into the nature of an individual. He also brings in his knowledge of channel palpation, pulse diagnosis, tongue diagnosis, and intuitive diagnosis. Any of these modalities used alone are effective diagnostic techniques, but used together they give an in-depth understanding of the totality of the patient's condition at the present moment, which allows for much more specialized and personalized treatments.

His discussion of treatment methods that correspond to Chinese medicine syndromes, disharmonies, and emotional symptoms is comprehensive and gives many tested options that are easy to find and therefore use, due to numerous charts. Of particular importance are his techniques of "Gathering the Qi" and "Soothing the Trauma Memory" protocols. And, he includes many other methods including three of his other specialties—shaking qigong, bloodletting and shamanic drumming—as powerful release techniques. His lifestyle suggestions show his adherence to classical Yang Sheng practices and remind those of us in Chinese medicine how important these practices are for strengthening the body in order to deal with trauma.

My personal favorite chapter is Chapter 5, "Prevention of Emotional Trauma." Prevention is at the heart of Chinese medicine and gives readers the understanding of how to build resistance and resilience to trauma. Prevention is also one of the cornerstones of ancient Chinese medical wisdom, where you treat disease before it arises. This gives people the ability to handle whatever life throws at them.

*Treating Emotional Trauma with Chinese Medicine* is a book that all Chinese medicine practitioners should read. I believe it will change how they practice in the best possible ways. This book highlights the potential of emotional trauma treatment and will inspire anyone suffering from trauma to see that there are techniques that work to relieve the effects of emotional trauma. The techniques offered in this book have been proven to work on the levels of Jing, Qi and Shen and achieve the goal of bringing back the peacefulness of a happy heart.

*Lillian Pearl Bridges, Founder of the Lotus Institute, Inc. and author of*
Face Reading in Chinese Medicine, *Seattle, WA*

# Acknowledgments

Teachers provide light to help a student navigate the path to their heart. Several aspects of this book materialized from the information shared by my beloved teachers. I thank Lillian Bridges for her encouragement, her amazing insights, and for inspiring me to teach. I am grateful to Master Zhongxian Wu for his instruction in ancient wisdom concepts and powerful shamanic qigong training. My daily practice of these powerful qigong forms made this book possible. The treatments and cultivation methods described in this book healed me personally and benefited hundreds of patients.

Thank you to Dr. Wang Ju-Yi and Dr. Wei-Chieh Young for imparting their abundant knowledge of channel theory, diagnostic techniques, and acupuncture treatments. During the process of completing this book, Dr. Wang passed away. He will always be remembered for his pioneering spirit and dedication to bringing healing to many. Several of the protocols presented within are directly from his teachings and I am truly grateful to have studied with him. I am also appreciative of the pulse diagnostic techniques taught to me by Brian LaForgia, L.Ac., and Brandt Stickley, L.Ac. Thanks to Susan Johnson, L.Ac., for her wonderful instruction on scalp acupuncture in the treatment of emotional trauma and to Nam Singh for his excellent lessons on Chinese nutritional therapy. I thank Yefim Gamgoneishvili, L.Ac., for teaching and mentoring me early on in my studies. Also, thank you to Pat Keenan for sharing her knowledge while I was interning for her in an outpatient psychiatric clinic in San Francisco.

I thank my colleagues for all their insights, especially Jason Robertson. His friendship and inspiration over the years, from studying together in China to debating over campfires, has fueled the continual expansion of learning and enjoyment of the medicine. I very much appreciated his jovial, razor-sharp critiques of the various drafts as he prodded me toward completion.

Thank you to all my students for their support and kindness along the way. Their dedication to the medicine continually encourages me to refine my treatments and teaching.

I am deeply grateful for all the years of learning and refinement gleaned from treating patients—the ultimate teachers. Also, big thanks to the patients who agreed to share their stories in this text—a generous act in the spirit of benefiting others.

We are all patients of life and this book would not be possible without my healers, Michael Haefler, Karen Davis, Jennifer Distrola, Wendy Childs, L.Ac., Charlie Ramsey, ChristiEl, Sherri Clark, and Alandra Napali Kai. I also want to thank another set of "healers"—my band mates Timmy Miles, Matt Williams, and Preston Koch for keeping punk rock'n'roll and my sanity alive in our band, Midnight Persuasion.

Thank you to my editor Claire Wilson and the lovely staff at Singing Dragon. Thanks to Kirsteen Wright for the marvelous illustrations, to Julian Holman for the contribution of his fantastic drawings, to Master Wu, Lillian Bridges, Dr. Wang, and Jason Robertson for sharing images from their books, and to Tammy Anderson, L.Ac., for creating the stunning and most accurate Facial Organ map available.

A big thanks to all who contributed excellent insights on the various drafts: Lillian Bridges, Jason Robertson, L.Ac., Master Zhongxian Wu, Alex Scrimgeour, L.Ac., Lesley Garber, M.D., Julian Holman, and Rick Breen, whose advice and tireless efforts improved my writing skills.

Thanks to my dad for his incredible emotional support, love, and guidance through life and the writing process. I thank my mom and sister for their love. Thank you to my kids, Dean and Julian, for sacrificing their time, helping with seemingly endless chores, and bringing laughter and fun into my life.

Thank you to Tammy Anderson for her expertise in editing and helping through this transformational process.

*CT Holman, III*

# Preface

Stillness allows for processing and transforming emotional trauma, ultimately awakening a person's potential. Lao Zi, in Chapter 15 of the *Dao De Jing,* emphasized the importance of stillness to transform energy in the question, "Who can be murky and use the gradual clarification of stillness? Who can be at rest and use the gradual arising of movement after a long while?" (Cleary 1989, p.16). When a person experiences trauma and is haunted by its memory, Chinese medicine stills the body and harmonizes the organ systems, establishing stability for the person to realize the magic held within. Analogous to the butterfly emerging from the chrysalis, the person emerges vibrantly transformed. The cells in the butterfly responsible for the metamorphosis are called "imaginal."

Imaginal cells are akin to the individualized wisdom present in all living things. Each person has "imaginal cells"—a potential of greatness, lying in wait for the light of a person's inner knowing to turn them on. Emotional trauma blocks a person's sight, sense, internal wisdom, and the activation of their unique gifts. Transforming the trauma, freeing the stagnation, and addressing the pathogenesis created by trauma enables a person to manifest their potential and step into their version of a butterfly. This progression serves as a catalyst for accessing excellence. Many great inventors, artists, and leaders point to some hardship or trauma they overcame to reach extraordinary achievement.

The cycle of birth, death, and renewal abounds in life, as well as in the practice of medicine. Attaining another level of proficiency requires wisdom, growth, insight, connection, and refinement. Chinese medicine continues to evolve. Every generation embraces and assimilates innovative ideas, while honoring the ancient theories utilized successfully over millennia. Following core concepts and lineages, newness emerges. Classical, traditional, and shamanic healing approaches presented in this text demonstrate Chinese medicine's synergistic capacity to resolve emotional trauma. Modern research, Western medicine theories, and integrated treatments enhance the ability to metamorphose trauma. Finally, mainstream acknowledgment of the magic stored by the divine feminine in cultures all over the world is growing. This renewed acceptance of mysticism by the general public fosters a creative approach to medicine. I credit a large part of my understanding of resolving trauma to this revolution in medicine.

I, too, have suffered from emotional trauma. Through learning ancient wisdom modalities, coupled with contemporary medical advancements, my healing process commenced. My past emotional traumas cleared. The experience acted alchemically to open my heart and inner knowing. This allows me to intuit imbalances in patients, especially in regard to the five minds, that is, the spirits of the organs. Connecting with my constitutional nature and using Chinese medicine, I guide patients through the transformation process to clear emotional trauma.

My heritage is Irish, Lithuanian, English, and German, and I access these pre-Christian, influential roots to facilitate healing. The Goddesses and High Priestesses in past generations utilized the healing power of herbs and other modalities to treat a variety of ailments, including emotional trauma. These women were respected leaders who worked in conjunction with the divine masculine. This balance has been disturbed over the last 2000 years, but a new alignment is now emerging. The time of embracing a new approach to medicine is here.

Jason Robertson (my good friend and colleague) told me, "I know you are enamored with the ancient way, but do not forget that Chinese medicine is alive, constantly evolving every moment." This reminder influences my practice of Chinese medicine and I present the information in this book with the intent to inspire the continuation of the dancing, growing, and refining of medicine in clinics everywhere.

The cover of the book was chosen in honor of my Chinese name, Hong Xi Ting, which translates as "red pavilion in the west." This shelter sits next to a reflecting pool. When the heart reflecting pool stills, a person realizes their innate wisdom. My Western name, Clarence (meaning light/clear), embodies the clarity gifted to me through the means of metamorphosing my trauma. May the information in this book inspire the reader and bring calm, healing light to those processing emotional trauma.

*CT Holman, III*
*Salem, Oregon, USA*
*February 18, 2017*

**Reference**

Cleary, T. (trans.) (1989) *Immortal Sisters: Secret Teachings of Taoist Women.* Berkeley: North Atlantic Books.

# CHAPTER 1

# Introduction to Emotional Trauma

A woman grabs her son and dives under a table. She huddles with him waiting for the enemy fire to cease. Seconds later, she realizes she is no longer in Iraq on active duty, but in her house and the neighbor's kids are setting off firecrackers.

Tires screech across the pavement. A man at a stoplight feels his neck tighten as a wave of fear sweeps over him. He prepares to be rear-ended yet again, but then sees it is just teenagers "hot rodding" down the street.

A husband and wife have a heated argument. The husband slams the door and storms out of the bedroom. The wife suddenly feels seven years old and experiences intense abdominal pains, just as she had when her dad left her when she was a child.

Across the globe, people seek medical care for health conditions caused by emotional trauma. The trauma and its memory create disruption of the natural body rhythms resulting in physical pains, organ diseases, and emotional imbalances. Resolving the trauma restores the body's natural ability to regulate and heal itself.

## Causes of Emotional Trauma

Chinese medicine recognizes the seven emotions as a major cause of disease when they upset the physiological regulatory functions of the body (Gongwang, Hyodo, and Quing 1994, p.123). An emotional trauma activates the emotions and, if unprocessed, lodges in the body, causing imbalances. Each time the person relives the trauma memory, the disharmony in the organs and acupuncture channels worsens. Digestive disorders, respiratory distress, cardiological conditions, chronic pain, and so on can all result directly from emotional trauma. Until the trauma clears, a person remains held back from accessing their full potential.

Everyone experiences emotional trauma at some point in their life, whether *in utero*, at birth, in childhood, in adolescence, or in adulthood. Trauma can be caused by a car accident, emotional upheaval (e.g., divorce, major move, job loss), a natural disaster, medical complications, childbirth, physical or emotional assault, a negative health diagnosis, losing a loved one, and many others. Trauma can be inherited as well. Chinese medicine unties the deep-seated knot of trauma and restores harmony in the body's systems.

The adage "what doesn't kill you makes you stronger" applies to emotional trauma. The Merriam-Webster Dictionary defines trauma as "*a:* an injury (as a wound) to living tissue caused by an extrinsic agent; *b:* a disordered psychic or behavioral state resulting from severe mental or emotional stress or physical injury; *c:* an emotional upset." The origin of the word trauma comes from the Greek word *traumat-*, meaning wound. Each person experiences and interprets events differently—what is traumatic for one person may not be for another. For those who are traumatized, the event needs to be processed and released from their consciousness. If the emotions relating to the event are not cleared, its memory continues to be triggered and patients develop what is known as post-traumatic stress disorder (PTSD).

PTSD, a diagnosis first established in 1980 (Van der Kolk 2014, p.19), was initially associated with combat trauma, but current research and development in Western medicine correlates PTSD to a variety of stressful events. Car accidents, assault, natural disasters, a mother experiencing a difficult delivery, and a major health event such as a heart attack are some of the events to possibly cause PTSD. A person exposed to (experiencing or hearing about) trauma may suffer from emotional distress, but not everyone will develop clinical PTSD. Risk factors of developing PTSD include: intensity and number of traumas, trauma experienced early in life, certain professions (military, first responders, etc.), a lack of a good support system, and genetic predisposition for mental illness (Mayo Clinic 2017). Emotional trauma and PTSD cause physiological imbalances, both emotionally and physically. Trauma has a common global effect on the body as well as a unique impact on each person based on their constitution.

## The Physiology, Diagnosis, and Treatment of Trauma

Emotional trauma—whether experienced, witnessed, passed down genetically, or even heard about second-hand—is a pathogen that creates disharmony (Figure 1.1). If left untreated, it leads to chaos in the body and affects the three treasures, Jing, Qi, and Shen (see the table below).

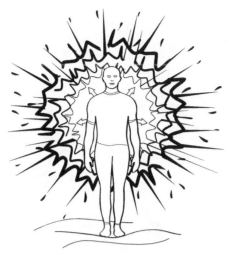

*Figure 1.1 Scattering of the Qi*
*Source:* Kirsteen Wright

## THE EFFECT OF EMOTIONAL TRAUMA ON THE THREE TREASURES

| | | |
|---|---|---|
| **Jing** | The material basis of the body and the fluid essence of the body's life force. | Disrupted, frozen, and/or depleted. |
| **Qi** | The energy animating the body. | Disordered, blocked, and exhausted. |
| **Shen** | The consciousness, emotional body, and thoughts. | Disturbed and unrooted. |

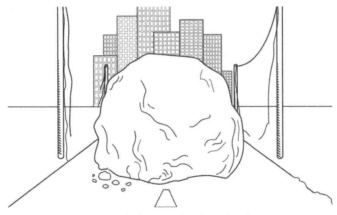

*Figure 1.2 Blockages in the Channel Pathways*
*Source:* Julian Holman

Organ systems and channel pathways are hindered or blocked (akin to a road block—Figure 1.2), resulting in various disruptions. These can be due to heat/fire, rebellious qi, qi/blood stagnation, and/or phlegm/damp accumulation. Until they are re-ordered, the channels and organs become depleted. Emotional trauma affects the body in three stages (see the table below).

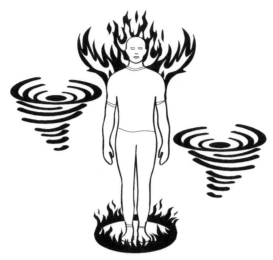

*Figure 1.3 Reliving the Trauma Memory causing Heat and Wind*
*Source:* Kirsteen Wright

**THE PHYSIOLOGICAL STAGES OF TRAUMA**

| | |
|---|---|
| **Stage One:** The Traumatic Event | The initial trauma scatters the qi (Figure 1.1), distresses the earth element, and disturbs the Shen. The pericardium tightens to protect the heart and the trauma becomes trapped, leaving the body unable to process the event. Emotions enter the body like wind, typically involving fear along with their constitutional emotional temperament. Blockages of Jing, qi, and blood occur throughout the body, leading to heat and/or cold and eventually an accumulation of phlegm/damp. |
| **Stage Two:** Reliving the Trauma Memory (PTSD) | The reliving of the trauma memory generates heat and wind (Figure 1.3). Emotions intensify and blockages increase. These blockages disrupt the flow of qi and cause rebellious qi. |
| **Stage Three:** Unresolved Trauma in the Body | The unresolved trauma exacerbates the blockages, heat, wind, cold, and phlegm/damp accumulation and depletes qi, blood, yin, and/or yang. A mixed excess and deficiency pattern is inevitable. If a patient is predisposed to heat, then the fluids are depleted, giving rise to yin deficiency. If cold was initially trapped in the body, then the yang eventually declines. The blockages in the channels and organ systems exhaust qi and blood. |

## *Diagnosing the Various Disharmonies*

Until these traumas are addressed, they continue to upset the harmony of the body's physiology, scatter the qi (the body's life-force), and reduce the body's innate ability to heal and regulate itself. Chinese medicine diagnostics provide insight into the various disharmonies involved.

Multiple diagnostics significantly increase the accuracy of understanding the root of the emotional trauma, ultimately allowing for swifter and more complete treatment. From Chapter 13 in the *Classic of Difficulties* (*Nan Jing*): "The inferior doctor knows one [diagnostic approach], the mediocre two, while the superior doctor can utilize all three. The superior ones can [cure] nine out of ten [illnesses], the mediocre ones [help] eight out of ten while the inferior doctor only [cures] six out of ten." (The three approaches are radial pulse diagnosis, diagnosis of the color of the skin [i.e., facial diagnosis], and channel examination.)

Sometimes a patient will simply know the source of their emotional trauma and communicate clearly how it influences their body. However, if the root is unclear and/ or suppressed, utilizing multiple diagnostics reveals the nature of the trauma. Five element, facial, channel palpation, pulse, tongue, and intuitive spirit diagnoses serve to give the practitioner a subjective means with which to understand the organ systems and channels needing treatment. The resolution of emotional trauma follows three distinct stages (see the table below).

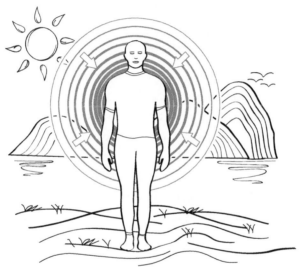

*Figure 1.4 Gathering the Qi*
*Source:* Kirsteen Wright

**THE STAGES OF TREATING EMOTIONAL TRAUMA**

| | |
|---|---|
| **Stage One:** Gathering the Qi | The patient's qi must be centered by supporting their earth element, stabilizing their Shen, regulating their pericardium, and releasing blockages—connect to "Mother Earth" (yin). |
| **Stage Two:** Soothing the Trauma Memory | The charge of the trauma memory must be soothed, the fire and wind reduced, and the Shen calmed by bringing down cosmic water—connect to "Father Sky" (yang). |
| **Stage Three:** Treating the Individual Imbalances | Each patient reacts differently to trauma and presents with unique signs and symptoms. After the qi is gathered and the charge of the trauma memory is reduced, these can now be addressed— harmonize the flow of energy between Mother Earth (yin) and Father Sky (yang). |

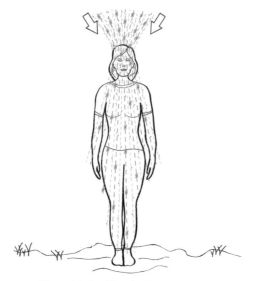

*Figure 1.5 Soothing the Trauma Memory*
*Source:* Kirsteen Wright

The treatment of emotional trauma begins with remedying overall shock to the body and then working on those specific channel and organ systems involved. "Gathering the Qi" (Figure 1.4) is the essential first step followed by "Soothing the Trauma Memory" (Figure 1.5). Finally, when the patient's general ability to regulate and nourish themselves is established, specific channels and organs affected for the individual are addressed. If treatments targeted at specific complaints (whiplash, digestive upset, memory loss, body pains, insomnia, etc.) are given while the patient is still in the throes of the trauma, the systems are in chaos and will not respond properly.

## Case Study: "Gathering the Qi" to Restore the Innate Healing Ability of the Body

A 67-year-old single woman, "Leonora," came to the Chinese medicine clinic with a wrist fracture. Falling on the lava flows in Hawaii, she incurred an open fracture (the bone protruded through the skin). The physical trauma was a significant shock affecting her emotions. She reported having an overwhelming feeling of vulnerability and poor concentration. The trauma triggered an underlying emotional condition of being alone in the world—Leonora had experienced several abandonments in the past. Her trauma scattered the qi and stirred up old patterns of feeling vulnerable, leaving her "out of sorts." Her qi first needed to be grounded and harmonized before any specific acupuncture points were used to treat her physical pain.

The first acupuncture treatment for this patient focused on gathering her qi and stabilizing her Shen. The patient returned the following week and reported a substantial reduction in feeling vulnerable and confused, reflecting a harmonious qi flow. She said the pain in her wrist had lessened. This treatment approach to gather qi improved her symptoms without using specific acupuncture points or Chinese herbs for pain. Harmonizing the qi allowed the innate healing of the body to flourish and subsequent treatments involved reducing heat and wind caused by the memory of falling and feeling helpless. Once the trauma memory was soothed, the heat depleting her yin was addressed in order to build bone strength and resolve kidney deficiency. Her trauma resolved and she implemented lifestyle modifications to prevent the future triggering of emotional imbalances created by her trauma memory.

---

The treatment protocol of emotional trauma is likened to helping an injured animal. If "Brandy," a Labrador, cut her paw on a wire and was lying on the ground in pain, she would need help. The dog would be scared if a person simply grabbed her paw to apply antiseptic, and might bite the helping hand. First, the person attending to Brandy must establish trust and energetically communicate their intention to help. Brandy would sense the person's good intentions and feel settled; she would be grounded. Next the person would gently pet and comfort Brandy to calm any fright, thereby soothing the memory of the trauma. At this point, when she was centered and relaxed, the person could treat her injured paw.

Chinese medicine treats disharmonies by utilizing multiple modalities such as acupuncture, herbal medicine, cupping (cups applied with suction to the skin to increase circulation), qigong (cultivating vital energy), nutritional therapy, drum healing (the use of vibrations to stimulate the channel pathways), heat therapy, and other supplemental treatments. In combination, these treatments work synergistically to efficiently accomplish the three stages of treatment. The individual then works to maintain harmony in the body to prevent the trauma memory from reoccurring.

## Triggering of the Trauma Memory

People seeking treatment for emotional issues are often suffering from past emotional trauma. A person reporting anxiety may have trauma as the root cause. Their anxiety may have begun after a certain event, or their underlying anxiety was exacerbated after an event.

## Case Study: Emotional and Physical Symptoms Resulting from Emotional Trauma

A 34-year-old woman, "Stella," reported having experienced anxiety since childhood. After moving to a new town, having a baby, divorcing, and starting a new job, her anxiety rose to a new level. Stella eventually settled into her new town, remarried, and found a less stressful job. However, her anxiety remained strong. She experienced increased body pain, digestive distress, and insomnia. It was only after being treated with Chinese medicine to address the different traumas that her anxiety was reduced and she could manage her stress. Stella adapted to changes with a new-found ease. Her physical symptoms were reduced and eventually stabilized. The protocols of grounding, soothing qi, and eventually focusing on specific constitutional imbalances helped resolve the root of her emotional and physical issues.

This is a common example of a reaction to a trauma bringing disorder to the system. Anxiety is one of the emotional manifestations that can occur. Fear, anger, depression, worry, sadness, and so on are all possible responses to emotional trauma and its memory. Each emotion relates to a specific organ system in Chinese medicine. The organ systems have several associations including the five elements and spirits/minds. The elements of water, wood, fire, earth, and metal help define each organ system and contain their own set of personality traits and mental attributes. The emotions and personality traits of a patient provide clues as to which organ system is disturbed by the trauma.

The age at which a trauma occurs influences organ systems (see the table below). If a patient reports experiencing an emotional trauma during childhood, the liver/gallbladder system requires attention to fully resolve the trauma.

**THE TIME A TRAUMA OCCURS AFFECTS CERTAIN ORGANS**

| Time Trauma Occurred | Element/Organ System Affected |
| --- | --- |
| Time *in utero* | Water/Kidney |
| Childhood through the teen years | Wood/Liver |
| Maturity | Fire/Heart |
| Later years of life | Metal/Lung |

### Processing Trauma

The skills needed to process trauma are learned through life experience. Having a nurturing childhood filled with love and encouragement enables a person to process and move through stressful events. After a traumatic event, a person must move through the "stages of trauma processing" (anxiety, aggression, insight, sorrow, and confidence) for them to fully clear a trauma (Raben 2011). Unfortunately, many people lack all the skills needed to process effectively, due to childhood trauma or to an absence of nurturing. When faced with a trauma, the person can become stuck in one of these stages, not fully processing the trauma. Until it is resolved, the charge of the traumatic event stays with them and revives each time it is triggered. In order to process trauma, Chinese medicine treatment supports the channels and organs, providing nourishment to address any deficiency in their childhood.

### Post-Traumatic Stress Disorder (PTSD) and Inherited Trauma

Each event provokes emotions, manifesting symptoms when a similar situation arises. When triggered, the individual "relives" the event and their qi is scattered. Until this initial trigger is cleared—or at least lessened—the body is vulnerable to future scattering of the qi, ultimately compromising the homeostasis of the body. PTSD and emotional trauma manifest differently in each person. People may respond with angry outbursts, violence, isolating themselves, and a whole variety of emotions (e.g., anxiety, depression, anger, grief, shame, guilt). These emotions point to imbalances in the organ and channel systems and, if not addressed, will continue to manifest themselves and cause disruptions in the qi.

Cellular research has proved that traumas are passed genetically—an ancestral qi imbalance. Certain markers on the DNA relate to trauma and continue down the family line. Children of Holocaust survivors growing up in relatively stable, peaceful environments can experience similar emotions and physical issues to those of their parents. The trauma memory has literally been passed down to them (Juni 2016). Until these trauma memories are treated, a person can manifest PTSD symptoms and pass these markers, including family karma, to the following generation. Now with modern science, one can see the link between the emotional body (Shen) and physical body (Jing).

"Sticks and stones may break my bones but words will never hurt me." This saying, for all its good intentions, falls short for many people—especially children. Emotional abuse is insidious and when experienced as a child can cause lasting scars, creating mistrust and timidity. Events, sensory stimuli, and authority figures, for example, can trigger the memories of abuse resulting in various reactions, causing both emotional and physical symptoms. This cascade of triggering involves any unresolved emotional trauma and intensifies faulty belief systems.

### *Emotional Trauma Creates Faulty Belief Systems*

Belief systems regarding how the world works develop during the formative years—birth to age seven. Trauma affects how each person views the world, hindering their ability to flourish and respond emotionally to their environment. This includes emotional trauma in the womb (in Chinese medicine birth age begins at conception—i.e., when a person is born they are one year of age). For children, PTSD symptoms can differ from adults. The National Institute of Mental Health website lists children's symptoms as: "Wetting the bed after having learned to use the toilet, forgetting how to or being unable to talk, acting out a scary event during playtime, being unusually clingy with a parent or another adult." The symptoms for teenagers are similar to those of adults, but "may develop disruptive, disrespectful, or destructive behaviors" (National Institute of Mental Health 2016) above the average levels for a teenager.

Forming faulty belief systems also creates conditioning patterns and cycles. These distress the body's physiology and imbed in the tissue memory. These patterns play out throughout a person's life unless they are addressed and cleared. Until resolved, the patterns trigger a person's trauma memory and continue to scatter their qi.

The cycling of patterns is a common phenomenon and tends to drive the emotional reactions and attitudes throughout a person's life. Belief systems and filters on the world influence decisions and relationships. Once the emotional trauma causing these beliefs and filters is addressed, a person can navigate life with improved clarity and maintain a better understanding of their life's purpose. The affected person always plays an active role in this transformation. As the trauma intensity reduces, the patient becomes empowered, freed from negative patterns. This process entails growing pains and requires a person to shift out of an ingrained pattern into a new way of being. Often, a person builds their identity based on the trauma, finding a sense of comfort in their story. This results in them developing difficulty in seeing a different path of life without being a victim of trauma; the trauma memory turns into a crutch. Attachments to the triggering of the memory go beyond conscious thought and reside at a cellular level. The trigger(s) become a form of addiction fed by certain lifestyle choices.

---

## Case Study: Transforming Destructive Behaviors

A 28-year-old woman, "Velma," sought treatment for depression. After a few acupuncture treatments, she felt safe to mention more personal information and disclosed that she suffered from an extreme eating disorder. She underwent treatment unsuccessfully in several residential facilities for bulimia. Her physician and family wanted her to return to a facility but she decided to try acupuncture. Acupuncture and other modalities reduced her PTSD and trauma connected with her eating. After several treatments, Velma found that making different choices was easy and eating became effortless. Velma reported feeling at peace with her body image and could better make plans for her career. She felt free from a pattern that had held her hostage and she could now step into the future with a sense of power. Her transformation was incredible and was likened to making it through the dark night into a new way of being. This is where shamanism is involved in the transformation of emotional trauma.

## Shamanism, Chinese Medicine, and Western Medicine

### Shamanism in Chinese Medicine

The term "shaman" refers to a practitioner engaged with the universal flow of change and who passes on this knowledge of the universal energy to others. For millennia, shamanism has contributed significantly to Chinese medicine. One phrase for Chinese medicine is 中醫 (*zhōng yī*) and the character for medicine/*yi*/醫 historically included the component 巫 *wū* (meaning shaman). This reflects the major influence of shamanism on Chinese medicine. Shamanism is not a religion, but a way of flowing with life and treating disharmony. For centuries, shamans served as the leaders of tribes in several cultures, including those in China. Before the development of the city-state, male and female shamans guided group decisions and offered counsel on many aspects of life—marriage, funeral rites, planting crops, where and when to move, healing, and more.

In China, Fu Xi is credited with being the shaman king who invented:

- Ba Gua (the eight trigrams)
- *Yi Jing* (*Book of Change*)
- Mathematics
- The Chinese calendar
- Chinese characters

- Naming and taming animals
- Making of fire
- Cooking of food
- The fishing net
- Riding of horses.

(Wu 2016, p.66)

Shamans understood the universal flow and respected the changes of life. Living a nomadic existence, people were subject to weather and the forces of nature, and relied on the shaman to guide them. As the city-states developed, people became sheltered from the effects of nature and the city-state established its own universe; the knowledge of the shaman was no longer needed. As politicians rose to power, the shamans lost their standing as leaders and were ultimately banished. In China, shamans retreated to the mountains and lived as hermits, within the rhythm of life.

Still, people considered shamans valuable and consulted them on various aspects of life, particularly healing. Although the writing of the classic texts of Chinese medicine occurred after shamans were supplanted in society, medicine still had connections to the shaman's ways of healing and watching changes. However, with each generation, medicine increasingly veered away from a spiritually based foundation. Moreover, in the "cleansing" of the Chinese culture during the Cultural Revolution, attention to spirit and the flow of nature was further removed. Nowadays, though, more practitioners are reclaiming the shamanistic roots and incorporating the principles into their practice of Chinese medicine.

## Defining the Term "Chinese Medicine"

Chinese medicine includes several aspects of medicine practiced in China over millennia. Shamanism, classical influences, traditional approaches, and modern medical research methods all comprise what is called Chinese medicine. This constantly evolves, yet the core principles and theories are still revered and used daily. Chinese medicine stands on the foundation of utilizing philosophies and treatments that prove clinically effective. These include anything from grounding a person's energy with shamanic drum healing treatments to activating a specific brain lobe with scalp acupuncture. Each of the treatments selected follows the principle of using differentiated diagnosis to understand and establish a clear healing intent. Integrating these with advances in Western medicine enhances the treatment outcome.

## Western Medicine and Chinese Medicine Working in Tandem

Modern Western medical brain research gives increased understanding about the effects of trauma on the physical body and has enabled Western medical providers to deeply understand the bio-medical causes of emotional trauma. This research supports the wisdom passed down by Chinese medicine ancestors. Interestingly, brain communication theories can be interpreted through the concepts of yin and yang and the three Dantians (the body's primary energy centers). Observing the similarities and differences in treating the complexity of emotional trauma from both Chinese and Western medicine viewpoints results in a greater comprehension of the condition. Examining emotional trauma from all angles improves the partnering of Western medical approaches (counselling and pharmaceutical medication) and Chinese medicine to successfully treat this multifaceted syndrome.

**WESTERN MEDICAL RESEARCH CORRELATING TRAUMA TO PHYSICAL DISEASES**

| Medical Journal (Date) | Research Finding |
| --- | --- |
| *Journal of Nutrition, Metabolism, and Cardiovascular Diseases* (2015) | Patients who experienced emotional trauma early in life were prone to obesity, diabetes, and cardiovascular disease (Farr *et al.* 2015). |
| *Journal of American Heart Association* (2016) | Women suffering from PTSD had a two-fold increased risk of venous thromboembolism (Sumner *et al.* 2016). |
| *BMC Psychiatry* (2016) | South African adults who had experienced several potentially traumatic events (PTEs) were studied for risk of chronic physical ailments. The research concluded that "PTEs confer a broad-spectrum risk for chronic physical conditions, independent of psychiatric disorders" (Atwoli *et al.* 2016). |

Patients taking antidepressant, anti-anxiety, and other medications *can* receive treatment with Chinese medicine. However, Chinese medical practitioners must be aware of the contraindications of combining pharmaceuticals with Chinese herbs if they choose to prescribe herbs for patients. Most herbal formulas (when taken two hours from ingesting a medication) are fine in combination with medication. Patients commonly see improvement in mood once they begin Chinese medicine treatment, though some patients believe they can simply discontinue medication—this is false. Patients should be monitored by their Western prescribing physician for dosage adjustments as necessary. Communication between Chinese medicine and Western medicine practitioners is optimal in fostering better care for the patient.

## Transforming Emotional Trauma and Fulfilling Destiny

Emotional trauma acts significantly on a variety of systems and emotions. It can become a part of a person's choices and chemistry and, if not addressed, limits the person's physical and mental ability. On a philosophical level, it restricts the person's full expression of their spirit on their life path. As Marcus Aurelius so eloquently stated in *Meditations*, "The soul becomes dyed with the color of its thoughts." Once the trauma clears, it is important to give the patient lifestyle suggestions in order to maintain their new balance. In the author's clinical experience, patients who utilize these suggestions grow and flourish into new ways of being.

> *Better to light one small candle, than to curse the darkness.*
>
> *Chinese proverb*

Chinese medicine treatment enables patients to uncover their light which illuminates the darkness resulting from emotional trauma. Their radiance helps to resolve the many traumas faced over a lifetime. As Carl Jung said, "I am not what happened to me, I am what I choose to become."

## Navigating the Dark Night

*Opportunities to find deeper powers within ourselves*
*come when life seems most challenging.*

Joseph Campbell

The ultimate goal of treating a person suffering from emotional trauma is to help them manifest their life path and fulfill their destiny—to educate the patient about the Chinese medicine treatment mechanism to enable them to engage in their transformation. This moves them from being a passive receiver to being an active participant. When the patient is aware of the Chinese medicine treatment intention, their understanding helps propel their progress. "The dark night of the soul" is about the heroine's and hero's journey to enlightenment.

The process of transforming emotional trauma serves as a catalyst for helping people move toward enlightenment—shifting a patient's perspective from seeing trauma as a wound to seeing it as a gift. If they can perceive the event as a method to shed limitations, they realize it ultimately allows them full access to Jing or essence. This journey can be difficult, and as Anaïs Nin explains, "Life shrinks or expands in proportion to one's courage."

A person must maintain a consistent heart of healing intention and virtue to be a practitioner of Chinese medicine. Persistence is essential no matter the turn of events in their life. This phrase relates to the patient *and* practitioner. Treating trauma can be a long process, and untangling the knot of a trauma memory takes patience. However, with dedication and tenacity the trauma can resolve and allow for a new level of engagement and harmony with life. Helen Keller elucidated, "When we do the best we can, we never know what miracle is wrought in our life, or in the life of another." Completing full transformation liberates the emotional energy of the organs and the overall spirit of the body; the person utilizes their full potential. Going through the dark night to get to the light exemplifies the interdependence of yin and yang.

---

## Case Study: Achieving Balance between the Divine Feminine and Divine Masculine

The divine feminine Mother Earth is associated with emotional depth and the wilderness. It symbolizes the untamed darkness which many people perceive as scary. In literature, particularly in fairy tales, it is viewed and depicted as a negative. The general Western cultural approach is to conquer nature. Over the last 2000 years, humans have turned away from exploring the mystery and spirit (divine feminine), including sidelining the spiritual aspects of Chinese medicine in lieu of intellectual pursuits (divine masculine/Father Sky).

However, mystery schools are re-emerging after existing in secrecy and their teachings are being brought into clinical practice. Combining the ancient mystical wisdom with the evolutionary progress gleaned from the scholarly advancements creates a truly integrated medicine (divine child). Achieving balance of yin and yang—incorporating both the spiritual and intellectual—brings full resolution to emotional trauma and allows a person to stand in harmony between heaven and earth (Figure 1.6).

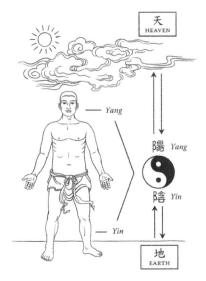

*Figure 1.6 The Human as a Vessel between Heaven and Earth*
*Source:* Reproduced from *Applied Channel Theory in Chinese Medicine* by Wang Ju-Yi and Jason Robertson with permission of the publisher, Eastland Press © 2008. All rights reserved.

Numerous qigong teachers and other spiritual practitioners speak of the importance of experiencing (and not just intellectually knowing) the practice. Through feeling and going "to the basement" to emerge into the light initiates true integration and resolution to the emotional trauma. Joseph Campbell elucidates, "It is by going down into the abyss that we recover the treasures of life. Where you stumble, there lies your treasure" (Osborn 1991). Joining the intellectual Father Sky energy with the dark wild of Mother Earth liberates the vessel of the human body to truly sing. Singing harmonious (yang) and dissonant (yin) notes with equal clarity allows the voice to completely ring out.

## *Light Shining Through*

The body can be likened to a flute between heaven and earth, producing a beautiful song when unobstructed. Processing emotional trauma can act as the mechanism to "trash out" (release and clear) what blocks the passageway in the flute. When the pathway is cleared, the flute can produce its true voice. Guiding a patient through emotional trauma releases the stagnation in the body and delivers the patient to a place where they can sing their song; they can walk their own path smoothly and unencumbered to fulfill their life's work.

People seeking treatment for trauma need inspiration and light to persevere. Maya Angelou shares an African saying: "When it looks like the sun is not going to shine anymore, God put a rainbow in the clouds." Throughout her life, she experienced many traumas, but when she remembered those people who were rainbows it kept her going. May the practitioners of Chinese medicine and all who seek to resolve emotional trauma be rainbows in life and help others unveil their brilliant light for all to witness and bask in.

## References

Atwoli, L., Platt, J.M., Basu, A., Williams, D.R., Stein, D.J., and Koenen, K.C. (2016) "Associations between lifetime potentially traumatic events and chronic physical conditions in the South African Stress and Health Survey: a cross-sectional study." *BMC Psychiatry 16*, 1, 214.

Farr, O.M., Ko, B.J., Joung, K.E., Zaichenko, L., *et al.* (2015) "Posttraumatic stress disorder, alone or additively with early life adversity, is associated with obesity and cardiometabolic risk." *Nutr. Metab. Cardiovasc. Dis. 25*, 5, 479–488.

Gongwang, L. (Editor, Translator), Hyodo, A. (Editor), and Quing, C. (Translator) (1994) *Fundamentals of Acupuncture and Moxibustion.* Coordinated by Chinese and Japanese Scholars at Tianjin College of Traditional Chinese Medicine & Goto College of Medical Arts and Sciences. Tianjin: Tianjin Science and Technology Translation & Publishing Corporation.

Juni, S. (2016) "Second-generation Holocaust survivors: psychological, theological, and moral challenges." *J. Trauma Dissociation 17*, 1, 97–111.

Mayo Clinic (2017) *Post-Traumatic Stress Disorder.* Available at www.mayoclinic.org/diseases-conditions/post-traumatic-stress-disorder/basics/risk-factors/con-20022540, accessed on 19 May 2017.

National Institute of Mental Health (2016) *Post-Traumatic Stress Disorder.* Available at www.nimh.nih.gov/health/topics/post-traumatic-stress-disorder-ptsd/index.shtml, accessed on 19 May 2017.

Osborn, D.K. (1991) (ed.) *Reflections on the Art of Living: A Joseph Campbell Companion.* London: Harper Collins Publishers.

Raben, R. (2011) "Stages of coping with stress: trauma management and acupuncture [Phasen der Stressbewältigung: Traumaverarbeitung und Akupunktur]." *Deutsche Zeitschrift fur Akupunktur 54*, 4, 13–17.

Sumner, J.A., Kubzansky, L.D., Kabrhel, C., Roberts, A.L., *et al.* (2016) "Associations of trauma exposure and posttraumatic stress symptoms with venous thromboembolism over 22 years in women." *J. Am. Heart Assoc. 5*, 5, p.ii: e003197.

Van der Kolk, B. (2014) *The Body Keeps the Score.* London and New York: Penguin.

Wu, Master Z. (2016) *Seeking the Spirit of the Book of Change.* London: Singing Dragon.

# CHAPTER 2

# Diagnostic Methods

When problem solving, viewing the issue from several angles reveals a more complete solution. If a practitioner looks at a disease pattern using only one lens or with blinders on, the whole presentation is missed. Understanding and utilizing several diagnostic methods leads to an accurate diagnosis, a fine-tuned intention, a focused treatment principle, and a quicker resolution of the emotional trauma. Moreover, the information gleaned from the various methods can be combined to monitor the progress and success of treatment. The following six diagnostic modalities are described for determining the roots of the emotional trauma:

- Five Element Diagnosis

- Facial Diagnosis

- Channel Palpation

- Pulse Diagnosis

- Tongue Diagnosis

- Intuiting the Five Spirits.

## FIVE ELEMENT DIAGNOSIS

Emotional trauma affects each individual differently. One of the core philosophies of Chinese medicine is that each person responds to a disease based on their personal constitution and their organ energy balance. Five element diagnosis provides insight into how a person's physiology is affected.

The five elements—water, wood, fire, earth, and metal—classify many aspects of a person's health, personality, development, and connection to the universal energy. Organs in the body are organized by the five elements and have minds and emotions based on this classification. The minds—or spirits—are the inner workings of a person through life, whereas the emotions are reactions to life. For example, a person gifted with insights and new ideas exhibits the spirit of fire. Typically, a "fire person" would tend to exhibit anxiety, sadness, and nervousness (Bridges 2012, p.293).

Each person possesses a varied proportion of all five elements. Most people will have a higher percentage of attributes of one or two elements, but rarely all of them equally. Discerning the primary element(s) assists the practitioner in comprehending the way emotional trauma affects an individual. For example, a "fire" person more commonly manifests anxiety and manic behavior, in contrast to a "metal" person who would gravitate toward grief and a sense of lacking (Bridges 2012, p.293). This is not to say that all people suffering grief have metal as their primary element. Observing their personality, emotional tendencies, physical attributes, pathology, and behavior all comprise the determination of the primary element(s).

Helping patients understand their elemental nature and aptitudes enables them to fully see themselves and realize their potential. With this knowledge, they are able to make specific dietary and lifestyle choices to transform the trauma and prevent future stressful events from affecting them. The following sections will summarize the various aspects of the five elements—their energetic nature, personality type, body type, health functions, and pathology. There are certain pathologies common to each element. However, pathologies are not exclusive to one element, and can cause different element imbalances. The elements have both generative and controlling cycles to achieve balance. Refer to Figure 2.1 to view the two cycles. An emotional trauma upsetting one element can reverberate in the other elements via these cycles.

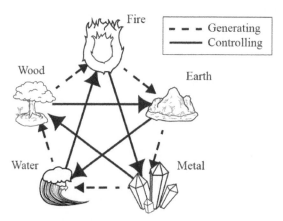

*Figure 2.1 The Five Element Diagram*
*Source:* Julian Holman

## Water Element
## Kidney and Urinary Bladder
### Hidden Power and Deep Emotions

Water holds hidden power. The great American Mississippi River embodies this aspect of hidden power. When looking at the surface of the river it appears calm and tranquil, yet under the surface whirlpools and strong currents reside. Author Tom Robbins elucidates, "Water dives from the clouds without parachute, wings or safety net. Water runs over the steepest precipice and blinks not a lash" (Robbins 2001). Water is the power within that contains the mystery of life. The water element begins the generating cycle of the Chinese five elements. Water is associated with the ability to rest within the flow of life. Simply being is something lost in the hustle and bustle of Western culture. Cultivating stillness increases the strength of the water element. As Lao Zi explained, "Be still. Stillness reveals the secrets of eternity." Water feels and absorbs deep emotions (Bridges 2012, pp.80–81). Any mysterious part of nature is seen as the water element. For example, the northern lights are one type of color and representation of water found on earth. The direction of water is north and associated with winter; its spirit animal is a combination of the Black Turtle and Black Snake (Wu and Wu 2016, p.83). In terms of a person's life cycle, water is the time *in utero* and where life cycles back into old age.

### The Kidneys and the Urinary Bladder

The kidneys and urinary bladder are the organs associated with water. The kidneys have four major functions: storing the essence/Jing; governing the bones; storing the will; and opening the ears (Wang and Robertson 2008, pp.120–123). Water is related to bones, and water people tend to sink in water due to their dense bones. Having a feeling "in your bones" relates to the deep-water aspect of emotion and the intuitive nature of water. In addition to dense bones, people endowed with a high proportion of the water element have wide hips, strong physical and emotional strength, large ears and chin, and thick flowing hair (Bridges 2012, p.252). Flowing downward and following the easiest path is indicative of water-type people, and observing this trait in a patient will give clues as to the depth of emotion felt by the patient.

ASPECTS OF THE WATER ELEMENT

| Personality | Emotions and Reactions | Common Symptomology | Cravings due to Imbalance |
|---|---|---|---|
| "Go with the flow" Great endurance Introspective Intuitive Exotic and sensual Enjoy lying down and found doing things in bed like eating, watching TV, and reading | Fear Willfulness Freezing Stubbornness Resisting flow (Bridges 2012, p.293) | Low back and knee pain Developmental issues Urinary problems Tinnitus Infertility Edema | Salty foods Marijuana |

## The Emotions Associated with the Water Element

Water emotions are fear and willfulness. Fear can either freeze or sink the body's energy, stopping a person's momentum in life. Willfulness, on the other hand, reflects in the body as stubbornness and resisting flow. If a person taps into their inherent wisdom and can see the situation clearly, the body's energy will unfreeze and stop sinking. When they allow the energy to take its natural course, the qi will flow again.

## Case Study: Fear Freezing a Person's Will

Trauma can scare a person to the point where they no longer carry out their normal activities or move forward on their path. A 60-year-old woman came in for Chinese medicine treatment weeks after being hit by a car while crossing the street. She suffered minor injuries, but no longer felt like walking to work. This woman had a strong constitution and, although she had never felt unsafe around cars previously, the trauma froze her ability to continue her normal routine. (For a complete description see Chapter 7, Case 3.) This blockage will continue until the kidney energy is bolstered to unlock her full potential. The kidneys store essence, also known as Jing, providing the life force for the body.

## Zhi (Will)—The Spirit of the Water Element

The ability of a person to stay with an idea and allow the body to manifest a dream or insight is Zhi (Wang and Robertson 2008, pp.121–122), the mind of the kidney. The *Jia Yi Jing* (*Classified Classic*) states in the first chapter, "That which gathers [and holds] intention is known as 'Zhi.'" For example, a person gets the idea they want to become an airplane pilot. The water or kidney strength determines if they can hold this path and stay with the idea. The Zhi is also associated with a person's connection to family and history (Maclean and Lyttleton 2010, p.99).

### Inheriting Trauma through the Water Element

Developmental issues or other inherited maladies relate to the water element. Jing is the root of the body (stored in the kidneys) and is passed from parents to child at conception. Emotional trauma experienced in previous generations carries through to the present life—via the kidneys—if not cleared. Examining family history can reveal a generational trauma. It can also reveal signs indicative of water pathology. As the classic Chinese proverb states, "A child's life is like a piece of paper on which every person leaves a mark." Even the Greeks understood this concept: "What we do now echoes in eternity" (Marcus Aurelius, *Meditations*).

Western medicine is now researching the implications of trauma from past generations in the field of epigenetics—"the study of changes in organisms caused by modification of gene expression rather than alteration of the genetic code itself" (Google Dictionary). As noted earlier, a trauma can be passed from parent to child via DNA (Yehuda *et al.* 2014)—the DNA is an equivalent to the Jing. Current findings confirm what several native cultures have already established, that is, the kidneys store emotional memories. If not resolved, these memories will be passed on to future generations. Working with the kidney organ system is one of the primary ways of clearing this energy.

## Wood Element
### Liver and Gallbladder

Lewis and Clark's[1] monumental expedition to the West displayed a healthy vigorous wood element. The pioneering spirit to drive forward and accomplish goals, despite the hard work and perilous dangers, embodies the wood element. Wood people are organized and love "to do," and their assertiveness may come across as pushy. The Nike slogan "Just Do It!" is the epitome of the wood element.

---

1   The Lewis and Clark Expedition from May 1804 to September 1806, also known as the Corps of Discovery Expedition, was the first American expedition to cross what is now the western portion of the United States.

## The Power of Change and the Wood Element

Wood is represented by thunder and change. Its direction is east and the spirit animal is the Green Dragon. Associated with springtime, the organs are the liver and gallbladder (Wu 2016, pp.109–111). The wood element needs to be moving, directing the blood, and keeping channel pathways open. The liver drains and dredges the pathways of qi (Wang and Robertson 2008, pp.160–162). When the pathways are blocked or blood is not directed to the correct location, anger can manifest itself. The anger can be in the form of depression when the qi is stagnated. The blockage can come from a person not acting, or overdoing and exhausting the qi so it no longer flows. The pressurized, blocked qi can rise, causing angry outbursts. An exaggerated sense of responsibility is a wood imbalance (Bridges 2012, p.293).

**ASPECTS OF THE WOOD ELEMENT**

| Personality | Emotions and Reactions | Common Symptomology | Cravings due to Imbalance |
|---|---|---|---|
| Passionate | Anger | Hypochondriac pain | Sour foods |
| Focused | Irritation | Eye issues | Alcohol |
| Assertive | Timidity | Indigestion | Drug use |
| Compassionate | Feeling of | Insomnia | Arguments |
| Intense | powerlessness (Bridges | Headaches/dizziness | Self-harm |
| Realistic | 2012, p.293) | Jaundice | |
| Dominant (Lotus | | Tinnitus | |
| Institute 2015) | | Tendon issues | |
| | | Weak immune system | |

## Decision Making and the Wood Element

Knowing how to manage the "doing" aspects of life is a role of the wood element. As in the example of the person wanting to become a pilot, there are several decisions and choices involved, for example which flight school to attend, which type of pilot to become, and when to start training. A harmonized wood element will weigh all the options, make the correct decision, and take action to accomplish each task on their way to achieving their goal. They have strong determination and courage to carry out their decisions (Wang and Robertson 2008, p.163). The wood element craves action and agitation to some degree; achieving this balance helps keep the element engaged. When a strong wood element is not active, the energy stagnates and can implode (Bridges 2012, pp.81–82).

## Case Study: Inverted Wood

A 38-year-old physical therapist, "Steven," came to the Chinese medicine clinic complaining of headaches which began after treating many patients. Steve felt like he was taking on their pain. From his face and body typing, he was diagnosed as primarily wood. Steve rarely expressed himself to others when experiencing pain and tried to "ride through it." He was not exercising—something a wood type craves. Essentially, his wood had inverted. Since Steve was not being active outwardly, he took on others' energy to fulfill the wood's need for agitation. His energy was pressurized and directed upward, causing headaches. Once Steve acted and moved his body, he no longer used other people's pain to activate his wood element.

### *The Hun (Ethereal Soul)*

The Hun lends the person the ability to take on difficult situations and crises (Wang and Robertson 2008, p.163). A healthy Hun gives the body courage to act when needed, which is necessary for a patient to process and move on from emotional trauma. The Hun is the mind of the liver and can be thought of as one's ability to clearly assess a situation and respond at the right time. If a building is on fire, a neighbor just might rush in to save a child without first evaluating the danger. They will be thought of as brave, but are foolhardy and could possibly suffer injury. A firefighter will first survey the building, find points of entry and areas that can be safely traversed, and then move into the burning building to perform a rescue. Great courage is needed to process and resolve emotional trauma. As Laura Ingalls Wilder explains, "The uplift of a fearless heart will help us over barriers. No one ever overcomes difficulties by going at them in a hesitant, doubtful way." To move forward through the trauma, courage is needed—along with a strong will.

Processing emotional trauma is likened to the dark night of the soul. To step up to the challenge, a strong Hun is required (Maclean and Lyttleton 2010, p.98). However, it is challenging to tease out the difference between the Hun and Zhi. The Hun makes the decision to move forward in a situation—fight or flight—and the Zhi provides the essence and stability to face a crisis. Both play a role when faced with a life-threatening situation. The *Nei Jing* states, "That which follows the spirit in its comings and goings is called the ethereal soul."

### Engendering Flexibility and the Wood Element

The wood element is commonly thought of as trees, but it also includes all plants such as vines, bushes, shrubs, and grass. A wood-type person can be either tall like a tree or short and full like a bush. Other wood physical characteristics are thick, full eyebrows, a prominent jaw, coarse hair, defined tendons, and active, hard bodies (Bridges 2012, p.252). The wood element possesses inherent flexibility and, by embodying this aspect, an emotional trauma becomes merely a stone that can be circumvented to allow a person to grow uninhibited on their path. This gentle yet powerful quality of wood is best described in the line from a poem in the Chinese astrology classic, *Di Tian Shui*. "Yi Mu Sui Rou" means gentle yin wood that has the flexibility to move around impediments to continue to grow forward (Wu and Wu 2016, pp.191, 199). A healthy wood element keeps the channel pathways free from the stagnation of trauma so that the patient can accomplish goals and thrive.

## Fire Element

## Heart, Small Intestine, Pericardium, and San Jiao

### The Sparkling Fun Fire Element

The spark of an idea spiraling up out of the darkness and illuminating the spirit with joy is the nature of the fire element. Fire is associated with the summer season, southern direction, and the Red Bird spiritual animal. Fire embodies play, movement, and enjoyment (Wu and Wu 2016, pp.59–65). Those with a fire personality are bubbly and spontaneous (Bridges 2012, p.158). Compared to their wood counterparts, they are somewhat disorganized, often unable to complete a task, excitedly jump from one thing to another, and have very active minds (Bridges 2012, pp.82–83).

Many patients with a dominant fire element find themselves in an inner conflict about accepting their fiery nature. The wood element is highly regarded in Western culture for its ability to do and accomplish tasks. A person endowed with fire can be shamed for being a dreamer and not following through with ideas. However, when "fire people" cherish their gift of insight and vision, they can contribute wonderfully to the world. They can make peace with themselves by understanding that manifesting their visions is not necessary. Helping a patient appreciate their inherent talents shifts their energy from muddled and tight to bright and relaxed.

There are four organs associated with the fire element and each plays a role in stabilizing the body after trauma and the trauma memory (see the table below).

## THE ORGANS ASSOCIATED WITH THE FIRE ELEMENT

| Organs | Functions | Relation to Emotional Trauma |
| --- | --- | --- |
| Heart | Commands the blood vessels. Circulates the blood. Stores the Shen (spirit) (Maclean and Lyttleton 2010, p.97). | Establishes proper blood circulation and clear perception after a trauma. Secures the Shen with yin and blood. |
| Small Intestine | Separates the clear from the turbid. Assists in the making of blood. | Helps to restore clear thought after trauma and build the blood. |
| Pericardium | Supplies blood to the heart. Regulates the thoughts and emotions going in and out of the heart, akin to a secretary deciding who will see the boss. Protects the heart from strong emotions and clears excess heat (Wang and Robertson 2008, pp.156–159). | Restores clear communication and proper functioning of the heart after trauma. Regulates the heat generated by a trauma memory. |
| San Jiao | Regulates heat in the body. Represents the infrastructure of all the channel pathways (Wang and Robertson 2008, pp.216–217). | Clears excess heat produced by trauma and the reliving of the trauma memory. Opens the pathways blocked by trauma. |

## *The Heart Mirror*

In Chinese medicine, the heart can be understood as a reflecting pool. A still pool accurately reflects a person's surroundings. Their perception of themselves, others, and the world is viewed with clarity. Thoughts, actions, and interactions are lucid and an individual can process and act with pure and true intent. The calm mirror brings harmony as one travels through life.

Emotions can be viewed as wind that travels through consciousness and stirs the waters of the pool. Brain researcher Jill Bolte Taylor asserts in her book *A Brain Scientist's Personal Journey* that an emotion exists for 90 seconds and, if not held in the consciousness, will simply pass (Bolte Taylor 2009). However, an emotion typically begins a cascade of thoughts and feelings and can build into a mighty wind that blows across the heart pool, stirring the waters of calm reflection. The more attention and energy given to the emotion(s), the cloudier the perception becomes. Emotional trauma creates turbulent winds that stir the heart pool. Until the trauma is addressed and resolved, there are underlying ripples, or in some cases waves, in the heart pool that continue to affect a person's perceptions.

The heart maintains proper circulation of the blood. If the blood becomes reckless or rough in movement, emotional issues arise. When the emotional trauma is triggered, a swell surges across the pool. For example, a combat veteran hearing a helicopter and thinking they are back in a war zone is an extreme misperception of reality. Not all emotional trauma affects the heart pool to this degree, but it does have an underlying influence. Resolving emotional trauma eliminates waves from the pool. A person may grow accustomed to the pool being active, but once the water is calm, there can be a shock effect. Even though the water becoming calm is a healthier reflection of reality, the patient will now see certain issues they may have been avoiding. This is likened to stilling the waters of a lake and seeing the trash on the bottom. The vividness can be overwhelming, so finesse on the part of the practitioner is crucial to allow for this adjustment. Many people can feel comfortable in their created reality and, if pushed too fast, they will retreat. Depending on the extent and length of the trauma, the ability for the pool to re-harmonize and settle varies for each person.

### The Great Insights of the Fire Element

The heart oversees insight and inspiration. A calm pool allows for accurate and purposeful awareness and innovation. When someone's pool is muddled or stirred, insights are lacking. The great inventors of our time and of years past rode the line between chaos and clarity, attaining leaps of insight unattainable by the common person. The inventor had a moment of clarity, as if the waters stilled between times of chaos. These moments are found when stirring the waters to transform and gain a new level of wisdom. This begs the question, "Does seeking to stir the spirit bring an evolution in consciousness?" What might seem a tragedy or trauma could be a stretching of spirit to move one into a new way of being. This fact alone can give anyone who has suffered an emotional trauma hope and confidence that the universe acts perfectly.

### Shen and the Fire Element

The Chinese character for Shen or spirit (both the modern and classical characters are provided below) can be interpreted as extending or reaching out. When people stretch themselves through internal psychological work or by gaining wisdom from overcoming a trauma, the spirit is activated. Connection to one's spirit is realized and strengthened.

Definition from *Shuō Wén Jiě Zǐ* (oldest extant dictionary):

神 *shén*

天神，引出萬物者也。从示申。

*tiān shén* Heavenly Spirit

That which draws down/through the 10,000 things [formed] from the constituent parts: 示 *shì* images suspended from Heaven and 申 *shēn* to extend or reach out

禍 (神)

A healthy functioning heart communicates these inspirational visions. Insight spirals up and is expressed with the tongue (the sensory organ associated with the heart). Emotional trauma hinders expression and the ability to form clear thoughts. Calming the spirit and strengthening the heart reestablishes clear expression.

**ASPECTS OF THE FIRE ELEMENT**

| Personality | Emotions and Reactions | Common Symptomology | Cravings due to Imbalance |
|---|---|---|---|
| Bubbly Charming Lively Imaginative Spontaneous (Bridges 2012, p.158) Expressive Curious Inventive (Lotus Institute 2015) | Over-excitement Scattered energy Anxiety Nervousness Over seriousness Insatiability (Bridges 2012, p.292) | Insomnia Nightmares Palpitations Dermatological issues Blood pressure irregularities (Bridges 2012, p.252) | Bitter foods Amphetamine-like narcotics Thrill-seeking activities |

## Case Study: Securing the Spirit

Emotional trauma has a profound effect on a person's Shen or spirit. A 33-year-old woman, "Beatrice," a pharmacist, suffered from panic attacks due to job stress and an assault three years prior. She recently started working at a new location. The demands of her job were intense and she frequently felt an overwhelming anxiety. Each time prescription orders would back up, she would lose sight of her surroundings and be transported to the past trauma. The first treatments focused on "Gathering the Qi" and "Soothing the Trauma Memory."

Once stable, determining her specific channel imbalances was addressed. Diagnostic evaluation revealed heart heat since she had a red tongue tip and a slightly red nose tip with a vertical line. The trauma memory flared heat, creating wind, stirring her heart mirror. HT-8 and KD-7 were stimulated to clear heart heat and to benefit fluids.

One week after this treatment, Beatrice was confronted by a mentally disturbed and intoxicated man threatening to attack her if she did not give him opiates. This event triggered her memory of the past assault when a man had tried to stab her in the throat. Beatrice was rattled, but held her ground and commanded the man away, and then alerted the authorities.

The treatments to stabilize her spirit kept her centered in an intense situation. Since the heart heat had been cleared, it did not flare up during the event. Her settled heart mirror allowed her to mentally remain in the present moment. Beatrice did not revert to the past event and panic, but responded according to the situation at hand. A healthy fire element has a rooted spirit that responds calmly in any circumstance.

# Earth Element
## Spleen and Stomach
### *The Homey Earth Element*

Entering a warm, cozy home, smelling freshly baked cookies, and being greeted with sweet smiles and warm hugs is the epitome of the earth element. Gatherings and sharing moments as a group, such as a family Thanksgiving holiday party, bring people and communities together. The earth element welcomes and receives (Bridges 2012, pp.84–85). The compass direction is appropriately the center. Earth has a nurturing spirit and is associated with the color yellow (like the rich, golden color of fertile fields of wheat). It does not have a fixed spiritual animal, but in Daoist traditions it is represented by the Yellow Phoenix (Wu and Wu 2016, p.67).

### *The Earth Element Pathology*

When the earth element is out of balance, the energy becomes cluttered and stuck. The organs of the earth element are the spleen and stomach. Yi (the mind of the spleen) is responsible for organizing logical thought in a smooth rhythm (Maclean and Lyttleton 2010, p.98). Stagnation occurs if processing ideas and intent changes from a steady momentum to over-thinking (i.e., "spinning the wheels in the mud") (Wang and Robertson 2008, pp.74–76). A person no longer feels centered and grounded once emotional trauma has created this stagnated environment. The trauma also impedes the spleen's function of transforming food and fluids into nutritive energy, thus compromising nourishment and stability (Maclean and Lyttleton 2010, pp.67–74). Physical symptoms, emotional reactions, and cravings manifest.

ASPECTS OF THE EARTH ELEMENT

| Personality | Emotions and Reactions | Common Symptomology | Cravings due to Imbalance |
|---|---|---|---|
| Consistent | Worry | Digestive distress | Nurturing |
| Faithful | Confusion | Nausea | Sweets |
| Grounded | Feeling uncentered | Low appetite | Starchy foods |
| Sentimental | Poor concentration | Bowel changes | |
| Easy-going | (Maclean and Lyttleton | Abdominal discomfort | |
| Enjoys sitting and | 2010, p.99) | (Bridges 2012, p.252) | |
| simply visiting | Indecision | Fatigue | |
| | Over- or under- | Fluid retention | |
| | nurturing | Over- or under- | |
| | Smother people with | nurturing | |
| | attention | | |

Support the earth element so it processes smoothly and maintains a healthy rhythm. This facilitates a patient's ability to take action and "trust their gut." Safety, trustworthiness, and processing thoughts with ease belong to a healthy earth element (Bridges 2012, p.293). Noting these transformations gives the practitioner confidence that the patient's earth element has been harmonized.

The following analogy relates to this disruption of flow. A woman is in a canoe on the bank of a river preparing to shove off into the current. Just as she pushes off and begins to move forward, she thinks of the past trauma. The trauma disturbs the ability to guide the canoe and it crashes into the rocks along the bank. The person realizes she lost control and redirects the canoe back into the water. She floats along for a few minutes, but again the thought resurfaces and she crashes back into the rocks on the bank.[2] Each time the trauma memory is relived, the person is thrown off course and out of the natural flow of life. Supporting the earth element centers the person and allows them to process thoughts and actions.

## Case Study: Rumination Causing Inaction

A 35-year-old patient had recently divorced and could not let go of thinking of his ex-wife. His path was bright, but thoughts of "how it used to be" kept derailing him from taking action and moving forward. Treatments to gather his qi were followed by treatments to soothe the intensity of the trauma memory, that is, continued thoughts of his ex-wife. After five treatments, the ruminations were significantly less frequent and intense. He could realize his path and, once in the flow, the impetus to act increased and he no longer had the re-occurring memories.

## Metal Element
### Lung and Large Intestine
#### Yin and Yang Balanced in the Metal Element

The metal element is an anomaly in Chinese medicine. It embodies an equal amount of yin and yang, whereas the other elements have either more yin or more yang (Bridges 2012, pp.85–86). In the environment, metal manifests as rock and metals, and it is also air. There are small metallic particles in the air that do not degrade or chemically break down (Environmental Protection Agency 2017). These microscopic pieces of metal float around us constantly. Essentially, the metal particles in the air

---

2   Analogy told by Martin Heskier of Heskier's One Tool, personal conversation with the author.

we breathe today remain from the air breathed by our ancestors. Metal provides a link to those who have lived before us—Jesus, Quan Yin, Buddha, Lao Zi, and Mary Magdalene, for example. As seen in the modern world in power lines and the internet, the metal element connects. It also refines, akin to smelting ore to gold (removing all the impurities). Fall relates to the metal element and the letting go of what no longer serves us. Metal expands (like the air across a valley) and cuts (like shears pruning away dead wood). This duality can make metal a challenging element to grasp. Metal is in the Western direction and its spiritual animal is the White Tiger (Wu and Wu 2016, p.75).

## The Sensitive Metal Element out of Balance

Metal-type people are highly sensitive and easily feel emotion. The sensitivity of the metal element is exemplified in cooking. Metal cookware heats up and cools down quickly. Using clay or wood will not replicate this sensitive reaction. Emotional trauma can have a profound effect on a metal-type person, especially grief (the emotion related to the lung). The lungs are the yin organ associated with the metal element and the most external of the five yin organs. Their rhythm of properly taking in a breath and distributing oxygen is compromised by the shock of trauma. This function is further hampered by the emotional reactions of the metal element (the wind under the wings is literally taken away), resulting in lung qi/yin deficiency or rebellious lung qi.

### ASPECTS OF THE METAL ELEMENT

| Personality | Emotions and Reactions | Common Symptomology | Cravings due to Imbalance |
|---|---|---|---|
| Sensitive | Grief | Coughing | Perfection |
| Orderly | Low self-esteem | Asthma | A hyper-clean |
| Precise | Sadness | Respiratory infections | environment |
| Refined | Feeling lack | Non-healing skin sores | Tobacco products |
| Idealistic | Literally takes the | Chemical sensitivities | Pungent foods |
| Gracious | air out of a person | (Bridges 2012, p.252) | |
| Careful | (Bridges 2012, p.293) | Weakened immunity | |
| Bossy (Lotus Institute 2015) | | Constipation | |

## Letting Go and Refining

The letting go aspect of the psyche (a function of the large intestine—the yang metal organ) is important for moving forward in life. The lungs and large intestine both suffer when a person is holding on to ideals or the past (Bridges 2012, pp.85–86). Constipation is a sign that the body is not letting go of what no longer serves it and can occur with reactions to emotional trauma. The lungs regulate qi flow, bringing strength to the body via oxygen.

The lung/metal energy is responsible for refinement. It cuts away and removes what is no longer needed, likened to whittling a piece of wood and creating a stunning sculpture. The following analogy illustrates an emotional trauma as a catalyst for refinement. Imagine a person traversing a stairwell from one level of being to a higher level of consciousness. The stairwell is noisy, full of echoes, and scary at times, but if the person keeps climbing they will eventually reach the next level and peace will surround them. The transition is difficult—and often overwhelming—but ultimately produces a more harmonious human being. Chinese medicine quiets the noise and confusion of the chaos during the time of transition. Working with the metal element to remove the trauma and letting go of faulty beliefs will enable the person to climb steadily on their life journey.[3]

## Case Study: Letting Go

A 36-year-old woman, recently divorced, complained of depression and feeling like she was constantly starting over. Chinese medicine treatment rooted her Shen and provided clarity. After a few treatments, she was able to identify her pattern of powerlessness and feeling vulnerable in life. Treatment then focused on helping her to let go of this faulty belief through strengthening the metal element. The woman courageously moved forward on her life path and took her licensing exam and landed a job at a medical clinic as the onsite supervisor—a large leap from where she was at the start of treatment. (For a detailed description of her treatment, see Chapter 7, Case 4.)

### Possessing Clear Boundaries and Instilling Confidence with a Healthy Po

Someone with strong lung energy displays confidence and a physical strength that inspires confidence in others (Wang and Robertson 2008, p.82). Harriet Tubman, an American slave in the southern United States, escaped slavery and led hundreds of other slaves to freedom via the Underground Railroad (Biography 2017). This "railroad" was a secret route from the Southern slave states to the Northern states, where slaves could be free. Using the Underground Railroad was incredibly dangerous and the journey to freedom was fraught with challenges. This trek took amazing stamina and heroism. The Po, or Corporeal Soul, is the mind of the metal element and gives the body the tenacity to accomplish tasks and strongly engage with the world (Maclean and Lyttleton 2010, p.98). Tubman had an amazing Po spirit, instilling

---

3    Analogy told by Clifton Harrison, personal conversation with the author.

confidence in such a large number of slaves who trusted her and displayed remarkable resolve to follow her to freedom.

The Po of the practitioner must be healthy and strong when treating an emotional trauma. This helps the patient to feel trust in the practitioner so that they more easily navigate their journey of transformation. Holding the space for transformation and expansion brings great healing. The Po also establishes clear boundaries between the individual and their environment (Maclean and Lyttleton 2010, p.98). A patient with a deficient Po has unclear boundaries, loses their individuality, and is hypersensitive. Benefiting the lung organ system corrects this imbalance and gives the patient strength to overcome emotional trauma.

## Summary of Five Element Diagnosis

*That the musical notes and tones become harmonious*
*through the relation to one another; and that being before*
*and behind give the idea of one following another.*

*Lao Zi*

The five elements work together to create a harmonious environment in the body. Each person has their own individual purpose and meaning that can be likened to "their song." When the elements are healthy and balanced, the patient's song resonates beautifully.

## FACIAL DIAGNOSIS

The face reflects the secrets within. Chinese facial diagnosis reveals emotions, personality, organ imbalances, past traumas, future obstacles, and personal strengths. This is one of the main diagnostic methods in Chinese medicine, practiced for centuries to observe the three treasures (Jing, Qi, and Shen) of a person. Features, lines, and colors all show how much a trauma has impacted an individual and their prognosis. These markers also change during treatment, providing indicators of progress and the effectiveness of treatment. The scope of this book focuses on the Lillian Bridges Family Facial Diagnosis Lineage System, and the various maps of the face used in this system will be presented below. (The reader is encouraged to study further with Lillian Bridges or her certified master face readers who hold seminars internationally—see Lotus Institute 2017.)

# Jing Level

## *The Facial Age Map*

The Jing is a person's essence, released throughout their lifetime. Face readers over the millennia have used a map to judge when Jing will be made available over a person's life span. Markers on the face show whether Jing was fully released or compromised at specific ages (Bridges 2012, p.40). This map is the Facial Age Map (see Figure 2.2).

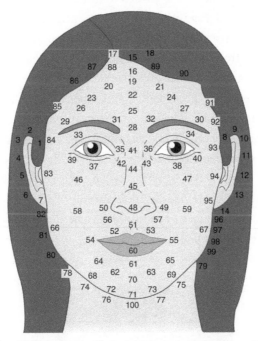

*Figure 2.2 The Lillian Bridges Family Facial Diagnosis Lineage System Facial Age Map*
*Source:* Reproduced from *Face Reading in Chinese Medicine*, Second Edition, by Lillian Bridges with permission of the publisher, Elsevier © 2003

The ears reflect the ages from *in utero* to age 13. Observing the cartilage on different areas of the ear reveals how the patient felt emotionally at different times in their youth. For example, the top of a man's left ear represents age one, and if the cartilage on the ear at that location is pinched, it means he felt suppressed at age one and his Jing was not fully available.

Markers to age 100 are found throughout the face. When a practitioner can determine each age in which Jing was affected, a pattern is identified and is frequently linked to a type of emotional trauma. These traumas are typically connected to an underlying belief system or thought process holding the person back from being fully present and operating in the world efficiently. This profound facial map enables a practitioner to use information about traumas at each age to develop a clear understanding of a patient's underlying emotional trauma.

## Case Study: Seeing a Disease Pattern Cycle

A 53-year-old woman, "Janis," sought treatment for her bouts of debilitating bronchitis that occurred every spring and fall. She hoped Chinese medicine could help her condition, as it worsened with moving to the northwest United States. She had moved to the northwest for its beauty and was working as an accountant. Janis liked the financial stability her job provided, but did not feel fulfilled and wanted to express herself in the world as a writer. A few years prior to the move, Janis had been diagnosed with celiac disease by her Western physician after suffering two intense bouts of hemorrhaging from her colon; its lining had completely sloughed off. Dietary changes successfully ameliorated her digestive problems.

When Janis first began Chinese medicine treatment, she was suffering from severe coughing fits, accompanied by wheezing, phlegm production, chemical sensitivity, fatigue, headaches, and insomnia. When examining her face using the Facial Age Map, she had markings at age three months and the years 4, 8, 11, 15, 19, 22, 25, 41, 51, 61, and 73 (refer to Figure 2.3). A picture of Janis ten years later with the markings still apparent showed that some had faded as a result of Chinese medicine treatment. Age markings can be seen at ages beyond the current age of patient during an exam, and in Janis's case there was a marking at 73.

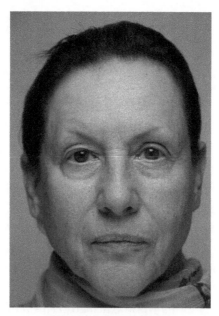

*Figure 2.3 Janis at Age 63*
*Source:* Steve Anchell Photography

**JANIS'S MARKINGS ON THE AGE MAP**

| Age | Event |
| --- | --- |
| 3 months | Severe case of measles where she almost died. |
| 4 | Moved to Germany with her family so her father could work as a spy. |
| 8 | Mom began drinking alcohol heavily. |
| 11 | Brother left home to join the U.S. military to be part of an intelligence agency. |
| 15 | Gang-raped as a virgin. (Later that year, her brother was assassinated.) |
| 19 | Quit using drugs (she had started using at age 14) and enrolled in college. |
| 22 | Started teaching at the high school she attended as a teen. |
| 25 | Married. |
| 41 and 51 | Had intestinal hemorrhaging. |
| 61 | At time of exam had a more significant line here, but with treatments it faded. |

The age markings followed roughly a four-year cycle up to her mid-twenties, and then changed to a ten-year cycle. Both patterns involved boundary issues, creating an imbalance. The metal element relates to establishing clear boundaries within the environment, and for Janis, her metal element was compromised due to her childhood illness. Measles is a respiratory infection and involves coughing and a whole-body rash (both relate to the metal element). Janis reported losing all her hair during the infection and her doctor believed she would not survive. She did survive, but with a depleted metal element. When residing in Germany, she was not allowed to interact with her dad in public, since he was a spy. This was confusing to her and she felt separated from her family. At age eight, she felt another level of disorientation due to her mother's drinking. Janis's disturbance about her mother being "sick" or "having the flu" added to her distorted understanding of boundaries. Then being gang-raped was a complete violation of boundaries which Janis dealt with by falling into heavy drug use and checking out of reality.

Janis shifted her energy by going back to school, teaching, and marrying in her twenties. This ended one cycle as she established a new level of boundaries. However, her metal element still showed weakness as intestinal issues and coughing were still occurring. Working as an accountant distracted her from her true passion for writing.

To address her metal element (lung/large intestine) deficiency, Janis was treated with Chinese medicine to strengthen the mother (earth) and daughter (water) elements of metal. The spleen and stomach were tonified, providing grounding, and the kidneys and urinary bladder were fortified to build her will. Treatments incorporated acupuncture, Chinese herbal medicine, nutritional counseling, shamanic drumming, qigong, and visualizations. In addition, Janis was encouraged to follow her dream as a writer and to publish a book.

Her dream was realized eight years later as she self-published a memoir of her childhood and teen years. Her lungs became stronger and all her symptoms were reduced to a level where she might get sick at times, but it would not lead to bronchitis. Before she started writing her memoir, Janis would suffer from frequent bouts of laryngitis. After treatments and while pursuing her dream, she rarely had laryngitis; she had reclaimed her voice. Interestingly, the age marker at age 61 faded as her metal energy grew stronger.

### Utilizing the Facial Age Map to Determine a Faulty Belief System and its Cycle

Emotional trauma commonly follows a repetitive cycle of a certain number of years, and age markers can be seen beyond a person's current age. When the belief pattern is addressed and changed, the markers at a future age will soften or disappear. The Facial Age Map provides clear information that identifies themes of emotional trauma and gives the practitioner a tool with which to form questions when interviewing the patient. Several types of markers are seen on the Facial Age Map, and in clinical practice the age markings can be grouped in decades over certain facial features. For example, the hairline represents the teenage years, the forehead the twenties, the areas around the eyes the thirties, the nose the forties, the lips the fifties, the chin the sixties, and the jaw the seventies (Bridges 2012, p.48). This simplified method quickly determines major affected areas and hones the diagnostic process.

### The Female and Male Difference on the Age Map

The left and right sides of the face are flipped for male and female based on yin and yang; that is, the left is male, so the male ages begin on the left ear and the female ages start on the right ear (Bridges 2012, p.43). The Facial Age Map is in Chinese ages, meaning that the Chinese believe the time *in utero* is so important that it counts as one year; thus, at birth a person is considered one year old. For Western ages, subtract one from the year on the Facial Age Map. Future references to the Facial Age Map in this book will refer to the Western age.

## Age Markings on the Ear (Ages Zero to 13)

The ear can present with a multitude of markings, each having its own meaning for the person. Markings can be found at one age, along a series of ages, or between several ages. They provide clues to the type of emotions felt at that age. Typically, there is a medium amount of cartilage and normal skin tone. One ear covers the ages from zero to six, which includes the time *in utero* and the other from seven to 13. The first segment of the ear is where time *in utero* can be seen and felt. This is the part of the ear that attaches to the cheek (left ear for the male and right ear for the female). It is important to palpate this area. A thick and wide attachment indicates the person had a healthy and uneventful time *in utero*. If the area is thin, some birth trauma probably occurred.

**DIAGNOSTIC SIGNS OF THE EAR CARTILAGE**

| Cartilage Quality | Diagnostic Significance |
|---|---|
| Missing | Patient felt like something or someone was taken away. |
| A notch | An accident, injury, or hospitalization. |
| Folded or pinched | Patient felt suppressed. |
| Thicker | A time when the patient felt strongly being cared for and loved; a happy time. |
| Less to none | Patient not feeling cared for or loved. |
| A dark spot | A traumatic event. |
| Bumpy cartilage | A turbulent time with many ups and downs. |

These markings can all be present or in any combination and, except for thicker cartilage, represent deep emotional trauma. For patients with exceptionally thick cartilage (indicating a highly joyful time), there is often a let-down, which may make subsequent traumas feel more painful. However, each person feels trauma differently, and what might be intense for one person is mild for another. When questioning the patient about the ages where markings are found, proceed gently and expect that some patients will be unaware of events early in their childhood—especially the early traumas that are preverbal (Bridges 2012, pp.43–46).

### Ear Markings in Janis's Case Study

On Janis's right ear (representing ages zero to six for females) there was a thick, strong area of cartilage at the *in-utero* area showing she was a wanted pregnancy (Figure 2.4). However, at the lower end region there was an indentation or dip indicating a hospitalization—her bout of measles. The cartilage was full until age three, revealing a happy time of nurturing. At age four, the cartilage was thinner and missing, representing the time in Germany and not being able to interact with her father in public.

On her left ear (ages seven to 13 for females) the cartilage at age seven was less thick and reflected when her mom started abusing alcohol (Figure 2.4). The lack of cartilage at age 11 pointed out the time when her brother left home.

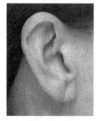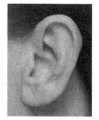

*Right Ear*                    *Left Ear*

*Figure 2.4 Janis's Ear*
*Source:* Steve Anchell Photography

## Age Markings on the Hairline (The Teen Years)

Markings on the hairline of clinical significance are indented or have areas of less hair. These markings are common, as many teens have experienced some form of emotional trauma. Specific ages are helpful to focus on when observing the hairline, and most patients will remember an event if the age is marked (Bridges 2012, p.47).

### Hairline Markings in Janis's Case Study

Janis had an inverted "V" shape in her hairline (Figure 2.5), marking the time when she was gang-raped and her boundaries were violated. The other ages in her hairline were smooth and showed that, although she had wild teen years, the hairline did not suggest any loss of Jing. This inversion was at age 15—an important developmental time in the female seven-year cycle. At around age 14, women become fertile. This developmental stage was halted in Janis's case. Because she was raped, her sense of being a "woman" in the world was violated. It was not until she reclaimed her power in her twenties that this stage was fully moved through and she stood in the world as a responsible adult. By becoming a teacher, she could see herself as an empowered woman and not as a vulnerable child in the world.

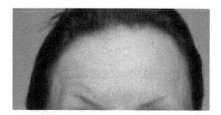

*Figure 2.5 Janis's Hairline*

## Age Markings on the Face

The face can have many markings, but to be relevant to the Facial Age Map, they must be horizontal lines, pits, or unusual colors (Bridges 2012, p.40). Any vertical or diagonal lines belong to the Facial Emotional Map and will be addressed later in the chapter (Bridges 2012, pp.59–60). Horizontal lines represent a block or partial infusion of Jing and show a past, present, or future trauma based on the age of the patient. The infusion of Jing is essential for the body to function efficiently. If compromised, this leads to disharmony. The lines can be significant or shadow-like and can fade as Jing is accessed.

### Markings on the Face in Janis's Case Study

There were three deep horizontal lines across her forehead at ages 19, 22, and 25 (Figure 2.3). These lines displayed her choices to become responsible and establish clearer boundaries in the world. Each line fully crossed Janis's forehead, demonstrating that the lessons learned at each age were complete.

She also had horizontal lines at ages 41, 51, 61, and 63, all of which showed some compromising of Jing. The line at 51 represented the breath of life and ties in to her lung issues. The line at 73 (coupled with dark areas) related to her need of establishing more boundaries. (This will be discussed further in Chapter 5.)

## Colors on the Face

Colors on the face show when Jing was affected and give clues to pathogens involved. Each color correlates with the five elements, indicating which organ system could be affected. The significance of colors on the face is as shown in the table below (Bridges 2012, pp.251 and 254).

**MEANING OF COLORS FOUND ON THE FACE**

| Color | Pathology/Emotion |
| --- | --- |
| Black | Blood stagnation and/or fear |
| Green | Toxicity and/or anger |
| Red | Heat and/or anxiety |
| Yellow | Putrefaction/phlegm and/or worry |
| White | Frozen and/or grief |

References to facial diagnosis are found throughout the classics, and Chapter 39 in *The Yellow Emperor's Classic* (*Huang Di Nei Jing*) states, "The five depots and six palaces (correspond to the face), they definitely all have corresponding sections. When inspecting the five colors there, yellow and red represent heat, white represents cold, green-blue color and black represent pain. This is the so-called from inspection one can obtain insight."

## The Facial Emotional Map

Putting on a "happy face" might fool the lay person, but a practitioner educated in facial diagnosis sees what a person really feels. The emotional make-up of a person is another aspect of reading the Jing on the face and is represented on the Facial Emotional Map (Figure 2.6). The emotions are seen on the face via diagonal and vertical lines.

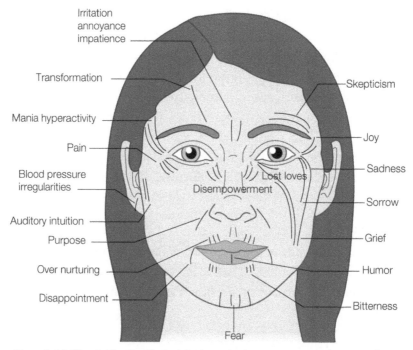

*Figure 2.6 Lillian Bridges Family Facial Diagnosis Lineage System Facial Emotional Map*
*Source:* Reproduced from *Face Reading in Chinese Medicine*, Second Edition, by
Lillian Bridges with permission of the publisher, Elsevier © 2003

During the practitioner's first encounter with a patient, detection of the emotions can be obvious. For example, if a patient is dealing with or has dealt with deep grief in their life, you can see this in lines traveling from the outer canthus down across the cheek bones. If deep personal grief, the lines will start from under the eye or from the inner canthus (Bridges 2012, pp.61–62). Observing these lines between treatments allows the practitioner to see if their treatment is effective. The lines will soften and clear as the emotional trauma is treated accurately.

## Two Sides of the Face

Many people present one image to the world while their true self is quite different. Rarely do people show all of themselves to the world:

The left side of the face is the true self. The right side is what people want the world to perceive. (Bridges 2012, pp.91–94)

Understanding and using this in detecting emotional trauma is powerful, as people hide or push away intense emotions; though these are not always "negative" emotions. For example, a 45-year-old woman had more lines representing happiness on the left side of her face than on the right, meaning she is happier than she shows the world. This could be a defense mechanism to prevent being taken advantage of or thought of as silly. In clinical practice, comparing these two sides assists with diagnosis as the person shifts their energy and steps into the world. A patient is considered more balanced when the two sides become similar.

## Qi Level

### The Facial Organ Map

Organ diagnosis is as "plain as the nose on your face." Each feature on the face represents an organ system (Figure 2.7). The physiology of the organs is determined by examining the facial features, colors, and spaces on the face.

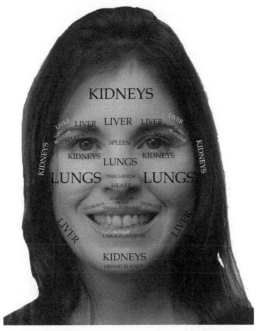

*Figure 2.7 Lillian Bridges Family Facial Diagnosis Lineage System Facial Organ Map*
*Source:* Photograph taken by Steve Anchell Photography, edited by Tammy Anderson

Emotions affect the functioning of an organ system, and the organ system affects the emotional body. Balancing an organ system improves the state of emotional health and reduces the emotional trauma. The face will change in regard to colors, and the features themselves can change shape as a patient is treated.

## Case Study: The Ever-Changing Face

A 38-year-old female patient, "Gretchen," presented suffering from fear resulting from divorce. Her chin was measured before treatment at a certain length. After a few years of qigong, acupuncture treatment, Chinese herbal prescriptions, and affirmations, Gretchen's chin grew. It is possible for bone to grow long after puberty. The chin represents the kidneys and bladder, and fear can affect these organs (Bridges 2012, p.252). As Gretchen stood confidently on her own and worked through her fear, her will increased, as shown by her chin growth.

The shape, skin color, and size of each feature all play a role in determining the physiology of the organ system and give clues about the emotions and how they affect the organ system. There will be several examples in Chapter 7; one example is the darkness in the temples representing depression (Bridges 2012, pp.261–262). Pictures of Robin Williams before he took his life show the darkness in the temples that also runs down the sides of his face.

**FACIAL FEATURES ASSOCIATED WITH CERTAIN ORGANS**

| Organs | Associated Facial Features |
| --- | --- |
| Kidneys and Urinary Bladder | Ears, under the eyes, chin, philtrum, and forehead/hairline |
| Liver and Gallbladder | Jaw, eyebrows, brow bones, third eye (the area between the eyebrows), and temples |
| Heart, Small Intestine, Pericardium, and San Jiao | Eyes, dimples, tips and corners of the mouth and eyes, nose tip, tongue tip, and upper lip line |
| Spleen and Stomach | Mouth, above the upper lip, under the nostrils, upper eyelid, bridge of the nose, and warehouses on the face (i.e., the fleshy areas of the face) |
| Lungs and Large Intestine | Nose, cheek bones, cheek area lateral to the mouth, area immediately below lower lip, and spaces on the face |

*Source:* Adapted from Bridges 2012, p.252

*Interpreting Colors to Diagnose Organ Pathology*

When a person is ungrounded and their earth element is compromised, the bridge of the nose will be pale (Bridges 2012, pp.275–276). Basic indicators provide understanding of the root causes of emotional trauma and which organs are most affected. Colors are helpful in seeing recent or temporary effects to the organ systems. (Refer to the table "Meaning of Colors Found on the Face" above.)

*Patients Exhaust their Dominant Element(s)*

Most people have one or two organ systems/elements that are primary and strong. These do the work—or pick up the slack—for the other less prominent and weaker systems/elements. Often, the feature(s) affected are the person's primary organ system. This dominant element is working overtime for another suffering organ system and it is important to identify the underlying organ system as the culprit for the imbalance.

## Case Study: An Exhausted Dominant Element

A water person (strong ears and chin) had darkness and swelling under her eyes. She reported experiencing excessive anger in addition to frequent urinary tract infections, insomnia, migraines, and teeth grinding. Her condition began after she was stressed at work due to working long hours. Her water system was suffering, but she continued doing excessive wood activity—working long hours and exercising vigorously every day. The patient's water system was being affected because her wood was asking for a lot of energy. Few symptoms showed in the wood element aspects of her face, but if only the water element was treated, her condition would not resolve. Both the wood and water elements needed to be addressed.

## Kidneys and Urinary Bladder

### Ears

The ears reflect the fundamental kidney strength and show the state of the Jing. The size of the ears determines the amount of risks an individual is willing to take. Patients with smaller ears usually require bolstering of the kidney energy to have the courage to work through and resolve old trauma. The tautness of the ear attachment to the skull determines the strength of the Zhi. To gauge a patient's level of tautness, hold and gently pull their ear. Softly attached ears show a need to increase the Zhi.

## Chin

Observe the chin for dimpling (Figure 2.8) or discolored areas to determine if fear is present. If the chin is small or "pushed in"-looking, the patient does not stand up for themselves and can be dominated easily (Bridges 2012, pp.258–259). If the chin is dark or lined (Figure 2.8(c)), a considerable amount of fear is being held in the body.

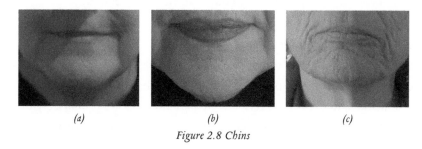

(a)                              (b)                              (c)

*Figure 2.8 Chins*

## Under-Eye Area

Swelling under the eyes represents unshed tears and unexpressed grief. A lighter color of the skin over the swelling indicates a recent, painful event. A patient with "three-sided eyes" (meaning there is white under the lower part of the iris—see Figure 2.13(c)) is pushing their body hard without enough water present, which can lead to heat. If there is redness on the lower eyelids, the patient is suffering from kidney yin deficient heat and the adrenals are exhausted. Darkness under their eyes (see Figures 2.10 and 2.11) signifies the kidneys are tired, and when the darkness covers the entire socket, there is severe kidney deficiency (Bridges 2012, pp.255–257 and 269).

## Forehead

An indentation across the width of the forehead, like a band, indicates despair. This is akin to a person placing their hand over their forehead in despondency, as if suppressing their will. The indentation is frequently coupled with dark, hollow temples and is a serious marker requiring precedence. This marker resolves with Chinese medicine treatment and, in some cases, within three treatments (Figure 2.9).

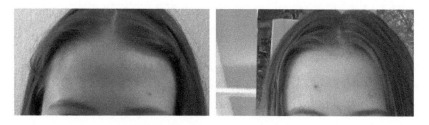

*Figure 2.9 Forehead Before and After Three Chinese Medicine Treatments*

## Liver and Gallbladder

### Temples

Indented temples are indicative of someone who enjoys altered states through drugs, alcohol, recreational means, or through creative and/or spiritual pursuits. Encourage some type of spiritual practice for this person to avoid emotional stagnancy. Darkness in this area (see Figures 2.10(c) and 2.11(b)) represents stagnation of liver qi and can indicate depression and/or addiction (Bridges 2012, pp.261–262).

### Eyebrows

A patient with thick eyebrows (Figure 2.11(b)) needs to engage in strong physical activity to keep their liver energy moving, otherwise the result is anger or depression (Bridges 2012, p.260). A person with eyebrows that are thin on the edges (Figure 2.10(c)) would benefit from asking for help from others to feel empowered. Patients with thinning or sparse eyebrows (Figures 2.10(a), 2.10(b), and 2.11(a)) are sensitive to toxins.

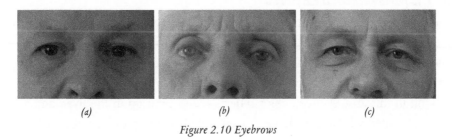

(a)                    (b)                    (c)

Figure 2.10 Eyebrows

The eyebrows are a primary area indicating how the wood element is managing energy. Referred to as the leaves on the tree, the thickness of the eyebrows shows how well a person filters toxins and indicates how much wood energy an individual has available to "do" in the world. An increase in neurological conditions is no surprise with the entire "Just Do It!" attitude in Western culture. People lacking a strong wood element easily overuse their wood energy and thus experience issues including tremors, insomnia, menstrual irregularities, and migraines. The condition of the eyebrows communicates to the practitioner the person's ability to exercise, take medication, and process toxins (Bridges 2012, p.260). For those practitioners who prescribe herbs, be aware of the amount of eyebrow hairs. If someone's eyebrows are thin, ask them if they are actively plucking or waxing. If not, a smaller dosage of herbs (if any) is warranted.

As the world becomes more toxic, there has been a rise in cases of chemical sensitivity, and those individuals with smaller eyebrows are most susceptible. Clinically, eyebrow hairs can grow, thus showing that the strength of the liver has increased. They can also change the direction in which they lie on the face—when growing upward, the person feels confident/self-assured (Figure 2.14). The outer eyebrow hair area is associated with the gallbladder and can also relate to the thyroid, giving clues as to the state of the wood system (Bridges 2012, pp.264–265).

## Case Study: Thinning Eyebrows

Facial diagnosis is a quick way to gain trust with patients. A 61-year-old male, "Burt," with Lou Gehrig's disease, apprehensively came in for an acupuncture treatment. His notably sparse eyebrows indicated the need to work on his liver energy, which was communicated to him shortly after he arrived at the clinic. A look of surprise came over his face and he reported that his MD had determined the same thing. With the understanding of how face reading was used to assess his condition, the patient gained trust in the Chinese medicine treatment. Over the months of treatment, his eyebrows did fill in.

### Third Eye (Area between the Eyebrows)

Redness in this area can represent heat and repressed anger in the wood system. Shadows or darkness show a lack of seeing into situations or motivations, and care should be taken in opening the third eye. If done too quickly, it can have a rebound effect. If someone is overusing their liver emotionally, there will be darkness or a hollowing in this area. A green color reflects toxins built up in the liver, and a white color is associated with a liver that is frozen and unable to process emotions or toxins (Bridges 2012, p.262).

### Heart, Small Intestine, Pericardium, and San Jiao

#### Tip of the Nose

A vertical line down the tip of the nose (Figures 2.11(b) and 2.13(b)) is referred to as "the human angel marking," and belongs to a person who is giving their "blood" to someone close to them. This can be the co-dependent spouse or caretaker or people who are meeting someone else's needs before their own. This marking is of concern in treating emotional trauma since the blood houses the emotions. If someone is not fully accessing their blood, their emotional stability is compromised. Redness on the tip reflects heat, paleness is heart blood deficiency, and purple or darkness (Figures 2.10(b) and 2.11(a)) is blood stagnation in the heart. A pinched nose tip reflects a tight heart and pericardium and a lack of joy (Bridges 2012, pp.266–270).

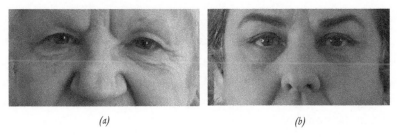

(a)                                    (b)

Figure 2.11 Nose Tips

## Dimples

Dimples on the cheeks represent charm and can be quite endearing. A dimple on the chin indicates an individual who seeks outside affirmation to feel comfortable with their choices and path. Encourage these folks to follow their inner desire, to find ways to strengthen their internal resolve, and not place strong emphasis on others' approval (Bridges 2012, p.176).

## Spleen and Stomach

### Mouth

The mouth signifies the strength of the earth element, which is the center of the body. When treating emotional trauma, the mouth helps identify how the earth is affected—color, shape, dryness (Figures 2.8(c) and 2.12(c)), and so on. A large lower lip indicates the person has desires for physical pleasure (good food, fine wine, high quality mattress) (Bridges 2012, p.188). If this is swollen, there can be issues with letting go and moving on from a trauma (Figures 2.12(a), (b), and (c)). A person with a tight upper lip (Figures 2.8(a) and 2.12(c)) should be encouraged to enjoy life more (Bridges 2012, pp.274–275). In contrast, a person with a large upper lip (Figure 2.12(b)) tends to exaggerate and be dramatic (Bridges 2012, p.187).

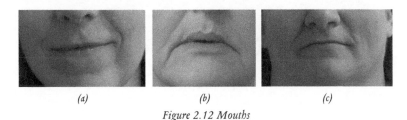

(a)                    (b)                    (c)

Figure 2.12 Mouths

*Above the Upper Lip*

Redness in this area represents heat in the stomach and can indicate wood overacting on earth, creating heat. Paleness in this area (Figures 2.8(b), 2.8(c), and 2.12(a)) is associated with cold and reflects poor diet and frozen earth (Bridges 2012, pp.276–277). Trauma prevents patients from being grounded and depletes earth energy, causing cold in the stomach.

*Warehouses*

These are places that have extra flesh and show an extra amount of earth. Extra flesh above the eyes (Figures 2.10(c) and 2.11(b)) displays a person's ability to "weather the storm," while someone with little flesh in this area (Figures 2.10(b) and 2.13(c)) feels suffering intensely (Bridges 2012, pp.273–274). This can be a key to understanding how someone is processing emotional trauma.

### Lungs and Large Intestine

*Nose*

The nose represents the lungs and, if it is red, there is inflammation and heat in the lungs. Trauma stirs up heat and, if coupled with grief, heat can become trapped in the lungs. If there are lines on the nose (Figure 2.13(a)), the fluids are seriously depleted (Bridges 2012, pp.283–284). A dusky-colored nose (Figures 2.13(b) and (c)) indicates blood stagnation in the lungs and can be associated with long-term grief caused by reliving a trauma memory.

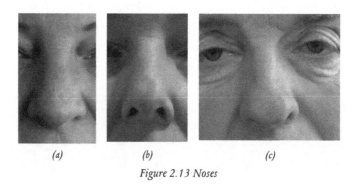

(a)        (b)        (c)

*Figure 2.13 Noses*

*Wei Qi Area*

The cheek area lateral to the mouth represents the wei qi, reflecting the immune system. Hollowness (Figure 2.12(c)) or lines (Figure 2.12(a)) in this area give the practitioner a clue as to the state of the immune system and the level of stress on the body (Bridges 2012, pp.284–285). Treating the wei qi area, if affected, speeds the recovery from emotional trauma.

# Shen Level

> *Be not afraid of growing slowly; be*
> *afraid only of standing still.*

*Chinese proverb*

The Shen, or spirit, is constantly in flux and changes within microseconds. The goal of treating trauma is to help the spirit move forward unencumbered. Emotional trauma disrupts and unroots the spirit and causes it to dampen and darken. Reliving trauma also disturbs the spirit; and during patient intake, changes in the Shen can and should be observed on the face. The Shen aspect of facial diagnosis is crucial to understanding trauma and which stage of trauma the patient is in. Observing the Shen on the face provides clues about which elements are involved and the severity of the emotional trauma (Bridges 2012, p.227). The color of the skin, the look in the eyes, and the appearance of light in the eyes present clues as to the state of the Shen.

## *The Colors of Shen*

The colors are the same as noted previously. When someone is stuck in a pattern and the issue resides at the organ level, an overall darker tone to the skin is seen. This represents an emotional trauma that has severely blocked qi and blood flow and is at a very deep level. The appearance of red in the face, also known as being a "hot head," relates to fire and yang rising and is an obvious indication of heat stirring the spirit. If the trauma is becoming toxic and affecting the body throughout the systems, a green tone to the skin is apparent. Often, the emotion will be accompanied with phlegm in the body, exhibiting a yellow skin tone. As people experience an emotional trauma that freezes their energy, white will be predominant (Bridges 2012, pp.229–234). These colors relate to the organs that are most affected: red, the heart; yellow, the spleen; and so on.

### THE SHEN IN THE EYES

| Shen of the Eyes | Meaning |
| --- | --- |
| "The lights are on but nobody's home." | Shock, frozen energy, or when the trauma has rendered the patient unengaged in life (Bridges 2012, p.229). |
| "Wild eyes" (darting/moving around quickly) | Fire rising and stirring the spirit (Bridges 2012, p.231). |
| Dull | Grief (Bridges 2012, p.234). |

### The Subtle Movements of Shen

The Shen is quick to change (Figure 2.14). In fact, practitioners will find it helpful to see what "makes a person tick" by observing the changes in the Shen in the eyes when asking patients questions. Watching the eyes is especially useful to identify triggers of the trauma memory. A patient's eyes get darker, narrow, teary, or close when touching on "hot button" issues. This reflects the heart mirror becoming clouded, limiting their ability to see or deal with an issue (Bridges 2012, p.227).

For example, when questioning a patient about their mother's family heritage and their eyes darken and their facial muscles freeze, this indicates an area of life that is sensitive to them. The patient will shut down rapidly when a specific topic is broached. Revealing and allowing the trigger to be seen takes great finesse by the practitioner and it is crucial they continue the line of questioning around the trigger. Gently allowing the patient to recognize their trigger(s) is a skill requiring grace. A transformation is initiated when a practitioner can allow the trigger to come into view. Once this happens, the trigger can begin to be processed and released.

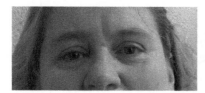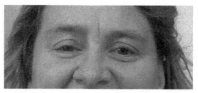

*Figure 2.14 Shen Transformation*

Some practitioners might view this line of investigation as "pushy." However, helping the patient through the forest of darkness into the light is quite beautiful and ultimately leads to great healing for the patient. The process is gentle if the practitioner's motivation is to truly assist the patient. The Shen or spirit of the patient will see the true intention and, if it is helping, then the patient will feel taken care of and safe.[4]

---

## Case Study: Using Shen Reading to Gain Trust

A 42-year-old woman, "Alexia," came in for Chinese medicine treatment and while sitting in the waiting area shared with the office manager that she had been "strongly encouraged" to seek Chinese medicine treatment. She expressed feeling apprehensive and, when asked by the practitioner to come back to the treatment room, she

---

4    Modern psychiatric research suggests that constantly focusing on discussing the old trauma is not effective. However, providing a safe place for patients to release feelings and explain the root of the trauma is helpful. This does not mean it is good to create a full-blown emotional reaction, but a gentle release is appropriate. Counseling is left to other professionals, as this does not fall within the scope of Chinese medicine.

mentioned her fear of needles. The practitioner told Alexia she did not have to receive acupuncture, but could simply sit down and talk about treatment options.

Alexia's Shen was frozen and dark, indicating her fear and stagnation (Bridges 2012, p.229), but she agreed timidly to just chatting. The practitioner, noticing her well-defined widow's peak, conveyed to the patient how creative and imbued she was with female yin power. This comment established immediate rapport. Her energy shifted instantly and she stated that she missed doing creative work as a graphic artist since moving to a new town. Alexia had experienced trauma with the move, and the reason for her visit was chronic fatigue and pain. Communicating the positive attributes about her personality and physical strength helped Alexia acclimate to the clinic. She felt safe being seen by the practitioner and her Shen relaxed and glowed within minutes of the meeting. She shared her past and soon was open to receiving acupuncture treatment.

---

The Shen of a person can detect the intention of another, as Shen can be felt as well as seen. This is the basis of intuition. Face reading allowed Alexia's spirit to see the practitioner's intention of helping. The power of Shen-to-Shen communication is especially palpable in moments like these and truly assists the treatment. Facial diagnosis is certainly not the only way to connect with the spirit of the patient, but it is a quick way to communicate that the patient is in a safe space.

Reading the Shen on the face provides a measurement of prognosis and treatment effectiveness. The brightness in the skin and eyes reflects clarity and harmony within. Typically, a healthy Shen is classified as clear, translucent, warm, and light. Each emotional state and trauma affects the Shen differently. The pictures of the case studies in Chapter 7 reflect examples of how the Shen changes. The goal of every treatment is to improve the state of a patient's Shen—to increase their glow.

## Summary of Facial Diagnosis

> *The face is the mirror of the mind, and eyes without speaking confess the secrets of the heart.*
>
> St. Jerome

Chinese facial diagnosis is a powerful tool in understanding the underlying cause and current state of emotional trauma. The three treasures are seen on the face and, when diagnosed in combination, yield great insight. Incorporating the information about the age(s) when a trauma occurred, the emotions involved, the health of the organ systems, and the state of the Shen provides detailed diagnostic information about the root of their trauma. The face is like a painting. The practitioner needs to see the whole picture to understand the root cause of the trauma—to "see the forest through the trees." Facial diagnosis is one of the many diagnostic techniques available to the practitioner. Combining it with other diagnostic methods, such as channel palpation, is essential for fully comprehending the pathophysiology of emotional trauma.

## CHANNEL PALPATION

*Music in the soul can be heard by the universe.*

*Lao Zi*

The music of the organs can be felt under the skin. Dr. Wang Ju-Yi likened the use of acupuncture points to tuning an orchestra. Thus when all players are in tune, a beautiful symphony is played. The 14 channels reflect the physiology of the organ systems and through palpation one can literally feel how the organ systems are functioning. Dr. Wang was a master Chinese medicine practitioner and teacher of channel palpation. The following discussion of channel palpation is based on his teachings, his textbook *Applied Channel Theory in Chinese Medicine* (Wang and Robertson 2008), and his students' contributions to this diagnostic technique. (The reader is encouraged to study further with Dr. Wang's senior apprentices/certified teachers who hold seminars internationally—see Wang 2017.)

### *Palpating the Channels to Determine the Diagnosis*

Dr. Wang always encouraged the practitioner to "put their mind in their thumb" and focus on what is felt under the fingertips at each of the three levels of the channel. The term, translated here as "mind" (心 xīn), is the same Chinese character more often translated as "heart." In both modern and classical Chinese, the two are often interchangeable. Thus, the practitioner is to use their clear heart perception to observe the changes in the channels. The technique is to softly or firmly (depending on the level of the channel palpating) press the tip of the thumb over each channel to detect nodules, weak areas, temperature changes, dryness, and tight areas. The non-palpating hand holds the limb firmly, opening the channel, allowing the pathway to be easily felt (Figure 2.15).

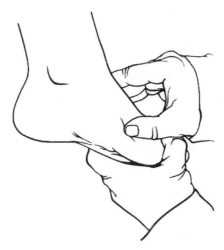

*Figure 2.15 Channel Palpation*

When diagnosing patients, palpation of the channels narrows the practitioner's focus and leads to pertinent questioning and examination. For example, if palpation of the arm yields palpation findings on the lung channel, attention to the metal element attributes, lung facial areas, and lung pulse can be observed. If correlating signs are detected by using other diagnostic methods, the palpation changes are clinically relevant. The channels are dynamic and provide information about the effectiveness of treatment. The nodules, weak areas, dryness, firm places, and so on should all resolve and smooth out as a person responds positively to treatment. Conversely, if a nodule hardens with treatment, this could point to greater qi and/or blood stagnation developing (Wang and Robertson 2008, p.345).

Over the years, Dr. Wang and his students have correlated certain findings on the channels with pathology in the body. Discerning these changes helps determine the etiology and ongoing dynamic of emotional trauma. Palpatory and visual changes along the channels can indicate both physical and emotional imbalances in the body. Deciding if the changes are associated with emotional trauma is done by cross-referencing with the other diagnostic techniques available in Chinese medicine.

### Diagnosing Emotional Trauma with Channel Palpation

Emotional trauma presents itself in various channels and can be felt through palpation examination. Nodules, temperature changes, softness, hardness, dryness, slipperiness, and tightness are some of the many findings referred to as channel changes, which give clues into how the channels are being or have been affected (Wang and Robertson 2008, pp.341–349). Palpation of the whole channel and the three depths of each channel can reveal how emotional trauma has affected an organ system. The intensity and duration of a trauma can be felt by the depth, tenderness, or hardness of the nodule, or in the number of changes along a channel. Typically, the deeper, harder, and more pronounced a nodule, the more chronic and more serious the condition (Wang and Robertson 2008, p.349). (*Note:* When treating a channel with a nodule, Dr. Wang taught that one should never needle the nodules, but just to the side of them.)

### Detecting Changes Unilaterally versus Bilaterally

Changes can be on one side of the body or bilaterally; for example, a nodule present at PC-4 on the right arm versus both arms. If the change is present on both limbs, the condition is of internal origin, compared with being one-sided, which generally indicates a musculoskeletal condition.

### The Organization of the Channel Palpation Section

For organization, the channels are listed in a six-level order starting with the yin channels, from external to internal, followed by the yang channels, also from external to internal. Channel palpation includes viewing and feeling the channel, followed by examination of individual areas and points. When palpating a patient, all the arm channels are typically palpated together, beginning with the yin arm channels, feeling from the jing-well points to the he-sea points. The legs are then examined in the same manner. The abdomen and the back are also palpated, yet less frequently. Practitioners must be mindful of palpating points above the knee and points on the abdomen since these are sensitive areas and can trigger memories of abuse.

The descriptions of findings on each channel will be in order from the jing-well points toward the core of the body. This list is meant to be a launching point for discovery and classification and is a humble offering.

## Arm Tai Yin Channel—Lung

The lungs are the closest zang organ to the outside world and is commonly affected by emotional trauma. It has an "opening" movement and serves as a buffer to the patient's environment, interacting with pathogens and warding off "invaders." These invaders include the winds of emotions. A healthy Po can establish clear boundaries within a person's environment. If the Po is weak, a traumatic event (a pathogen) is more likely to disturb the physiological functioning of the lung system: associated emotions lodge in the body.

Differentiating the heart organ from the lung organ system is important in understanding their roles in response to trauma. The heart is like a still pool reflecting the person's environment, which can be stirred once the emotions enter the body.

A rooted Shen protects the heart-reflecting pool from a traumatic event and it will remain still. The lungs play a defensive role and when weak will be disturbed by the trauma. In either case, channel changes will indicate how extensively the trauma disrupted the organ system.

### Trauma Memories Found on the Lung Channel

Often, nodules felt on the lung channel are the residue of old emotions. The channel can have higher-than-average palpable "memories" and it is crucial that the practitioner inquires about the health history of the lungs: pneumonia, loss of a loved one, childhood asthma, and so on. Grief is the predominant emotion to affect the lungs, but several emotions can lodge in its system. Since the lungs act as a defender, when the patient experiences trauma, the entire lung channel can have a feeling of tightness or bumpiness throughout.

**LU-10:** Examination of LU-10, the ying-spring point, can reveal red skin, pale skin, darkness, and engorged blood vessels. The redness represents heat, pale is cold or deficiency, and the darkness and engorged vessels are indicative of stagnation.

**LU-7 vs. LU-6:** Tenderness and nodules in the LU-7 area can relate to an external pathogen (Wang and Robertson 2008, p.365) possibly from a recent emotional trauma that has not yet lodged deeply into the body consciousness. LU-6 relates to an acute emotional reaction or, since it is a xi-cleft point, could also be associated with blood stagnation and emotional trauma affecting blood flow. Both relate to acute issues. The trauma can clear quickly and a resolution of nodules at these areas is rapid. However, LU-6 can relate to tissue memory and there are times when an emotional trauma memory is found here. Darkness seen in this area indicates a chronic lung condition (Wang and Robertson 2008, p.364).

**LU-5 vs. LU-3:** Observing swelling at the he-sea point, LU-5, reflects general qi stagnation in the body (Wang and Robertson 2008, p.363). Chapter Eight in the *Ling Shu* states, "The lung holds the office of prime minister and is the issuer of management and regulation" (Wang and Robertson 2008, p.52). The lungs govern the qi. When a person suffers emotional trauma, the flow of qi is disturbed, which can be felt especially at LU-5. Tenderness and/or nodules will be detected here when an emotional trauma is causing inflammation or heat (Wang and Robertson 2008, p.363). Typically, palpation is done from the jing-well to the he-sea points, though findings at LU-3 are helpful in diagnosing emotional trauma. LU-3 is tender or has a slippery nodule present in the case of mental disassociation or strong grief. The pinyin name is Tian Fu, meaning celestial storehouse. When activated, it can treat emotional imbalances affecting the lungs such as depression, sadness, and confusion. However, not all lung conditions are rooted solely in a lung disharmony.

## Case Study: Using Comprehensive Diagnosis to Determine the Underlying Cause of the Condition

A 56-year-old male, "George," came in reporting a chronic cough. Palpation revealed a slippery nodule at LU-5. His initial diagnosis was lung heat from a pathogen and points on the lung channel were treated. The patient returned with no relief and similar treatment approaches continued, assuming the chronicity of the condition warranted additional treatments. The patient returned with no reduction of the cough.

Upon re-evaluation, George shared that, before the cough began, he had an argument with a woman who was a prominent member of the chamber of commerce; she had threatened to have him removed from his position as president. Anger, stemming from liver congestion, was the main emotion involved and seemed to be injuring the lungs. In the five element overaction cycle, liver can insult the lungs. The liver and gallbladder channels were checked to see if there were any relevant palpatory changes. LV-5 (the luo-connecting point) had tenderness and slippery nodules present. GB-38 (the jing-river point) was tight and tender when pressed. This confirmed wood overacting on metal. Treatment focus changed to address the liver and gallbladder channels. Acupuncture on the yin/yang pair LV-5 and GB-38 cleared the inflammation in the lungs and his cough resolved. Stimulating LV-5 moves qi, and GB-38 frees liver qi stagnation and stops a cough.

This case demonstrates how inflammation at LU-5 gave a clue that heat and inflammation were present in the lungs and indicated the lung channel was affected. However, as Dr. Wang always emphasized, it is important to not simply treat the channel with the palpation changes, but to look deeply into the interaction of all the channels to determine which points to treat.

## Leg Tai Yin Channel—Spleen

The leg tai yin channel is one of the primary channels to palpate when treating emotional trauma. An emotional trauma scatters the qi, un-centers the person's energy, and disrupts the earth element. The spleen organ system is tantamount to gathering energy. This in turn provides the grounding for a person to navigate stressful events in life. Nodules can be found throughout the spleen channel after an emotional trauma and provide great insight into the effect on the spleen and earth aspect of the body.

**SP-3:** Small, slippery nodules or a dip in this area support the diagnosis of spleen channel deficiency (Wang and Robertson 2008, p.371). At times, there will be nodules between SP-3 and SP-4. Tran Viet Dzung identifies "SP-3.5" as a point to treat over-thinking (Dzung 2004). Patients with compulsive or loop thinking will have nodules at this "SP-3.5" area. The side of "SP-3.5" to needle is chosen by the amount of qi deficiency or trauma in the blood. If a patient is weak, choose the SP-3 side, but if they have blood stagnation or issues with the Chong mai (penetrating vessel), then needle on the SP-4 side of the nodule. This technique is effective to alleviate rumination on the trauma memory.

**SP-4:** The Chong vessel opening point will have nodules when there are issues with the blood. The blood, housing the spirit, is connected to emotions, and palpating SP-4 can help indicate the magnitude of effect on the blood by an emotional trauma. The channel changes are usually identified by firm or slippery nodules. When checking the area from SP-3 to SP-4, several sweeps with the thumb near the bone are needed to feel all the subtleties. Changes at the point can also show if an emotional trauma is trapped or originates in the Chong vessel.

**SP-6:** Weakness here is common in patients reliving the trauma memory. The qi and blood are exhausted, and this can be detected with an indentation at this point (Wang and Robertson 2008, p.372). SP-6 is one of the main points to needle after an emotional trauma and will gather the qi and re-order the blood. Typically, once the blood and qi are re-ordered and gathered, the weakness at SP-6 resolves. The three leg yin channels cross at SP-6. Thus, a palpation change at SP-6 indicates an issue with one or more of the leg yin channels—not only spleen involvement. A change here requires the practitioner to employ other diagnostic techniques to understand its significance.

**SP-8:** Representing the gynecological area, nodules here relate to issues with menstrual irregularities, fibroids, ovarian cysts, and so on (Wang and Robertson 2008, p.372). Emotional trauma associated with sexual abuse or repression of sexuality can cause channel changes in this area. Nodules that are softer, closer to the surface, or movable typically represent a trauma that is recent and less intense (Wang and Robertson 2008, p.345).

**SP-9:** Emotional trauma can upset the fluid metabolism and can be detected by the presence of nodules at SP-9. Trauma can scatter the qi, inhibit the fluid metabolism, and create damp accumulation. Nodules at SP-9 indicate fluid accumulation (Wang and Robertson 2008, p.371).

**SP-10:** Heat in the blood commonly occurs with emotional trauma, and tenderness at SP-10 helps to confirm this diagnosis. Clinically, SP-10 is needled with SP-8 for gynecological issues to clear heat if there is a sexually related emotional trauma. SP-10, used on its own, clears general heat due to trauma.

## Arm Shao Yin Channel—Heart

The arm shao yin channel is an obvious channel to check since the heart stores the spirit. Changes on this channel indicate that an emotional trauma has penetrated the pericardium and is housed in the heart. Great care must be taken to slowly feel the channel as nodules tend to be subtle (like grains of sand), primarily in the HT-7 to HT-4 area (Wang and Robertson 2008, p.373). Several palpation checks are required to detect the minute yet significant changes. Dr. Wang located the arm shao yin channel toward the arm jue yin channel in the deep empty space between the flexor carpi ulnaris and the flexor digitorum superficialis.

### THE SIGNIFICANCE OF NODULES ON THE HEART CHANNEL

| Point | Point Designation(s) | Usual Meaning of Nodule |
|-------|----------------------|-------------------------|
| HT-8 | Ying-spring | Heat |
| HT-7 | Source and shu-stream | Qi stagnation/heat |
| HT-6 | Xi-cleft | Yin deficiency |
| HT-5 | Luo-connection | Blood stagnation |
| HT-4 | Jing-river | Qi stagnation |
| HT-3 | He-sea | Disruption in circulation |

Dr. Wang described changes on the heart channel as relating to the conductivity of the heart organ, as opposed to changes on the pericardium channel which represent issues with the blood flow to the heart muscle (Wang and Robertson 2008, pp.157–158). Therefore, when palpating both the heart and pericardium channels, a practitioner differentiates how an emotional trauma has affected the heart. The pericardium is the heart protector and shields the heart from emotional disturbance. If the trauma penetrates this barrier, nodules will be present on the heart channel, indicating possible circulation issues due to conductivity.

## Leg Shao Yin Channel—Kidney

The leg shao yin channel stores the Jing (essence) and holds many clues as to the causes and effects of emotional trauma. Fear, a frequent result of emotional trauma, can freeze or sink the qi, causing kidney deficiency, reflected in palpation findings along the kidney channel.

| Point | Palpatory Findings | Significance |
|---|---|---|
| KD-2 | Vessels | Heat and/or blood stagnation (often due to an acute or chronic head injury) |
| KD-4/ KD-5 | Tenderness | Deficiency |
| | Nodules | Problems in the urinary system |
| KD-3 | Tenderness and/or dip in the tissue | Deficiency |
| KD-7 | Nodules or an indentation | Heat has depleted the yin (Wang and Robertson 2008, p.381) |

**KD-9:** Nodules or tenderness at KD-9, the xi-cleft point of the Yin Wei mai (Linking vessel), can reflect an accumulation of toxins (Wang and Robertson 2008, p.381) in the physical system, correlating toxins and old emotional trauma. More research is needed to confirm this hypothesis.

## Arm Jue Yin Channel—Pericardium

Chapter Eight in the *Su Wen* refers to the pericardium as the secretary; what comes and goes to the heart is protected by the pericardium. The pericardium controls the flow of emotions to and from the heart while regulating its blood supply (Wang and Robertson 2008, p.357). Tightness is commonly found along the entire channel following an emotional trauma. Specific points on the channel will reflect heat, phlegm, qi stagnation, and/or blood stagnation. Frequently, a combination of nodules is present. Nodules on the pericardium channel respond quickly to treatment and generally resolve with one or two acupuncture treatments.

| Point | Palpatory Findings | Significance |
|---|---|---|
| PC-7 | Nodules and tightness | Heat |
| PC-6 | Nodules | Qi stagnation (Wang and Robertson 2008, p.382) |
| PC-5 | Tightness and nodules | Phlegm<br>Emotional disturbance (Wang and Robertson 2008, pp.382–383) |
| PC-4 | Tightness and nodules | Blood stagnation (Wang and Robertson 2008, p.382)<br>Recent trauma, unless there are deep firm nodules indicating the pattern is chronic (Wang and Robertson 2008, p.383) |
| PC-3 | Tenderness | Throat pain or inflammation (Wang and Robertson 2008, p.383)<br>Inability to express due to a trauma |

## Nodules between Channels

Sometimes changes are located between channels. A cluster of nodules is generally found around the area between LU-6 and PC-4 immediately following a verbal assault or confrontation. The patient will report great heaviness in the chest along with a mix of sadness and anger. Needling distally in the empty space right next to the palpation change is effective at reducing chest pain and calming the spirit. By the end of a treatment, the nodule or change will usually have resolved, depending on the acuteness of the trauma. Jason Robertson, senior apprentice of Dr. Wang and certified teacher of the Wang palpation system, frequently finds nodules in this area in patients who sit all day with their shoulders rolled forward, unable to breathe fully with the diaphragm. This scenario commonly leads to feelings of frustration. In these cases, there is not an emotional trauma, but a physical cause. Utilizing questioning and other diagnostics will tease out the root of the nodules. For both etiologies, the nodules in this area tend to resolve quickly with proper treatment.

# Leg Jue Yin Channel—Liver

The leg jue yin channel maintains a harmonious movement of qi by keeping all the channel pathways open (Wang and Robertson 2008, pp.160–161). An emotional trauma blocks this flow, and the extent of impact can be determined through palpation of the leg jue yin channel. The liver is referred to as "the general" and an emotional trauma constrains the general, resulting in disruption of qi flow. A hasty decision by the practitioner to use the liver channel to treat emotional trauma can be erroneous if there are not indicators present. Palpation of the leg jue yin channel is one of the best diagnostics to determine if the liver is significantly affected.

**PALPATORY FINDINGS ON THE LIVER CHANNEL**

| Point(s) | Palpatory Findings | Significance |
|---|---|---|
| LV-2 | Tenderness | Heat |
| LV-3 | Tenderness with nodules/thick tissue | Qi stagnation (Wang and Robertson 2008, p.388) |
| | Soft nodules | Deficiency |
| LV-5 to LV-6 | Nodules and tenderness | Qi and blood stagnation (Wang and Robertson 2008, p.389) |
| LV-8 | Dip or tenderness | Blood deficiency |

## Case Study Revisited: "George" with the Lingering Cough due to Emotional Upset

Identifying the slippery nodules found at LV-5 was crucial in the case of the 56-year-old male, "George," who complained of a lingering cough (mentioned earlier in the arm tai yin channel section). During re-evaluation of his case, palpation of the channels on the leg revealed nodules at LV-5 and spurred questioning as to whether he had experienced any recent emotional upset. He told the story of a chamber of commerce member threatening his job. This information led to reformulating the diagnosis and treating the condition as wood insulting metal. The new diagnosis was quickly confirmed as George felt improvement with breathing after acupressure was applied to LV-5. Acupressure is an effective diagnostic tool for selecting points to needle—it works to test points that help both musculoskeletal and internal medical conditions.

## Arm Tai Yang Channel—Small Intestine

Separating the positive thoughts from the negative is one function of the arm tai yang channel. As the small intestine separates the clear from the turbid, heart function improves. Due to its yin-yang relationship, the small intestine channel plays a large role in clearing trauma from the heart, which maintains a peaceful outlook on life. Singer-songwriter Willie Nelson points out, "Once you replace negative thoughts with positive ones, you'll start having positive results" (Nelson with Pipkin 2006, p.vii).

**SI-3 vs. SI-4:** Understanding if the channel is in a state of excess or deficiency is quickly determined through palpation of SI-3 (the shu-stream point) and SI-4 (the yuan-source point) (Wang and Robertson 2008, p.376). Changes at SI-3 indicate excess, and changes at SI-4 indicate deficiency.

**SI-4 to SI-6:** Nodules between SI-4 and SI-6 indicate neck, shoulder, and scapula musculoskeletal problems (Wang and Robertson 2008, p.375). Tension from emotional trauma can be reflected here.

### *Master Tung Acupuncture Points on the Small Intestine Channel*

**Xin Men (Heart Gate) 33.12:** This point is located 1.5 cun distal from the tip of the olecranon process and is used to treat physical heart conditions (Young 2005, p.48) and opposite-side hip, groin, and sacral pain (Young 2005, pp.49–50). A slippery disc-like nodule at 33.12 can indicate an emotional trauma affecting the heart. Treat this area by needling just distal to the nodule. Instruct the patient on how to locate the point and have them press on the point several times daily for self-care.

**Gan Men (Liver Gate) 33.11:** This point is located midway between the wrist crease and the olecranon process. It is used to treat liver disease when needled on the left arm (Young 2005, pp.48–49). Sometimes, due to emotional trauma, tenderness in this area can indicate imbalances in the liver organ. Careful differentiation using other diagnostic modalities reveals the pathology.

## Leg Tai Yang Channel—Urinary Bladder

The leg tai yang channel is the first line of defense against pathogens invading the body and traverses the largest amount of surface area on the body. Emotional traumas are pathogens. A harmonious and healthy leg tai yang channel protects the body from vulnerability to emotions. The urinary bladder channel connects to all the organs via the back shu points, and thus is commonly used to regulate, balance, and treat the emotions. Tenderness or weaknesses at the back shu points indicate deficiency of organ energy (Wang and Robertson 2008, p.379). If nodules are present at an organ back shu point, the trauma could have affected the organ at the cellular level. Emotions lodged in the channel can cause neck and/or back pain.

**UB-65 vs. UB-64:** Palpating the points UB-64 and UB-65 can help determine how the trauma has affected the channel. Nodules at UB-65 relate to excess, as opposed to nodules at UB-64 indicating deficiency (Wang and Robertson 2008, p.378).

**UB-40:** Fear or stress can affect the leg tai yang channel, resulting in patients reporting pain in the low back. Observation of blood vessels at UB-40 helps to identify long-term fear that caused stagnation in the urinary bladder channel.

---

Case Study: Treating Night Terrors with the Outer Back Shu Points

Dr. Wang described a case of a nine-year-old boy, "Geo," who experienced disturbing dreams, bordering on night terrors. The boy would frequently sleep walk. Dr. Wang instructed Geo's parents to perform acupressure on the outer urinary bladder points (especially at UB-42, UB-44, UB-47, UB-49, and UB-52) to calm his spirit. The technique effectively resolved Geo's night terrors and sleep walking.[5]

The author finds this approach clinically applicable for treating children with emotional trauma who have night terrors.

---

Western psychology recognizes that dreams represent the subconscious; terror (or other intense emotions) can become part of dreams if they are locked in the body. Patients

---

5    Personal teaching from Dr. Wang Ju-Yi to the author.

with PTSD have a higher rate of nightmares (Thünker and Pietrowsky 2012). Studies directly correlate the intensity of anxiety and depression symptoms of patients with PTSD to the strength and frequency of nightmares (Jevtović *et al.* 2011). In addition to stimulating back points on the outer urinary bladder channel, the "Soothing the Trauma Memory" protocol utilizes scalp points, which activate this channel to treat nightmares.

## Arm Shao Yang Channel—San Jiao

The san jiao organ system represents all the channels in the body. (For a detailed description of this concept, refer to Wang and Robertson 2008.) Palpatory changes are frequently found on this channel due to the global impact an emotional trauma has on the body. Several small or large nodules can be present, indicating blockages in the channel system at large. Trauma often causes inflammation, and this can be detected by a generalized bumpiness, which signifies heat accumulation (Wang and Robertson 2008, p.384). A person who has been in a recent car accident would commonly present with this palpatory finding in their san jiao channel.

Once a trauma is trapped in the body, the san jiao can reflect when a trauma memory is cycling. The shao yang channel is a pivot between the external and internal yang channels and is where pathogens become trapped. An emotional trauma that "invades" the body, but has not penetrated the internal pathways, can lodge here. Palpation of the san jiao channel helps determine trauma of this nature.

**PALPATORY FINDINGS ON THE SAN JIAO CHANNEL**

| Point(s) | Palpatory Findings | Significance |
|----------|--------------------|--------------|
| SJ-2 to SJ-3 | Nodules and tenderness | Heat and/or qi stagnation affecting upper body (Wang and Robertson 2008, pp.384–385) |
| SJ-4 | Tenderness | Yang deficiency (Wang and Robertson 2008, p.385) |
| SJ-5 | Nodules and tenderness | Wind-heat or qi stagnation (Wang and Robertson 2008, p.385) |
| SJ-6 | Nodules | Qi stagnation (Wang and Robertson 2008, p.386) |

**SJ-5 vs. SJ-6:** Emotional trauma generating heat can be subtle—undetected in the face, tongue, or pulse. A mild heat accumulation in the channels can be easily triggered by the trauma memory. Palpating the area between SJ-5 and SJ-6 quickly determines if there is more heat or qi stagnation present in the channel system. Changes in the shao yang channel also indicate excess conditions in the jue yin. Heat and stagnation can be diagnosed by palpating both the san jiao and gallbladder channels. For example, heat in the liver can be detected in nodules at SJ-5, compared with qi stagnation showing at SJ-6. The gallbladder channel also reflects changes in the liver.

# Leg Shao Yang Channel—Gallbladder

Trauma can disorder thinking and decision-making. Palpation of the leg shao yang channel measures the extent of the trauma on the gallbladder function. Emotional trauma scatters the qi, rendering the patient unable to make decisions and move forward in life. Feelings of resentment can affect the gallbladder channel and constrain the Hun. The state of the Hun can be assessed by palpating the gallbladder channel due to its connection with the liver—the yin paired channel.

**GB-41:** If there is heat accumulation in the gallbladder channel, there can be tenderness at GB-41 (Wang and Robertson 2008, p.386). In addition to heat, because GB-41 is the opening point on the Dai (Girdle) vessel (Deadman and Al-Khafaji 1998, p.460), changes here can relate to emotions disturbing the Dai vessel.

**GB-40:** The gallbladder channel is paired with the heart channel in the same moving pivot channel pairing (see page 122). Observation of GB-40 is helpful in diagnosing heart deficiency caused by emotional trauma. Puffiness at this point indicates deficiency and, if nodules are present, the deficiency is chronic, coupled with qi stagnation (Wang and Robertson 2008, pp.386–387).

**GB-39:** A dip or weak feeling at the meeting point of the marrow represents deficiency (Wang and Robertson 2008, p.343) and can be an indicator of how emotional trauma has affected the shao yin channel. Emotional trauma, especially that involving fear which weakens the kidneys, can lodge deep in the body—into the marrow. Needling GB-39 supports the kidneys and treats atrophy disorders (Deadman and Al-Khafaji 1998, p.457). Therefore, activating the point helps the body to shore up strength and release fear. Also, due to the gallbladder and heart connection, fear creating heart deficiency can be reflected at GB-39 by a dip or weakness in the tissue. (*Note:* In this system, GB-39 is located anterior to the fibula.)

Conversely, if nodules are present at GB-39, there is qi/blood stagnation in the channel. Anger or frustration affect the wood element and can imbed in the leg shao yang channel. A common example is a patient having a stiff or painful neck following an argument. Needling GB-39 releases this emotional block. Such an argument is not usually a significant traumatic event, but there can be long-term resentment that is triggered. For example, a patient wanting to shield herself from a trauma memory could tense up in her neck.

**GB-38:** Examine for nodules or weakness. The point frees the congestion in the liver channel (yin-yang channel pairing connection) and is also the jing-river point on the gallbladder channel. Thus, it can treat a cough and open the voice.

**GB-34:** This point relates to the qi flow of the gallbladder. Tenderness at this point indicates channel stagnation as opposed to pain specifying stagnation in the organ (Wang and Robertson 2008, p.387). Once the stagnation is cleared, the patient's ability to make choices and move forward is restored. The tenderness should reduce at each patient visit, reflecting treatment effectiveness.

## Arm Yang Ming Channel—Large Intestine

The yang ming channel has the most qi and blood, and both the arm and leg channels commonly have several changes reflecting emotional trauma. Tenderness, nodules, and pulsing are all indicators of the status of qi and blood (excess or deficient) in the arm yang ming channel. Palpation changes found along the arm yang ming channel often indicate the large intestine emotional pattern of having trouble "letting go."

**LI-4:** This point is commonly tender on most people and thus sensitivity is not helpful in differentiation. However, small nodules in this area can give clues as to emotional trauma affecting the heart. The second metacarpal bone can be viewed as a microsystem for the body, where the point two-thirds distally represents the chest/heart. When needled it treats insomnia due to emotional etiology.[6]

**LI-5:** Differentiating the pulsing found at LI-5 will determine excess or deficiency; that is, strong pulsing indicates excess, and weak pulsing shows deficiency (Wang and Robertson 2008, pp.366–367). Clinically, when a person is holding onto a trauma and not letting it go, they can suffer with constipation detected by a strong deep pulse at LI-5. If the strong pulse is on the surface, this relates to an external condition (Wang and Robertson 2008, p.367) and could indicate a recent trauma.

**LI-10 and LI-11:** Several small nodules along the arm yang ming channel, from the jing-river point to the he-sea point, are common. Typically, these nodules show inflammation or blocks in the channel (Wang and Robertson 2008, pp.366–367). Nodules concentrated at LI-11 indicate heat accumulation, whereas a weak feeling at LI-10 reveals deficiency (Wang and Robertson 2008, p.368). The chronic reliving of a trauma exhausts the qi in the large intestine channel, reflected by nodules, tenderness, or weakness at LI-10.

---

6    Personal training with Wei-Chieh Young and Susan Johnson, L.Ac.

## Case Study: Resolving Crohn's Disease with the Large Intestine Channel

A 23-year-old male, "Cecil," sought acupuncture treatment for his Crohn's disease. He had been dealing with severe intestinal symptoms for three years and was now housebound. Cecil's bouts of diarrhea, fatigue, and abdominal pain had become constant and he was depressed about not being able to engage in life. His initial diagnosis was lung and spleen deficiency, and treatment was focused in the tai yin channel. Treating the he-sea and yuan-source points gave mild relief. However, he could only be away from his house for a few hours. Coincidentally, Yefim Gamgoneishvili, L.Ac., senior apprentice under Dr. Wang, visited the clinic around the time of Cecil's treatment.

Mr. Gamgoneishvili palpated the arm channels and discovered several large nodules on the arm yang ming channel. Cecil was given a new diagnosis of heat accumulation in the yang ming channel. Utilizing points on the yang ming and jue yin channels, he experienced great relief. During this stage of treatment, Cecil became aware of old emotional trauma he had been holding on to. With the new treatment approach, he felt it clear and had the courage to engage more fully in life; his condition stabilized. Five years after this course of treatment, he was an artist working in the community, reporting strong energy, and eating and drinking previously irritating foods and fluids in moderation.

## Leg Yang Ming Channel—Stomach

The leg yang ming channel (associated with the earth element) can reveal both excess and deficiency changes resulting from trauma. Traumas frequently cause tension in the digestive system, and nodules at certain points reflect this excess condition. The depth and firmness of the nodules shows the chronicity of the trauma. Conversely, indentations and weakness in the tissue are frequently palpated along the channel due to a depletion of energy. Reliving the trauma memory drains the qi and blood, causing the stomach to exert energy to maintain and support the needs of the body. This exertion can result in an overall deficiency in the stomach organ system.

The stomach channel supports the pericardium channel due to the same moving closing channel pairing (see page 122). Nodules, tenderness, and weakness at areas in the stomach channel provide hints to the effect of the emotional trauma on the pericardium. Because of its yin-yang pairing connection with the spleen channel, palpated changes on the stomach channel can reflect when the spleen is disrupted by trauma. Utilizing other diagnostics determines which channels are affected.

**ST-44 to ST-43:** In cases of strong emotion affecting the qi and blood flow, nodules are felt throughout the channel. A "bumpy" stomach channel can signify wood overacting on earth and cases of emotional trauma held in the stomach. Tenderness and nodules between ST-44 and ST-43 suggest heat and qi stagnation (Wang and Robertson 2008, p.368). Nodules at ST-43 can also specify cold, indicating that the trauma has frozen the energy in the digestive system. To discern whether the nodules are from heat or cold, other diagnostic methods are needed. In some cases, a stick-like change is present at ST-43 that crosses over to the liver channel.

## Case Study: Recognizing the Significance of Stick-Like Nodules

A 54-year-old woman, "Yolanda," with work stress and migraines, sought treatment with acupuncture. On the first visit a large stick-like nodule was noticeable. It traversed the leg jue yin and yang ming channels at the level of ST-43. The nodule seemed to signify qi stagnation, causing her migraines. Her stress and headaches were managed with acupuncture, but the stick-like nodule remained. This appeared to be a tissue memory associated with stress. Treatment to control her headaches continued. She had a lot of resentment and anger toward her job and felt her supervisor was demanding and overbearing. She struggled to maintain a life outside work, while working 60-hour weeks. After her headaches were stabilized she discontinued treatment. A year later she returned, diagnosed with breast cancer.

Dr. Wang explained stick-like nodules as indicators of inflammation in the channel or in a specific area of the body related to the channel (Wang and Robertson 2008, p.347). Since both the liver and stomach channels go to the breast, and resentment is a key emotion in breast cancer (Beerlandt 1993, p.153), this stick-like finding should have triggered a thorough diagnostic work-up. A large stick-like nodule on any channel is significant.

The patient had been through chemo and radiation treatments. By the time of her return, the stick-like nodule was reduced by 75 percent. As treatment continued, the stick-like nodule remained, but was smaller and represented a memory. There was a tendency for Yolanda to develop inflammation and toxins, and her treatments incorporated regulation and clearing heat when necessary.

This change is sometimes found on women with breast cancer. Another patient with breast cancer—Stage Three in the right breast and Stage Two in the left breast—had stick-like changes across ST-43 to LV-3 on both feet (with a larger stick-like change on the right side). A third patient with breast cancer in the left breast presented with a stick-like change only on the left foot. Having a stick-like change in this area does not confirm or relate solely to breast cancer but it is a helpful marker to give clues as to whether the patient might have this type of disease.

## Resentment and Over-Nurturing

Resentment is one emotion underlying breast cancer and is about not letting go. The stomach takes in food, ferments it, and then lets it go to the spleen to be transformed. Finding a stick-like nodule at ST-43 to LV-3 could reflect a woman harboring resentment. Resentment tends to constrain the energy and create pressure—frequently resulting in wood overacting on earth. Chronic pressure in the system will lead to a mixed excess and deficiency condition.

Another emotion involved with breast cancer, and cancer in general, is over-nurturing (Bridges 2012, p.253). After experiencing emotional trauma, patients can hold the faulty belief that they need to give all of themselves to others in order to be loved. Nodules and/or weakness in the tissue on the stomach channel can reflect this tendency. Over-nurturing drains the energy of the earth element, causing deficiency.

**ST-39 to ST-36:** This area is helpful in determining excess and deficiency conditions in the stomach, large intestine, and small intestine. A thickening of tissue or nodules identifies qi stagnation, and engorged blood vessels indicate blood stagnation. Finding engorged vessels in this area and bleeding them is incredibly effective at treating blood stagnation due to an emotional trauma. Patients commonly report an immediate lightening of their spirit and openness in their chest. (For a detailed description of this technique refer to "Bloodletting" in Chapter 3.) If a dip or weakness in the tissue is present in ST-36, there is an overall qi and blood deficiency; whereas if present at ST-37 or ST-39, it can be qi deficiency in the large intestine or small intestine respectively (Wang and Robertson 2008, p.370).

**ST-34:** Emotional trauma can create coldness in the stomach channel, and nodules at ST-34 can confirm this condition (Wang and Robertson 2008, p.370). Tenderness and pain at ST-34, the xi-cleft point, signify blood stagnation. Acupressure on this point is a helpful part of a self-care program for those who have wood overacting on the stomach. When the patient has stress that causes stomach pain or cramping, pressure on the point can quickly resolve the physical complaint.

**ST-25:** Examination of ST-25 assists in determining the state of fluids, qi, and temperatures in the digestive system. Emotional trauma disturbs the Yi and the processing of nutrition. A pulsing indicates accumulation of fluids. Tenderness or tightness shows excess in the channel, and if it is weak or soft at this point then there is deficiency (Wang and Robertson 2008, p.370). Feel the upper and lower abdomen with the back of the hand to test if there is heat or cold present (Wang and Robertson 2008, pp.339–340).

# Ren Channel—Conception Vessel

Emotional trauma unsettles the yin and blood. The Ren vessel is responsible for collecting the yin and blood and for the development of the fetus (Wang and Robertson 2008, p.289). Therefore, trauma (including trauma experienced *in utero*) can be diagnosed and treated with this vessel. Three zones are especially useful: the area from R-4 to R-6, the area around R-9, and the area between R-11 and R-13.

**R-4 and R-6:** Palpating the area from R-4 to R-6 (regularly utilized to treat deficiency) displays both excess and deficiency patterns. Hardness shows blood stagnation, weakness or softness means deficiency, a strong pulse indicates accumulation of fluids and/or cold stagnation, and nodules mean cold phlegm (Wang and Robertson 2008, p.393). R-4 is a primary point to increase yuan qi, tonify kidney yang, nourish kidney yin, and benefit essence (Deadman and Al-Khafaji 1998, p.502). R-6, compared with R-4, primarily tonifies qi rather than nourishing yin and blood (Deadman and Al-Khafaji 1998, p.505). Depending on the changes found, and other diagnostic signs, either or both of these points address deep-seated trauma and build the body's energy to transform the trauma.

**R-9:** This point regulates water in the body (Deadman and Al-Khafaji 1998, p.509). A strong pulse in this area indicates an accumulation of fluids, and stimulating R-9 effectively resolves the accumulation.

---

## Case Study: Dissolving a Cyst with R-9

A 58-year-old woman, "Catalina," complained of right leg pain that was electric, intense, and worse when she turned over in bed. Her diagnosis was qi and blood stagnation in the urinary bladder channel, treated using the Master Tung point pair of 22.05 Ling Gu and 22.04 Da Bai, along with SI-3. Catalina reported some reduction in the pain after five treatments, but the pain was still intense. She went to her medical doctor for a work-up. The MD said she had a cyst at L5-S1 that was pressing on a nerve. His treatment was to aspirate and, if unsuccessful, surgery would be required. The patient wanted to try a few acupuncture treatments before any Western medical procedure.

Catalina communicated her Western diagnosis, which led to a more extensive Chinese medicine diagnostic work-up, including palpating the Ren vessel. Palpation revealed a pulsing at R-9 and at R-6. R-9 was added to the acupuncture treatment. Catalina shared that she had suffered great stress from dealing with her husband's mental state. Fear was a common emotion she had felt over the last few years. This information prompted the addition of using KD-16 along with R-9, Ling Gu, Da Bai, and SI-3. KD-16 was treated due to its location, ability to regulate the qi, stop pain, and address conditions where kidney yang deficiency curtailed fluid circulation. The patient returned the next week reporting the pain was gone. This treatment was continued for four sessions and she continued to be pain-free. Catalina saw her MD for a follow-up exam. The MD reported that the cyst had been resolved, thus obviating the need for surgery.

It is amazing that simply adding R-9 made such an impact; it shows the power of the point. The emotional effect of her fear possibly caused the cyst. Now years after this series of treatments, her back remains pain-free. Even though she does not report pain in her back, continued acupuncture treatment to address fear along the kidney channel and other channels ensures that fluid does not reaccumulate.

**R-11 to R-13:** A softness at R-11 reflects deficiency in the digestive system and is used in treatments to bolster the qi. The center of the body is R-12. Being the primary point to regulate stomach function (Deadman and Al-Khafaji 1998, p.511), it grounds and gathers energy in the body and is one of the points in the "Gathering the Qi" protocol. Palpation changes at this point can indicate excess or deficiency. Detecting a strong pulse between R-12 and R-13 indicates an excess condition affecting the spleen and/or stomach (Wang and Robertson 2008, p.393). Feeling softness or tender nodules between R-12 and R-13 shows spleen deficiency, including chronic stomach problems. There can be an issue with the proper ascending and descending action of the spleen. As described in Wang and Robertson (2008), "Lack of proper transformation, over time, leads to dampness and possibly heat accumulation that can be palpated in the area" (pp.393–394). This indicator helps determine if the emotional trauma is causing an excess or deficiency pattern in the earth element. Simply feeling and pressing this area centers and grounds patients and, for those who are needle-sensitive (especially children), gentle acupressure can be an effective treatment.

## Du Mai—Governing Vessel

The Du vessel governs the yang channels. Changes on the vessel can reflect emotional trauma on a systemic level since the channel connects with all the six regular yang channels and is used to treat a lack of movement anywhere in the body (Wang and Robertson 2008, p.290). The Du vessel can also indicate specific organ involvement. Palpation changes at the level of each organ denote the particular organ system affected and are similar to the urinary bladder channel in this regard (Wang and Robertson 2008, p.390). Tenderness, thickening, and nodules can be found in the spaces between and on the vertebras. The nodules relate to heat and qi stagnation in the respective organ system closest to the change.

## Case Study: Treating Digestive Disorders with the Du Vessel

A 52-year-old man, "Kwan," sought Chinese medicine treatment, suffering from indigestion and stomach pains that worsened with stress. Acupuncture treatment began in the supine position addressing wood overacting on earth, but yielded minimal results, primarily because in hindsight the position prevented examination of the Du vessel. Kwan mentioned mid-back pain that seemed to correlate to his stomach pain. Palpation along the Du vessel revealed tenderness, a thick area, and nodules between DU-6 and DU-9. His urinary bladder channel in this area was tight but didn't show changes. Needling DU-6 and DU-10 opened the channel, dispelled heat, and cleared the changes. Kwan reported significant relief, and the symptoms resolved after three treatments. He was feeling good and was released from treatment.

For the next several years following his initial acupuncture session, Kwan continued to have a great deal of frustration and tension due to his job. He explained it was "just life." Kwan's pains would return every six to nine months, and each time a few treatments of the Du vessel would resolve the stagnation and heat.

---

Treating the Du vessel for organ involvement is helpful in situations when the radial pulse diaphragm position is inflated from a shock or "heartbreak." Dr. Leon Hammer, teacher of the Shen/Hammer pulse system, finds that suppressed feelings cause this inflated quality in this pulse position (Hammer 2001, p.451). To confirm this type of emotional trauma, palpate the area from DU-8 to DU-9. If there are nodules present, needling the Du vessel on either side of the affected area will transform the repressed emotions. Jason Robertson finds that nodules between DU-8 and DU-9 along with nodules between PC-5 and PC-6 indicate a pericardium pattern. This relates to what was found in the Kwan case.

## Summary of Channel Palpation

Acupuncture channels flowing smoothly produce beautiful music. Palpating the songs of the channels reveals which organ systems are in tune and which need attention due to disturbance from emotional trauma. As the trauma memory is released, the channel coordination is improved and a harmonious symphony resonates. Combining channel palpation with other diagnostic methods allows the practitioner to conduct the treatment of the body with ease. Pulse diagnosis is another technique relying on "listening" to the organs to know how best to transform trauma.

## PULSE DIAGNOSIS

### General Pulse Diagnosis Information

See the inside through the windows on the outside. Chinese medicine asserts that the external body reflects the internal environment, and the sound of the radial artery pulse provides immense information about the physiology within the body. Several family lineage pulse systems are in use throughout the world and they do share commonalities. A pulse that feels slippery can indicate fluid accumulation or heat. A choppy pulse indicates blood stagnation. These basic ideas clarify the nature of the pattern and determine which organs are involved as a result of an emotional trauma. However, if the practitioner incorporates the subtleties of the pulse, they have a better assessment. There are particular pulse qualities associated with emotional trauma, and each lineage has its own interpretation.

The specific pulse (radial artery) qualities presented below are from the Shen/ Hammer Pulse Diagnostic Lineage, a system requiring comprehensive training to fully understand. (For additional information about this lineage technique refer to Hammer 2001 and study with a certified pulse teacher—see Dragon Rises 2017.) This offering assists those proficient in this lineage and serves as a launching point for those interested in the system.[7]

### Specific Pulse Qualities and Presentations

#### Tight and Rapid

An emotional shock is sudden and causes the patient to physically tense up and eventually repress the trauma. This creates a tense quality in the pulse. Heat is usually present and the pulse is rapid. Hammer explains that a person with a repressed trauma is controlling their emotions and holding their breath. Over time, this leads to a flat quality in the pulse (Hammer 2001, p.213). A flat quality indicates that the qi is unable to reach an organ (Hammer 2001, p.211).

---

7   The lineage was taught by John H.F. Shen to Leon Hammer. Brian LaForgia studied under both Dr. Shen and Dr. Hammer and is the person who primarily taught the author. The author is not a certified teacher in the Shen-Hammer Lineage but has studied under LaForgia (Certified Shen-Hammer Lineage teacher) for several years, having taken beginning and intermediate pulse courses. The author also completed a six-month internship under Brandt Stickley (Certified Shen-Hammer Lineage teacher and apprentice under Leon Hammer), and used this pulse lineage system clinically for over nine years. The author is not an expert but, through both LaForgia's and Stickley's teachings and clinical experience, has insight to offer in regard to diagnosing emotional trauma through the pulse.

## Slippery

A slippery quality is most known for indicating damp and phlegm accumulation, but can also be detected when the heart is disturbed by trauma and circulation is affected (Hammer 2001, p.315). A slippery pulse is also found if heat stirs the blood (causing turbulence) (Hammer 2001, p.735) and when emotional trauma drains yin (Hammer 2001, p.137).

## Choppy

The choppy quality of the pulse is commonly known to reflect blood stagnation and is often found in cases of trauma. This quality can exist across the whole pulse or at specific positions (indicating the organ affected by the emotional trauma) (Hammer 2001, p.365).

## Deep

A deep pulse represents a deficiency and can indicate a chronic condition (Hammer 2001, p.269) such as unresolved emotional trauma depleting the Zheng qi (upright qi). The pulse will rise as the trauma clears and is a great determiner of treatment efficacy. If a pulse becomes deeper, the qi is decreasing (Hammer 2001, p.216).

## Feeble Absent and Empty

An old, deep-seated trauma causes both pulse types, with the feeble absent quality preceding the empty quality (Hammer 2001, p.251). These pulses are associated with qi and blood deficiency—the empty quality being more serious and belonging to the "qi wild" category (discussed below) (Hammer 2001, pp.216 and 246). When the organ energy is exhausted, the pulse separates and disperses with pressure (Hammer 2001, pp.216–219). If the deficiency is not treated, an empty pulse (felt at the superficial level but disappearing with pressure) is detected (Hammer 2001, p.247). The empty pulse indicates a serious condition and requires immediate attention.

Organ exhaustion is common with unresolved traumas and the reliving of trauma memories. Deciding which organs need attention can be challenging, but becomes obvious if a particular organ position has an empty quality. One scenario, when this quality is found, is when a certain organ system is working overtime to correct a disruption by an emotional trauma. The organ is exhausted from trying to maintain balance in the body. For example, there is an empty pulse in the proximal position because the kidneys are struggling to sustain harmony, ever since a childhood trauma. An empty pulse can also be detected when an emotion has depleted an organ system; for example, grief exhausting the lungs.

## Muffled

The muffled pulse is appropriately named as it represents a muffling or dampening of energy. The quality feels as if a blanket or cloth is on top of the artery (Hammer 2001, p.226). Many pulse diagnosticians say they listen to the pulse, not feeling it, and the quality is literally a muffled sound. The muffled quality indicates serious illness (Hammer 2001, p.226). The life of the spirit is hindered. Depression causes a muffled pulse in the left distal position, that is, the heart position (Hammer 2001, p.227).

## Scattered

Frequently, after a serious traumatic event, the pulse will be scattered, reflecting the dispersing nature of trauma. The pulse quality has a discontinuous rhythm and represents deficiency of qi, blood, yin, and yang (Hammer 2001, pp.256–257). The "Gathering the Qi" protocol resolves this quality and restores order.

## Blood Unclear/Blood Heat/Blood Thick

Blood unclear, blood heat, and blood thick are qualities aptly named since they refer to the progression of heat and/or toxins accumulating in the blood (Hammer 2001, p.478). This quality is found by pressing the fingers to the organ (deepest) depth of the pulse and then slowly lifting them to the surface. If the pulse strength increases and hits against the fingers as they are lifted to the surface depth, this indicates blood unclear/heat/thick (Hammer 2001, p.479).

The intensity of the overflowing strength of the pulse as one lifts to the surface directly correlates with how severely the blood is affected, that is, toxins are at an advanced stage. Blood unclear is the mildest condition, and blood thick is the most advanced (Hammer 2001, p.478). Emotional trauma stuck in the body has the potential to generate heat. These pulse qualities are effective indicators.

## Change in Intensity

Emotional trauma disturbs the heart and affects circulation (Hammer 2001, p.137), giving the pulse an inconsistent wave (Hammer 2001, pp.37–38). If the instability of the wave is consistent, there is a blood circulation issue. If the instability is inconsistent, the issue is qi circulation (Hammer 2001, p.38). The heart yin is commonly drained by trauma, changing the stability of the wave, along with causing a red face and pale hands (Hammer 2001, p.137).

## Hesitant

The hesitant wave quality feels as if the pulse has lost its wave shape and has a sudden sharpness rather than a gentle rolling. It indicates a mild heart yin deficiency caused by obsessive thinking (Hammer 2001, pp.126–127). This quality is becoming increasingly common and is found in students and others who have a strong cerebral emphasis, that is, "heady people" (people who are constantly thinking and processing) (Hammer 2001, p.126). Thus, patients who ruminate on their trauma and continue to relive the memory frequently have a hesitant pulse. As the trauma memory is soothed and the patient can let it go, this quality clears.

## Qi Wild

Qi Wild is an umbrella phrase to include several pulse qualities indicating yin and yang separation. Two of these are mentioned above—empty and scattered. These represent extreme weakness and a dispersion of the body's energy (Hammer 2001, p.128). Emotional trauma can have a serious impact on the body, depleting it over time. When these pulses are detected, attention to harmonizing the yin and yang is needed. Fortunately, the "Gathering the Qi" and the "Soothing the Trauma Memory" protocols, followed by tonification treatments, effectively address these pulse conditions and stabilize yin and yang.

## Rough and Smooth Vibration

A vibration in the pulse shows instability of energy and agitation of heart qi (Hammer 2001, p.368). The quality is like a buzzing and can be felt with the fingers stationary on the pulse (Hammer 2001, p.367). The vibration quality is often confused with the choppy quality. A delineating difference is that the choppy quality is felt as the fingers are rolled over the pulse (Hammer 2001, p.367). The level of instability is measured by the quality of vibration, rough indicating a higher level. Vibration quality represents a kind of shock to the body (Hammer 2001, p.368). As the intensity of the emotional trauma lessens, this quality will clear. Patients suffering from insomnia, stress, and worry typically have either a smooth or rough vibration.

## Bifurcated or "Split" Pulse

The bifurcated or split pulse (an uncommon finding) is sensed when feeling two pulses side-by-side at the radial artery. This represents abandonment at an early age, consuming thoughts of death, an experience of personal horror, or near-death experiences (Hammer 2001, p.380). The left and right wrists signify subtle differences about death. The left reflects a person having consuming thoughts about their own death, whereas the right reflects thoughts of someone else's death. Thus, suicidal people have this pulse on the left side. Emotional trauma can be intense, cause suicidal thoughts, and, when reflected in the pulse, show the severity of the case. Morbid thoughts involving loved ones, friends, and co-workers, for example, resulting from emotional trauma, would be felt on the right side, reflecting intense thoughts surrounding death.

### Spinning Bean

The spinning bean (commonly indicating severe fright or terror) is a rare pulse detected between or on the side of a main pulse position. It has a tight, wiry, and swirling feeling that tends to hit the finger with urgency (Hammer 2001, p.375). The spinning denotes a significant physiological disturbance caused by a significant trauma. Sensitivity is crucial when asking the patient about having a fright. If done graciously, the patient feels relieved to express their traumatic event. The intensity in the spinning bean may reduce as they talk about their experience, and the quality is expected to reduce with each successful treatment—reflecting the diminishing of stored terror in the body.

### Presence of the Diaphragm Position

The diaphragm position is considered present if there is an inflated quality detected when rolling the finger proximally from the distal position and distally from the middle pulse position. This can be found on one or both wrists (Hammer 2001, p.450). If the diaphragm position is present—more commonly on the left side—this indicates a broken heart or repressed anger over an event (Hammer 2001, p.579). When a person experiences a shock or fright, they quickly take a breath and hold it, essentially locking the trauma in the diaphragm. As noted in the channel palpation section describing the Du vessel, needling points around the seventh thoracic vertebra clear this pulse finding.

## Summary of Pulse Diagnosis

Chinese pulse diagnosis is a helpful sounding board with which to compare the findings of other diagnostic methods. For example, when finding a blood unclear pulse quality paired with tenderness at LV-2, and a deep red tongue, heat in the blood is confirmed. Another example would be verifying the diagnosis of heart/pericardium stagnation with the following signs: a person has the diaphragm pulse position present, a pinched nose tip, nodules and tenderness at DU-9, a history of an acrimonious separation, and duskiness in the tongue tip. Pulse diagnosis is one of the most common diagnostic techniques used in Chinese medicine clinics, along with tongue diagnosis.

## TONGUE DIAGNOSIS
### General Tongue Diagnosis Information

A farmer observes the soil to determine the health of their crops. If the soil is dry and cracked, water is needed. Comparatively, a dry, cracked tongue shows a body that is dehydrated. The tongue is an organ displaying all the qualities of the other organs within, and Chinese medicine evaluates tongue color, shape, and coating to deeply understand the health of the body. Distinctive qualities of the tongue presented below are included to support the diagnosis of an emotional trauma. Basic qualities are not included in this chapter, such as red (indicating heat), less coat (showing deficiency of fluids), or pale (meaning coldness and/or blood deficiency), but all help in determining the pathogens involved in trauma. (Many of the descriptions of qualities listed below come from Barbara Kirschbaum's 2000 book, *Atlas of Chinese Tongue Diagnosis*, and the reader is encouraged to reference her text and view the numerous pictures.)

### Specific Tongue Signs Relating to Emotional Trauma
#### Hammer Tip

The hammer tip is the shape wherein the tongue has a line to the tip with the two sides of the tongue joining at the tip. This is found in patients who have heart deficiency and a sensitive heart (Kirschbaum 2000, p.111). If there is a line at the tip, the patient has constitutional heart deficiency (Kirschbaum 2000, p.107). There can also be an indentation at the tip without a line, reflecting a temporary heart deficiency. Patients with this tongue shape might have a heightened level of sensitivity to their environment, enabling them to perceive energy on a subtle level. Helping to establish clear boundaries will benefit their energy reserves and maintain strong Zheng qi.

#### Rough Edges and Curled-Up Edges

Rough edges on the sides of the tongue indicate a tired and overworked liver. Not to be confused with scallop/teeth marks on the tongue, the rough edges appear lacerated and can reflect an overwhelmed liver striving to clear blocked qi from emotional trauma. These rough edges are frequently found in patients who lead stressful, overscheduled lives and don't sleep well. It is also common in those who have been exposed to many toxins, through recreational drugs, multiple pharmaceutical prescriptions, or environmental poisons. Patients with rough edges are prone to chemical sensitivity and to weak immune systems. If the edges are curled up, this signifies liver qi stagnation (Kirschbaum 2000, p.134).

### Coating on One Side

Coating on one side of the tongue indicates either a shao yang syndrome (on the left side) or liver stagnation (on the right side) (Kirschbaum 2000, p.186). This finding can help verify if the emotional trauma is trapped in the shao yang level or if it has affected the body at the organ level.

### Engorged or Pale Veins

The state of the blood is reflected under the tongue and provides insight into the spirit. Engorged veins under the tongue denote blood stagnation (Kirschbaum 2000, p.6). Treatments to regulate the blood commonly clear the engorgement quickly. Monitoring changes in the degree of engorgement provides a means to measure treatment effectiveness. Sometimes this area can be pale (indicating blood deficiency) and can take several treatments to amend.

### Dip in the Back of the Tongue

Assuming the patient is holding their tongue in the relaxed position, a dip in the back relates to constitutional kidney deficiency or it can be a sign of yin deficiency (Kirschbaum 2000, p.57). Emotional trauma will likely affect the kidney organ system in patients with this diagnostic sign.

### Puffy in the Center of the Tongue

A tongue with a puffy center area indicates stagnation and fluid accumulation in the earth element. Patients with wood overacting on earth commonly present with this sign.

## Case Study: Fluids Impeding the Spirit

"Jackie" suffered from chronic depression and felt worthless (the condition began at age ten when she was enrolled in public school). She had intense panic attacks and was unable to work, rarely leaving her house. Jackie was taking medications for depression and anxiety, but they offered minimal relief. She was constantly worried, resulting in nausea and a low appetite. Jackie had several organ spirit deficiencies: a weakened Yi, a frozen Zhi, and a destabilized Po. Jackie's inaction and poor dietary habits depleted her Yi, generating phlegm/damp accumulation with phlegm heat misting her heart. Jackie's Zhi was suffering, due to stagnation in her earth element that had exhausted her water element. Her lack of movement caused blood stagnation and strained her lung qi, which exhausted her Po. Jackie's energy field was perceived as extremely sensitive and disconnected. Helping her to regain her spirit was paramount. Jackie's tongue was red and dusky (heat accumulation and blood stagnation) with a thick green and white coating (phlegm damp accumulation with heat). She had an indentation on the tip (as opposed to a line to the tip), reflecting temporary heart deficiency (Figure 2.16).

Treatments focused on stabilizing her spirit and transforming phlegm. The "Gathering the Qi" acupuncture protocol was modified (PC-5 and SP-9 were substituted for PC-6 and SP-6) to address the phlegm. A gentle Shamanic Journey Drumbeat was used to calm her spirit. Jackie was instructed to adopt basic Chinese medicine dietary recommendations and was encouraged to return to her hobbies (quilting, baking, and gardening).

After three treatments, Jackie reported that she had gone to the park, was quilting, had lost weight, was feeling confident, had minimal panic attacks, and felt courageous enough to take care of a friend's son. Her tongue coating cleared, the dusky color reduced, and the indentation on her tongue tip lessened. Jackie continued to improve and after a few more treatments started working as a seamstress. She felt increasingly confident in public and had not experienced any strong anxiety attacks.

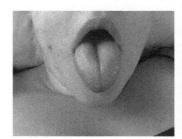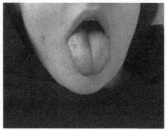

*Figure 2.16 Jackie's Tongue Before and After Three Chinese Medicine Treatments*

## Summary of Tongue Diagnosis

Chinese medicine tongue diagnosis provides an additional layer of confirmation of the root cause of emotional trauma, and is yet another method to illuminate a practitioner's intuition. The clearer the practitioner is about the cause, the better their ability to be grounded and centered, to hold a strong healing space for the patient, and to effectively treat trauma. It also opens the windows of awareness to perceive the subtleties in a patient's spirit.

## INTUITING THE FIVE SPIRITS

Great inventors and healers throughout time have relied on intuition as their guide. The five spirits in Chinese medicine (Zhi, Hun, Shen, Yi, and Po) are used to put words to the sensations and gut feelings a person has when encountering another. The emotions can be palpable when a patient first walks into the clinic, feeling scared about acupuncture and seemingly timid. Children are especially emotionally forthcoming and wear their emotions on their sleeves. Most people can tell when a child is scared, sad, or angry. However, adults frequently put on masks to conceal their emotions. During an intake, these masks are removed and the spirits dance before the practitioner. Their energy field can be interpreted using the understanding of the five spirits to reveal imbalances caused by emotional trauma.

### *Illuminating Intuition through Diagnostic Techniques*

The diagnostic methods in Chinese medicine guide intuition. Utilizing the signs verified by skills such as facial, pulse, channel, and tongue diagnosis, a practitioner's sixth sense is illuminated and feelings about a patient's imbalances are perceived. When a patient feels protected and senses good intention, they feel comfortable showing their true self. In a safe healing space, the patient's demeanor is genuine; they are not acting out a role. Reading a patient's body language, voice tenor, energy, and so on allows for any imbalance to be correctly detected. Diagnosing with intuition is about tuning in to the primal ability to sense the spirit of another.

---

## Case Study: Activating the Healing Process with Intuition

A 56-year-old man, "Reggie," sought Chinese medicine treatment to improve his energy levels. Through sensing the imbalances in his five spirits, it was determined that his Shen was not active enough in his life and Reggie needed to enhance creativity within his career. This insight was facilitated through facial diagnosis.

On Reggie's forehead was a deep, vertical indentation. This indicated that the sides of his ancestry were dramatically dissimilar, that is, his parents were two very different people. The marking was explained to Reggie using the example that his mother was very practical and his father was an artist. Reggie's eyes widened and he exclaimed, "That's true!" The practitioner was unaware of this fact and was simply giving a random example to describe the meaning behind the facial sign. Interpreting the facial diagnostic signs activated the practitioner's intuition and he sensed Reggie was not fully embodying his creative nature. Reggie had been working as a computer programmer, using the analytical skills passed down by his mother, but was in a creative slump at work—not utilizing his inventive talents. Reggie said he had incorporated many innovative ideas into his work in the past. When he talked about his creations, his Shen lit up, his eyes sparkled, his skin glowed, and his voice lifted.

Understanding the facial diagnostic sign on his forehead acted as a gateway through which the practitioner's intuition was accentuated, taking the healing to another level. By explaining the imbalance to him, Reggie's energy shifted instantly and his transformation began. Treatments of acupuncture, Chinese herbal medicine, shamanic drum healing, and others could then be added, but the healing process was already well underway.

Each practitioner possesses unique ways of interpreting a patient's energy field. For example, a practitioner who is a longtime yoga teacher or dance instructor can see how a patient holds their body and translate that into how their spirits are aligned. A practitioner who is very metallic in nature (highly sensitive) can feel the stability of spirits. These aptitudes provide a distinctive means for the practitioner to deduce the state of the patient's spirit health and must be self-monitored to balance their specific way of seeing/feeling/sensing with the other diagnostic techniques.

### Sharpening the Diagnosis through Insights

Each spirit communicates specific qualities of imbalance that can be intuited and addressed. Blockage at any stage of processing trauma can be detected in the patient's energy field. When the spirit imbalance is determined through diagnostic techniques (including intuiting the five spirits), an accurate diagnosis and treatment plan will allow for navigation toward resolution of the trauma.

## Zhi

The Zhi provides the will to live (Maclean and Lyttleton 2010, p.99). A patient whose Zhi is unstable and frozen exudes a sense of fear—lacking hope and courage to take on life and face their fears (Dechar 2006, pp.278–279). Their energy registers as frozen and unengaged. They cower or startle easily. When conducting the intake, the patient's lack of drive will be palpable and their reaction can be analogous to hitting a "raw nerve." As treatment progresses, the practitioner will feel an inner strength coming from the patient. They will be at ease and stable as a feeling of determination comes emanating from their core.

## Hun

An unbalanced Hun will be either ungrounded or constrained. If a patient's Hun is ungrounded, they feel timid and indecisive (Dechar 2006, p.202; Maclean and Lyttleton 2010, p.98). The patient gives off aimlessness and their energy can be easily "pushed over." As the Hun is settled, confidence and direction is sensed in their demeanor. They make choices with ease and display poise.

A patient with a constrained Hun gives off a confrontational energy (Maclean and Lyttleton 2010, p.98). They are quick to argue and frequently obsess on issues that seemingly constrain them (Dechar 2006, p.202). Their energy emits anger and yet feels stuck—akin to the sense of a "caged animal." However, when the Hun is freed, the patient displays peace, radiating with settled energy.

## Shen

A destabilized Shen results in confusion and panic (Maclean and Lyttleton 2010, pp.97–98), rendering the patient unable to perceive clearly. Their energy feels restless and muddied and, upon being interviewed, their personality does not match their description of themselves. They are unable to recognize what is best for them, are non-self-reflective, and give off a sensation of "blah" and "unoriginality" (Dechar 2006, pp.179–180). After treatments to secure the Shen, the patient beams with clarity and sparkles. They almost bounce when coming into the clinic and exude lightness. They are inspired, display joy, and shine—lucidness and depth is seen in their eyes.

## Yi

The Yi can suffer from constraint or destabilization. A person ruminating will impart a feeling of melancholy and heaviness. The character "Eeyore" from *Winnie the Pooh* is an example of the mopey sensation felt when a person's Yi has stagnated (Maclean and Lyttleton 2010, p.99). The patient might develop new ideas but is unable to put them into action (Dechar 2006, p.244); they are fixated on their trauma. When the Yi is freed, the patient is unencumbered and processes with grace. They radiate a sense of action and seem free of their trauma.

A weakened Yi results in an inability to act, with an additional sense of losing interest quickly (Maclean and Lyttleton 2010, p.99). Similar to those with a constrained Yi, they are unfocused. The weakness of the Yi leads to comforting with food and there is a "neediness" felt in their energy. When interviewing the patient, it is obvious they are having difficulty processing their traumatic experience and adopting values from the lessons learned (Dechar 2006, p.244). However, when the Yi is strengthened, the patient embodies focus and action; their energy is moving and rhythmic.

## Po

The Po can become scattered or constrained. When the Po is weak, the patient wants to "climb into a hole" and withdraw from life. They are extremely sensitive, fragile, and disconnected (Maclean and Lyttleton 2010, p.98). The patient frequently suffers from physical symptoms as a result of taking on someone else's problems (Dechar 2006, p.247). When the strength of the Po is restored, the patient exudes confident and grounded energy. They seem engaged with the world and able to deal with its changes.

If the Po is constrained, the patient's energy is depressed and sorrowful (Maclean and Lyttleton 2010, p.98). They are not moving forward in life but are trapped by the sadness of their trauma (Dechar 2006, p.247). However, when the Po is liberated, the patient beams with lightness and establishes strong boundaries. They freely immerse themselves in their environment and are stable and self-assured.

## Summary of Intuiting the Five Spirits

The practitioner's five spirits must be harmonized to detect their patients' imbalance(s)—each play a role in the process of intuiting. The practitioner's Shen perceives the imbalance; their Hun takes the perception and formulates the nature of the imbalance. Their Po provides them with the sensitivity to sense and feel the energy of the patient. Their Yi processes the diagnosis and brings the treatment plan into action. Their Zhi gives them the drive to act on the diagnosis, resolve the imbalance, and ultimately to clear the trauma.

## SUMMARY OF DIAGNOSTIC METHODS

Observing the body with a variety of diagnostic tools allows the practitioner to see the effects of an emotional trauma from many angles. As Abraham Maslow explained, "it is tempting, if the only tool you have is a hammer, to treat everything as if it were a nail" (Maslow 1966, p.15). This broad perspective enables a fine-tuned diagnosis to be made and provides an efficient system to monitor the progress of treatment. Using these multiple diagnostic methods yields an amazing amount of information and borders on the overwhelming. Determine the *main* pattern (e.g., excess heat) and begin treating it.

Each diagnostic clue can be tallied as part of a checklist to determine the primary organ(s) and channel(s) involved. When the diagnosis is established, the practitioner formulates their treatment principle and decides which of the several Chinese medicine modalities to utilize.

## References

Beerlandt, C. (1993) *Key to Self-Liberation.* Beerlandt Publications.

Biography (2017) *Biography of Harriet Tubman.* Available at www.biography.com/people/harriet-tubman-9511430, accessed on 19 May 2017.

Bolte Taylor, J. (2009) *A Brain Scientist's Personal Journey.* New York: Plume.

Bridges, L. (2012) *Face Reading in Chinese Medicine* (Second Edition). London: Churchill Livingstone Elsevier.

Deadman, P., and Al-Khafaji, M. (1998) *A Manual of Acupuncture.* Hove: Journal of Chinese Medicine Publications.

Dechar, L.E. (2006) *The Five Spirits.* New York: Chiron Publications/Lantern Books.

Dragon Rises (2017) *Dragon Rises Seminars.* Available at www.dragonrises.org, accessed on 22 May 2017.

Dzung, T.V. (2004) *Teaching.* Bastyr University, Washington, DC: VHS video release.

Environmental Protection Agency (2017) *Particulate Matter (PM) Basics.* Available at www.epa.gov/pm-pollution/particulate-matter-pm-basics#PM, accessed on 19 May 2017.

Hammer, L. (2001) *Chinese Pulse Diagnosis, Revised Edition.* Seattle: Eastland Press.

Jevtović, S., Gregurek, R., Kalenić, B., Brajković, L., *et al.* (2011) "Correlation of sleep disturbances, anxiety and depression in Croatian war veterans with posttraumatic stress disorder." *Coll. Antropol. 35,* Suppl. 1, 175–181.

Kirschbaum, B. (2000) *Atlas of Chinese Tongue Diagnosis.* Seattle: Eastland Press.

Lotus Institute (2015) *Five Element Primer Brochure.* Available at https://lotusinstitute.com, accessed on 22 May 2017.

Lotus Institute (2017) *Master Face Reading Certification Program.* Available at https://lotusinstitute.com, accessed on 22 May 2017.

Maclean, W., and Lyttleton, J. (2010) *Clinical Handbook of Internal Medicine, Vol. 3.* Sydney: University of Western Sydney.

Maslow, A.H. (1966) *The Psychology of Science: A Reconnaissance.* New York: Joanna Colter Books.

Nelson, W., with Pipkin, T. (2006) *The Tao of Willie: A Guide to the Happiness in Your Heart.* New York: Gotham Books.

Robbins, T. (2001) *Even Cowgirls Get the Blues.* Harpenden: No Exit Press.

Thünker, J., and Pietrowsky, R. (2012) "Effectiveness of a manualized imagery rehearsal therapy for patients suffering from nightmare disorders with and without a comorbidity of depression or PTSD." *Behav. Res. Ther. 50,* 9, 558–564.

Wang, J.-Y. (2017) *Applied Channel Theory.* Available at http://channelpalpation.org, accessed on 22 May 2017.

Wang, J.-Y., and Robertson, J. (2008) *Applied Channel Theory in Chinese Medicine.* Seattle: Eastland Press.

Wu, Master Z. (2016) *Seeking the Spirit of the Book of Change.* London: Singing Dragon.

Wu, Master Z., and Wu, K. (2016) *Heavenly Stems and Earthly Branches—TianGan DiZhi*. London: Singing Dragon.

Yehuda, R., Daskalakis, N.P., Lehrner, A., Desarnaud, F., *et al.* (2014) "Influences of maternal and paternal PTSD on epigenetic regulation of the glucocorticoid receptor gene in Holocaust survivor offspring." *Am. J. Psychiatry 171*, 8, 872–880.

Young, W.-C. (2005) *Tung's Acupuncture*. Taipei: Chih-Yuan Book Store.

# CHAPTER 3

# Treatment Methods (Primary and Secondary)

Many hands make light work. Chinese medicine capitalizes on this approach by treating all conditions using multiple treatment modalities. This bounty of methods increases the rate of recovery and allows for flexibility. If a patient has an aversion to one of the modalities in Chinese medicine, there are plenty of other methods to use. Patterns respond differently to the variety of modalities available, but a well-versed practitioner has a firm grasp on each modality with which to offer the best treatment.

Emotional trauma affects the body in a profound global manner, potentially creating stubborn and deep-seated belief systems requiring an integrated treatment approach to fully restore. A person is born with a certain rhythm and essence, which can be disturbed by trauma. Emotional trauma—especially occurring in the formative years—molds a person's beliefs and ideas about the external environment. Recurrent thoughts and behaviors become "normal" and routine, driven by the trauma(s). The constant triggering of old emotional patterns can easily throw the system out of balance again and again. The challenging nature of breaking these patterns requires the combination of multiple treatment methods to "keep the body guessing," which ultimately shifts the ingrained nature of a trauma.

## PRIMARY TREATMENT METHODS

### Acupuncture

Many celebrated individuals credit their success to various traumas they have experienced. Walt Disney reflected, "All the adversity I've had in my life, all my troubles and obstacles, have strengthened me" (Disney and Miller 1957). Acupuncture impressively transforms the adversity of trauma, bringing an individual closer to their full potential. Protocols are necessary to properly resolve the trauma and begin with centering a person's energy and reducing the intensity of the trauma memory. After this, the affected channels and the specific points on those channels are selected for treatment to address the distinctive way the patient is affected.

### Activating the Acupuncture Points

Emotional trauma creates blockages in the channel pathways. The stimulation of acupuncture points has been used for millennia to re-establish harmonious flow in the channel and organ communication systems, producing profound healing. The points are openings, which provide access to the internal environment. *Applied Channel Theory in Chinese Medicine* defines acupuncture points as "places on the body surface from which there is transformation and transportation of information, regulation of channel and organ function, irrigation of surrounding tissues, and connectivity to the channel system as a whole" (Wang and Robertson 2008, p.422). Pathological patterns upset the body's homeostatic balancing system and cause disease. The *Huang Di Nei Jing* states "bu tong ze tong," meaning if there is blockage in the body there is pain.

### Acupuncture Emotional Trauma Treatment Protocols

- Gathering the Qi

- Soothing the Trauma Memory

- Individualized Treatments.

Utilizing a three-tiered treatment approach successfully resolves emotional trauma. The "Gathering the Qi" and "Soothing the Trauma Memory" protocols are described in detail below. The support for each point's use is given along with its precise location. The section outlining the third tier covers channel selection and point designations to treat individual patterns. It is imperative to begin treatment at the macro level. If a practitioner starts with details such as a complaint of headache after a divorce, the effectiveness is compromised.

## "Gathering the Qi" Protocol

| "Gathering the Qi" Protocol |
| --- |
| • Centering the Qi by Benefiting the Earth Element |
| • Stabilizing the Shen |
| • Regulating the Blood |

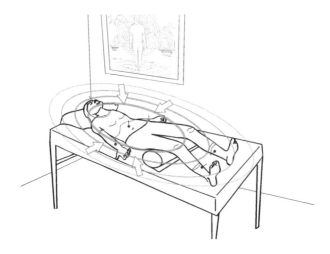

*Figure 3.1 "Gathering the Qi" Protocol*
*Source:* Kirsteen Wright

| Acupuncture Prescription |
| --- |
| • Yin Tang M-HN-3 |
| • Nei Guan PC-6 |
| • Zhong Wan R-12 |
| • San Yin Jiao SP-6 |

### Centering the Qi by Benefiting the Earth Element

An emotional trauma is like dropping a boulder into a still pond. This scatters a patient's external and internal regulation systems and the qi no longer flows harmoniously. Addressing the scattered qi restores the proper functioning of the body's channels and organs. Li Dong Yuan, the founder of the Spleen and Stomach school, believed the body needed a well-functioning earth element to perform efficiently. All organs are crucial, but the post-natal qi-building ability of the spleen and stomach provides the vital energy to fuel all the organs. Until the earth element (the spleen and stomach organs) is harmonized and functioning well, the entire body is at a deficit. Gathering the qi resumes the nutritive capacity of the earth element (Figure 3.1).

The spleen and stomach exist in the center of the four directions, and the other organs belong to either north, east, south, or west (see Figure 3.7). As the energy flows through the directions by the hour, month, year, 12-year cycles, and so on, the other organs rely on the center for harmonious movement to function properly. Trauma compromises the transformation, transportation, and distribution of the post-natal qi by the earth element, resulting in poor channel and organ function. After a car accident, for example, as tempting as it might be to use specific points for whiplash, the earth element needs to be re-ordered for proper communication and functioning of the channels.

The "Gathering the Qi" treatment relies on points primarily connected to the eight extraordinary vessels. These channels affect the body in a broad sense and affect the qi on all levels, from the wei qi to the yuan qi. The eight extraordinary vessels provide the means to process and move forward when faced with change (Farrell 2016, p.42). The protocol "mothers" the patient by connecting them with the earth and by utilizing the Ren vessel. (For a more detailed account, see "The Eight Extraordinary Vessel Points" later in this chapter.)

**CENTERING THE QI BY BENEFITING THE EARTH ELEMENT**

| Yin Tang M-HN-3 | Nei Guan PC-6 | Zhong Wan R-12 | San Yin Jiao SP-6 |
|---|---|---|---|
| • Located where the "Seat of the Stamp" is found and, when open and clear, it allows the patient to grasp the bigger picture and center their energy (Bridges 2012, p.149). | • The internal pericardium channel connects with the middle jiao (Deadman and Al-Khafaji 1998, p.367).<br>• Regulates the qi flow in the stomach (Deadman and Al-Khafaji 1998, p.377).<br>• The pericardium channel has the same closing movement as its paired Stomach channel (Young 2005, pp.xxxiv–xxxvi). | • Located in the center of the body, thus centers the whole system.<br>• Mothers the body by activating the Ren mai to build self-love (Farrell 2016, p.80).<br>• Connects with the stomach.<br>• Mu/alarm point clears accumulation.[1]<br>• Connects to the third chakra—a patient's personal power (Judith 2015). | • On the leg tai yin channel associated with the earth element.<br>• Provides nourishment of the post-natal qi akin to providing a tree with healthy soil to root in.<br>• Benefits the Yi and establishes a steady pace.<br>• Regulates and nourishes the blood, giving a person a feeling of being in their body and centered. |

1 Personal communication with Jason Robertson about Wang Ju-Yi's interpretation of mu/alarm points.

### Stabilizing the Shen

The shock of the trauma frightens the spirit. "Gathering the Qi" establishes a peaceful environment for the spirit to feel safe to reside in—the heart opens. Centering the qi and harmonizing the blood creates calm in the body and the spirit is secured (Figure 3.1). When a person can shift their perception about the trauma, the enormity of its impact is reduced. Each point in the protocol has the function to settle the spirit, allowing the body to function efficiently and improve the communication between the channels and organs.

**STABILIZING THE SHEN**

| Yin Tang M-HN-3 | Nei Guan PC-6 | Zhong Wan R-12 | San Yin Jiao SP-6 |
|---|---|---|---|
| • Calms the Shen and settles agitation of the body, mind, and spirit.<br>• Affects the frontal lobe of the brain and assists in healthy brain communication (Zheng *et al.* 2012), thus regulating the fight-or-flight response and calming the spirit. | • Calms the spirit and the heart (Deadman and Al-Khafaji 1998, p.277).<br>• Links with the heart and acts like a secretary safeguarding the Shen.<br>• Opens the Yin Wei mai to calm the Shen (Farrell 2016, pp.101 and 103) and brings the patient into the present (Farrell 2016, p.106). | • Activates the Ren mai to improve the capability of letting go of trauma and accepting their present situation (Farrell 2016, p.85).<br>• Activates the small intestine to promote clear thinking (is a meeting point with the SI channel) (Deadman and Al-Khafaji 1998, p.511). | • The crossing point of the spleen, liver, and kidney channels and thus harmonizes all the three minds (intent, courage, and will) to support the Shen.<br>• Nourishes the blood, thus stabilizes the Shen. |

## Regulating the Blood

Emotional trauma causes the pericardium to tighten, restricting the flow of blood to the heart and ultimately the ability to process the trauma. Engaging the points in the "Gathering the Qi" protocol restores circulation and unlocks the trapped trauma to serve as a catalyst in the alchemical transformation. Regulating the blood also begins to remove stagnation and restore harmonious rhythm in the body. Restoring the blood flow gathers the emotions and re-orders a person's circulatory system. The nourishment of blood to the channels is imperative for bringing the body back into balance.

**REGULATING THE BLOOD**

| Yin Tang M-HN-3 | Nei Guan PC-6 | Zhong Wan R-12 | San Yin Jiao SP-6 |
|---|---|---|---|
| • Pacifies wind (Deadman and Al-Khafaji 1998, p.566), thus calms the Hun and harmonizes the channel flow.<br>• Located in the liver area by facial diagnosis, thus benefits the liver and Hun to calm the spirit. | • Activates the jue yin channel to regulate blood (Wang and Robertson 2008, pp.161–162).<br>• Releases tightness in the pericardium.<br>• Regulates the blood flow in and out of the heart.<br>• Opens the Yin Wei mai to regulate the blood in all the "nooks and crannies." | • Regulates rebellious qi and thus has an indirect effect on the blood circulation. | • Regulates the blood.<br>• Benefits the Yi and establishes a steady pace.<br>• Associated with the chest in the Master Tung microsystem (Young 2005, p.xxviii) and links to the heart and lung to harmonize the rhythm of the qi and blood. |

## Point Location and Needling Technique

Each point has a traditional location, but input from teachers and experience informs clinical location. Feeling for the space of the point is essential. The traditional location directs where to look, but the fingers ultimately do the discovering.

### YIN TANG MH-N-3

Yin Tang is traditionally found "at the glabella, at the midpoint between the medial extremities of the eyebrows" (Deadman and Al-Khafaji 1998, p.565). However, needling the point 0.3 cun above the midpoint between the eyebrows, at the location of Master Tung point Zhengjing 1010.08, provides an enhanced calming effect. Zhengjing has similar indications to Yin Tang, but treats a wide variety of mental disorders (Young 2005, p.140). A 1 cun needle is used at this point inserted to ⅓–½ cun (connecting Zhengjing to Yin Tang) and causes a gentle pressure sensation. By inserting the needle to this depth, it activates a larger aspect of the facial diagnostic liver area and thus enhances the calming of the spirit, pacification of wind, and third eye functions. (When inserting a needle at Yin Tang or at any point, if a sharp or burning sensation is felt by the patient, then the needle must be withdrawn and re-inserted.)

### NEI GUAN PC-6

The traditional location of PC-6 is "on the flexor aspect of the forearm, 2 cun proximal to Daling PC-7, between the tendons of palmaris longus and flexor carpi radialis" (Deadman and Al-Khafaji 1998, p.376). In this system PC-6 is found in a slightly different location. It is located proximal to the vein that is closest to 2 cun proximal to PC-7, diagonally crossing the tendon of palmaris longus and flexor carpi radialis. This distance from Daling PC-7 differs for each person, and careful examination of the vessels is needed. Insert a 1 cun needle slightly radial in the space between the tendons, not exactly in the middle. This elicits a gentle electrical sensation to the fingers and, if done gently, the patient also feels the sensation travel up the arm to the elbow. A retained needle gives a heavy pressure sensation.[1]

### ZHONG WAN R-12

The location of R-12 varies and can change between treatments on the same patient. The traditional location is "on the midline of the abdomen, 4 cun above the umbilicus and midway between the umbilicus and sternocostal angle" (Deadman and Al-Khafaji 1998, p.511). However, find it by palpating this general area for a "tight" sensation. A 1½ cun needle is inserted at the point to obtain a distended pressure feeling.

---

1   Personal teaching to the author by Dr. Wang Ju-Yi.

The intention of the practitioner is to draw all the energy to the center, regulate the qi, and settle the patient.

### SAN YIN JIAO SP-6

SP-6 is clinically found slightly proximal to the traditional location of "3 cun superior to the prominence of the medial malleolus (on the medial side of the lower leg), in a depression close to the medial crest of the tibia" (Deadman and Al-Khafaji 1998, p.189). Palpating this area reveals the correct location of the point, typically detecting an indentation and opening. Insert a 2 cun needle perpendicularly to produce a distended ache which ideally travels distally and proximally along the medial leg.

*Summary of the "Gathering the Qi" Protocol*

Use the above protocol to treat both acute and chronic emotional trauma. Other point combinations exist to regulate channel flow and bring stability to the organ systems, like Taichong LV-3 and Hegu LI-4 or Chize LU-5 and Yinlingquan SP-9. However, they lack the capacity to ground the spirit and center the patient's qi, if used on their own. Stimulating points on the heart and kidney channels calms the spirit, but fails to adequately address the body globally. Gongsun SP-4 (the command point of the Chong vessel) liberates deeply held traumas that, if released before the qi is organized, exacerbate the tightening of the pericardium. Guanyuan R-4 and Qihai R-6 strongly tonify the body and, if used in the beginning phase, would also increase the constricting of the pericardium by feeding the excess condition. These point combinations are appropriate once the qi is gathered and the trauma memory is soothed.

## *"Soothing the Trauma Memory" Protocol*

| **"Soothing the Trauma Memory" Protocol** |
| --- |
| • Bringing Down Cosmic Water to Clear Heat and Dispel Wind |
| • Soothing the Spirit |
| • Increasing Perception |

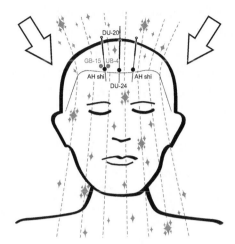

*Figure 3.2 "Soothing the Trauma Memory" Protocol*
*Source:* Kirsteen Wright

---

**Acupuncture Prescription**

- Baihui DU-20
- Shenting DU-24
- Ah Shi 2 cun lateral to Shenting DU-24 (*between Chu Chai UB-4 and Tou Lin Qi GB-15*)

The point prescription was taught to the author by Susan Johnson, L.Ac., who learned the protocol from Dr. Xue-Jian Lin.

---

### Bringing Down Cosmic Water to Clear Heat and Dispel Wind

The initial shock of the trauma creates a highly charged memory that, when triggered, causes the patient to relive the memory and re-experience the trauma. The triggering of the memory brings the emotions connected to the trauma into the patient's consciousness and generates movement. This creates a charge in the body that ignites fire and stirs internal wind. In pre-inner classic traditions, mental disorders were caused by wind entering through the brain (Deadman and Al-Khafaji 1998, p.578). To effectively clear the heat and dispel the wind, cosmic water is needed to release heat and fill the vessels to expel wind. Cosmic water is discussed in many qigong practices and is accessed from the heavens. Stimulating acupuncture points on the scalp brings the cosmic water down from the heavens to clear the charge of the trauma memory (Figure 3.2).

The Du vessel, known as the "sea of the yang channels," contains points along the channel frequently used to clear heat (Deadman and Al-Khafaji 1998, p.558). Tran Viet Dzung teaches the use of the points in the scalp and hairline to bring down the cosmic water and cleanse the fire (Dzung 2004). Moreover, the forehead, in facial diagnosis, is the sea of yang and represents the kidney and ancestral connection. The ancestors are connected to the cosmic qi, and their influence on a person—according to the Lillian Bridges Facial Diagnosis Lineage—is found on the forehead (Bridges 2012, pp.19–21). Therefore, needling the points on the scalp can bring the cosmic qi of the universe to the body. Faces commonly change once the scalp needles are placed. The face softens and wrinkles fade, in addition to an increase in Shen. The skin will glow from the inside and the face takes on a serene look. These transformations reflect the water cooling the fire.

### BRINGING DOWN COSMIC WATER TO CLEAR HEAT AND DISPEL WIND

| Baihui DU-20 | Shenting DU-24 | Ah Shi 2 cun lateral to Shenting DU-24 |
|---|---|---|
| • Indicated for crying, disorientation, fright palpitations, sadness—all symptoms of reliving the memory (Deadman and Al-Khafaji 1998, p.552). <br><br> • Nourishes the sea of marrow (the deepest part of the body where trauma memories are stored) (Deadman and Al-Khafaji 1998, p.552) and, by nourishing it, clears heat. <br><br> • Known as Tian Shan, Mountain of Heaven (Deadman and Al-Khafaji 1998, p.553). In qigong it is the opening to the heavenly qi, thus cosmic water. <br><br> • Subdues yang rising and pacifies wind (Deadman and Al-Khafaji 1998, p.552). <br><br> • Located at the highest point on the body—directs rising yang downward. | • Treats mania (Deadman and Al-Khafaji 1998, p.558), thus clears heat. <br><br> • Pacifies wind; in pre-inner classic traditions, mental emotional disorders were caused by wind entering the brain (Deadman and Al-Khafaji 1998, p.558). | • UB-4 expels wind (Deadman and Al-Khafaji 1998, p.259). <br><br> • UB-4 treats heat in the body (Deadman and Al-Khafaji 1998, p.259). <br><br> • GB-15 calms internally generated wind and subdues rising liver yang (Ching 2016, pp.583–584). <br><br> • GB-15 connects with the Yang Wei vessel that harmonizes the provision of yang to the regular channels (Wang and Robertson 2008, p.293), hence cosmic qi. <br><br> • GB-15 is on the shao yang channel that clears heat. |

## Soothing the Spirit

Activating the Du mai "fathers" the patient to soothe their fears and give them courage to move forward on their path (Farrell 2016, pp.90, 93, 94, and 97). Their self-love is intact from the "Gathering the Qi" treatment and attention is now placed on building the patient's fortitude in moving on from the trauma. Activating the scalp points connects the patient with Father Sky. Dr. Lin, the teacher of the protocol, used this point combination to treat PTSD and other conditions including depression, anxiety, and insomnia.

SOOTHING THE SPIRIT

| Baihui DU-20 | Shenting DU-24 | Ah Shi 2 cun lateral to Shenting DU-24 |
| --- | --- | --- |
| • Benefits the brain and calms the spirit (Deadman and Al-Khafaji 1998, p.552).<br><br>• Builds the "father energy" to stand tall with confidence.<br><br>• Strengthens the spine for upright posture; the patient believes in themselves (Farrell 2016, p.97).<br><br>• Activating this point—the heavenly qi pours in to "trash out" the old energy that is disturbing the Shen.[1] | • Calms the spirit (Deadman and Al-Khafaji 1998, p.557).<br><br>• Connects to the urinary bladder channel (the channel that traverses all organs/spirits) and resets and cleanses the spirits of all the organs. | • UB-4 treats agitation and fullness of the heart (Deadman and Al-Khafaji 1998, p.259).<br><br>• UB-4 pacifies any emotions that are imbalanced (UB channel travels through the organs).<br><br>• GB-15 calms the spirit (Ching 2016, pp.583–584). |

1 Master Zhongxian Wu, Lecture for the Lifelong Qigong Program.

## Increasing Perception

Reliving the trauma memory upsets the heart mirror and perception. If a person's perception is distorted, they will believe the trauma is currently happening. The heart mirror needs to be stilled by settling the spirit. The points in the "Soothing the Trauma Memory" protocol soothe the spirit and treat emotional imbalance. "The head is the supreme leader, the place where man's spirit concentrates" (Sun Si Miao, from the *Thousand Ducat Formulas*) (Deadman and Al-Khafaji 1998, p.532). In Western medicine, the charge of reliving the trauma memory disturbs the frontal lobe (where memories are stored) and excites the nervous system (Bremner 2006). The Du vessel "has the closest relationship with the brain" (Deadman and Al-Khafaji 1998, p.557). Points along the Du vessel influence the frontal lobe and assist with clear brain communication so that the nervous system is not falsely activated (Zheng *et al.* 2012).

The front lobe of the brain is called the pre-frontal cortex. The center of the pre-frontal cortex—the medial aspect—oversees the person's inner experience of themselves (Van der Kolk 2014, p.69). The lateral pre-frontal cortex regulates an individual's understanding of their environment (Van der Kolk 2014, p.69). Thus, needling all three points (DU-24 and the two Ah Shi points) actuates a person's complete experience. They can see themselves and their external surroundings with clarity.

## INCREASING PERCEPTION

| Baihui DU-20 | Shenting DU-24 | Ah Shi 2 cun lateral to Shenting DU-24 |
|---|---|---|
| • Anterior pathway of the Du vessel connects with the heart (Deadman and Al-Khafaji 1998, p.553). | • Location relates to the pre-frontal cortex that is responsible for accurately perceiving reality. | • UB-4 acts like a shield (tai yang is the most external channel), deflecting triggers (person stays present). |
| • Has close relationship with the brain (Deadman and Al-Khafaji 1998, p.553). | • Connects with the stomach channel, therefore benefits the earth element to stabilize perception. | • GB-15 connects to Yang Wei mai—moves a person forward (Farrell 2016, p.112) and unfreezes fear so they accept their present situation (Farrell 2016, pp.115–116). |
| • Indicated for emotional conditions causing a disturbance between the heart and the brain (Deadman and Al-Khafaji 1998, p.553). | • Connects to the Mud Ball Palace (brain) and benefits brain communication. | • UB-4 and GB-15 activate the transformation lines on the facial diagnostic map and improve perception. |
| • Connects with all the yang channels and the liver channel (Deadman and Al-Khafaji 1998, p.552)—facilitates free movement in the channels and clear communication. | | • Zhi Liang Huo uses points for thoracic issues (Hao and Hao 2011, pp.5 and 59), thus activates Shen and Po. |

## *Point Location and Needling Technique*

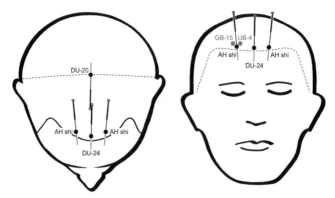

*Figure 3.3 "Soothing the Trauma Memory" Protocol Acupuncture Points*
*Source: Kirsteen Wright*

### Baihui DU-20

Find DU-20 by drawing an imaginary line from the tops of the ears to the crown of the head and feeling for the depression in the area. When pressed, the patient will sense a distending intensity. Thread a 2 cun 30-gauge needle transversely toward the back of the head (the needle lays flatly on the scalp). A pressure-like sensation is common. If the patient feels a lasting sharpness or senses a headache, the needle must be reinserted.[2] Stimulate all scalp needles with a rubbing action rather than with twisting or thrusting. First, insert the needle just under the skin of the scalp to 1½ cun. Then one hand holds the needle firmly while the other hand gently massages the area of the scalp over the needle with one or two fingers.

### SHENTING DU-24

The traditional location, "At the top of the head on the midline, 0.5 cun posterior to the anterior hairline and 0.5 cun anterior to Shangxing DU-23" (Deadman and Al-Khafaji 1998, p.557), is appropriate. However, with aging, hairlines change, but the point location remains the same. Palpate for the depression at the point and transversely thread a 2 cun 30-gauge needle toward the forehead. When stimulated, it produces a dense qi sensation that travels toward the eyes—this is the cosmic qi. Some classical texts contraindicate this point for needling (Deadman and Al-Khafaji 1998, p.557). However, needling this point is incredibly effective and is an essential part of this protocol.

### AH SHI POINTS 2 CUN LATERAL TO SHENTING DU-24

These Ah Shi points are found approximately 2 cun lateral to DU-24 (between Chu Chai UB-4 and Tou Lin Qi GB-15), in a groove or notch in the skull that travels slightly diagonally toward the inner canthus (Figure 3.3). They are typically located within the hairline, but like DU-24 are outside the hairline for those patients with receding hairlines. For each point, a 2 cun 30-gauge needle is transversely threaded forward toward the inner canthus. Activating these points produces a heavy qi sensation that moves down the forehead. This sensation is a result of the cosmic water coming down to cleanse the body and soften and cleanse the memories of the trauma.

### *Overall Benefits of the "Soothing the Trauma Memory" Protocol*
### ACTIVATING THE "TRANSFORMATION LINES"

Another hint at the effectiveness and purpose of the Ah Shi points on the scalp comes from information on the Facial Emotional Map. Transformation lines on the map are located on the forehead, angling up from the eyebrows toward the corner of the forehead. Needling the points located between UB-4 and GB-15, and angling them toward the inner canthus, resembles the trajectory of the transformation lines. These lines, not present on all people, represent someone who has gone through the dark night and experienced transformation to some degree (Bridges 2012, pp.72–75).

---

2   Thicker-gauge Chinese needles are preferred over the thinner Japanese counterparts. However, for body points 34-gauge Japanese needles are effective. The scalp needs to be penetrated through the thick skin. Thin needles tend to bend or simply irritate the tissue. The needle does need to go through the dermal layer into the connective tissue and not penetrate the Aponeurosis layer. If the needle goes into the Aponeurosis layer, the patient will feel an intense sharp sensation.

## CLEARING INHERITED TRAUMA

Many traumas are inherited and can be cleared by facilitating the circulation and movement of qi and blood through the "sea of yang"—the forehead. The vertical position of a protuberance on the forehead delineates the generation of ancestry. That is, the closer to the hairline, the further back in the ancestral line. Which side of the forehead it is determines whether the inheritance is from the mother's or father's side. For instance, if someone has a rounded aspect on their upper right forehead, they have an extra inheritance from their mother's lineage (Bridges 2012, pp.19–21). If that protuberance is high on the forehead, the inheritance comes from several generations back. A protuberance does not necessarily indicate a trauma; rather, it shows the amount of inheritance from the mother and father. Therefore, by needling these Ah Shi points with a 2 cun needle (covering a large portion of the ancestral area), the qi is being initiated and moved through several generations. This movement soothes any residual trauma in the family lineage by bringing cosmic qi through the area.

## Case Study: Benefiting the Water Element

A 55-year-old woman, "Ronda," came for treatment of mid- and low back pain. Low back pain is often a sign of water involvement. Ronda reported that she had fallen down a flight of stairs into the basement thinking she was opening a door to the bathroom. The fall had happened over ten years earlier. After several visits of receiving acupuncture on local points in the thoracic area, she felt comfortable to express the emotional impact of her injury. Ronda said the shock of the fall was significant and was followed by months of rehab and intense pain. She said it had left an emotional scar that created a fear of being dependent in the world. This emotional state became a central issue she dealt with in everyday life.

The acupuncture treatment approach was changed from treating the local area to working distally and focusing on the PTSD. The new treatment emphasized soothing the trauma memory, strengthening the water element, and reducing fear.

After the new treatment approach, she reported significant pain reduction in her mid-back; her pain became minimal and easy to manage. She also found the fear and anxiety were no longer impacting her life, and the triggering of the past trauma was considerably reduced. By nourishing the water element and shifting the focus from simply clearing the blockage in the channels with local treatment, she obtained complete resolution and engagement in life. The "Soothing the Trauma Memory" protocol activated the pre-frontal cortex, helping her stay in the present moment without fear taking over her life.

*Supplementing the "Soothing the Trauma Memory" Protocol*

The scalp points in this protocol are used in combination with a few select body points depending on the state of the qi. Part of the "Gathering the Qi" protocol (PC-6, R-12, and/or SP-6) is sometimes combined with the "Soothing the Trauma Memory" protocol to continue grounding the patient's energy. After the patient is sufficiently centered, begin incorporating other points. Choose points based on the general body physiology, such as opening points of the extraordinary vessels or major points that have broad effects, like ST-36, KD-3, LI-4, and SP-9, for example. Once the trauma memory is lessened, choose points to target specific channels.

## Case Study: Flexibility of the "Soothing the Trauma Memory" Protocol

A 47-year-old man, "Pete," reported suffering from low back pain. He went to see his medical doctor for an evaluation and was immediately rushed into surgery due to a fractured vertebra in his lumbar area. Gas was administered and Pete did not feel it was effective. He tried to tell the surgeon, but was unable to communicate. Pete said his brain was functioning and his mind was racing. He heard the emergency signals of his vitals and the nurses exclaiming "his blood pressure and heart rate are extremely high" before passing out. As he went under sedation, Pete reported he felt as if he was out of his body looking down from above at the situation.

When he awoke, Pete (a strong, robust prison guard) felt scared and disoriented, which continued for days after the surgery. He came in for Chinese medicine treatment nine days after the trauma. His Shen was dark and he appeared dazed and confused. The "Gathering the Qi" treatment was administered. Nineteen days later, he returned and felt settled, but said paint smells triggered the trauma memory. Pete stated he was grounded and he appeared calmer with a lighter Shen. However, his trauma memory was triggered and he felt an underlying sense of fear. His energy was centered and now it was appropriate to use the "Soothing the Trauma Memory" protocol, adding SI-3 and UB-62 to activate the Du and Yang Qiao vessels to reduce his back pain. KD-6 and KD-16 were included to open the Yin Qiao vessel and support his kidney energy to reduce fear.

Pete came in for a follow-up nine days later feeling settled and reported minimal triggering of the trauma memory. At this point, specific local treatment was appropriate. Needling UB-20 and UB-25, along with electric stimulation, was applied. This pair was added to the point combination of LU-5 and SP-9 to regulate channel energy. UB-23 and KD-6 were also used to continue tonification of the kidneys and to open the Yin Qiao vessel. Afterward, the patient was free of the sensitivity to paint smells.

Following the protocol order of first "Gathering the Qi," then "Soothing the Trauma Memory," and finally working with specific channels yielded the best results. Without being grounded, a treatment focused on an individual organ could aggravate the patient's qi flow and increase scattered qi.

### Choosing when to Advance to the Next Stage of Treatment

The treatment protocol for emotional trauma follows the above approach but should be customized based on the patient. Generally, starting with the "Gathering the Qi" protocol for at least one to three treatments is recommended. However, some patients who have experienced trauma are grounded and the qi is settled. In these cases, proceeding with the "Soothing the Traumatic Memory" approach is warranted. This stage of treatment is imperative to get to the depth of the trauma and prevent surges of wind and fire in the patient.

When transitioning a patient from the "Gathering the Qi" stage to the "Soothing the Trauma Memory" stage, a blending of both treatments is suitable. For example, for a patient whose qi has started to settle, but still shows signs of an ungrounded Shen, combine DU-20 and DU-24 with PC-6, R-12, and SP-6. If the memory is strongly triggered and the qi is scattered again, return to solely using the "Gathering the Qi" treatment.

When the qi is settled and the trauma memory has been soothed, then specific channels can be treated. Remain flexible when carrying out the third protocol (individualized treatments). The patient might relive the trauma memory while undergoing treatment for specific organ imbalances. The "Gathering the Qi" protocol would be the appropriate treatment to revisit at that time. If the patient's energy was not scattered by the memory but the memory was still intense, use the "Soothing the Trauma Memory" protocol. The ability to dance between the three stages of treating emotional trauma is vital to resolve the condition.

### Strategies for Selecting a Channel

Once the qi of the patient is centered and the memories are soothed, the practitioner may then place attention on the specific channels and organs affected by the trauma(s). Everyone responds to trauma uniquely, and the elements, organs, and channels will be affected differently. When the "dust is settled," detailed diagnosis can be determined to reveal which systems are most out of balance. The goal of this section is to supply the reader with theories, not "cookie cutter recipes," to use in the complex treatment of emotional trauma.

Before considering acupuncture point combinations to treat the patient's specific imbalances, the channels must be selected. Since each person reacts to trauma differently, deciding which channel to treat with acupuncture can be challenging. Often, the channel at the root of the diagnosis is not the one needled. Delving into detailed channel theory is beyond the scope of this text; however, mentioning a few strategies sheds light on the point prescriptions listed in Chapter 4.

### The Channel Most Affected

This straightforward approach involves the practitioner treating the channel most affected by the emotional trauma. For example, a patient suffers grief after their mother dies and experiences a lingering cough, sadness, allergies, fatigue, and constipation. The practitioner treats the main channel involved, the lung channel. This strategy is effective for recent trauma which has not entered the other channels.

### The Yin-Yang Paired Channels

Channel selection based on the yin-yang pairing is a classic method to treat the channel and organ system involved. The yin-yang pairing refers to the internal and external pair, for example lung and large intestine channels. The channels can be selected individually based on excess or deficient conditions or used in tandem to treat a pattern consisting of both excess and deficient aspects. Typically, if the channel has an excess condition, the yang channel is treated. For example, a liver channel excess condition would be treated using the gallbladder channel. If the gallbladder channel is in excess, the gallbladder channel is again treated.

For deficiency conditions, select the yin channel. A deficiency in the heart channel or the small intestine channel would be treated using the heart channel. The detailed diagnostic work-up determines if the channel is in a state of excess or deficiency. Reliving a trauma commonly creates both excess and deficient patterns. Generally, when a patient seeks care, the trauma is old, has entered several channels, and has affected the organ systems. For example, a practitioner addressing a pattern of heat combined with blood deficiency could use ST-44 to clear heat (excess) and couple it with SP-6 to build blood (tonify).

### The Same Name Channel Pairs

This selection process refers to needling the same name arm and leg channel, for example tai yin. A patient with a deficient lung channel diagnosis benefits from a treatment utilizing points on both the lung and spleen channels. Treatment of the tai yin channel synergistically activates their mutually dependent relationship. Because these channels have a functional synergy, a hidden trauma is released easily. For example, the heart channel can be used to clear heat upsetting the heart. But if the kidney channel is added to the treatment (utilizing the entire shao yin channel), the fire water balance is activated, offering a complete approach to transform trauma.

### The Same Moving Resonance Channel Pairs

The same movement pairing originates from the *Nei Jing* and is an essential part of the Master Tung family lineage system (Young 2005, p.xxxiv). The leg and arm channels are paired by opening, pivoting, or closing, and have a yin-yang paired relationship in addition to the same movement. For the purposes of this text, the pairing will be referred to as the "same moving resonance channel pairing." The word "resonance" will be replaced by "opening," "pivot," or "closing," depending upon the channel action. The opening moving channels are the tai yin and tai yang. The pivoting channels are the shao yin and shao yang. The channels that have a closing movement are the jue yin and the yang ming. Each of these channels are paired by their movement, their yin or yang paired channel, and by the arm and leg. Each movement has two pairs. For example, the arm tai yin channel is paired with the leg tai yang channel, that is, the lung and urinary bladder channels are the opening moving yin-yang arm-leg pair. The leg tai yin channel is paired with the arm tai yang channel, that is, the spleen and small intestine are the opening moving yin-yang arm-leg pair.

**OPENING MOVEMENT—TAI YIN AND TAI YANG**

| | |
|---|---|
| Hand: Lung channel | Foot: Urinary Bladder channel |
| Hand: Small Intestine channel | Foot: Spleen channel |

**PIVOTING MOVEMENT—SHAO YIN AND SHAO YANG**

| | |
|---|---|
| Hand: Heart channel | Foot: Gallbladder channel |
| Hand: San Jiao channel | Foot: Kidney channel |

**CLOSING MOVEMENT—JUE YIN AND YANG MING**

| | |
|---|---|
| Hand: Pericardium channel | Foot: Stomach channel |
| Hand: Large Intestine channel | Foot: Liver channel |

Many classic acupuncture prescriptions use this pairing; it is often taken for granted and simply interpreted as "experiential point pairings." For example, the classic point prescription to treat inflammation in the skin is: LI-11, SP-10, and UB-40. The use of LI-11 and SP-10 are somewhat obvious since they clear heat in the blood. However, UB-40 is a rather odd point included in the prescription. The urinary bladder channel is paired with the lung channel due to its opening movement paired relationship. The lung governs the skin, and by needling UB-40 the skin is cleared. Another example is the classic "Four Gates." LI-4 and LV-3 are part of the closing movement pair of the arm yang ming and the leg jue yin. Needling these points together causes a powerful circulation of qi and blood, and their relationship enhances the effect deep in the body. This powerful approach clears deep-seated trauma.

*The Five Element Cycle*

The five element relationships between channels provide clues into pathology. Selecting the channels based on the generating or controlling cycle successfully helps resolve trauma. Reliving the trauma memory depletes the body's energy and can cause deficiency of the earth element. A patient ruminates on an old trauma, which further drains the spleen organ energy. The spleen channel (earth element) is deficient and needs support. The fire element generates earth, and points on the heart channel support the earth. HT-7, the source point, benefits the fire element generating earth. The classic prescription of HT-7 and SP-6 exemplifies this idea. This channel selection strategy is also effective for excess conditions, in which case the controlling cycle or the generating cycle is helpful.

For example, a trauma has created heat in the liver channel (wood element), resulting in angry outbursts. The heart channel (fire element) can be used to vent the heat. Points on the heart channel, such as HT-8, vent the heat stirring the emotions and release the intensity of the trauma. The metal element controls the wood element and points on the lung channel can be selected. LU-11 or LU-5 both clear heat and can reduce heat rising from the liver into the lungs.

Paying attention to the harmony of the elements is essential in treating trauma. The emotions experienced by patients give clues to the channels and organs affected. The patient relives the trauma, exacerbating the situation. As the seasons change and different elements are activated, the emotions are liable to change, as are the channels and organs affected. Understanding the heavenly stems and earthly branches provides another level of treatment effectiveness.

*Heavenly Stems and Earthly Branches*

Time and space are vital to martial arts. Without proper timing and space, a martial artist's skills are ineffective. A martial artist could be the strongest and most powerful person on the battlefield, but if the timing of their punches and kicks is off, they will lose to a lesser opponent. If they are not within reach of their opponent, they might have superior technique, but it is moot since they are not in the correct space to engage their adversary. As in all aspects of life, this idea applies to Chinese medicine.

Selecting channels based on the heavenly stems and earthly branches follows the flow of the universal energy. There are many styles using the stems and branches, and the one presented in this text selects channels based on the energy present each month. Roughly every 30 days, different channels and organ energies are active. This is discussed in detail in the stems and branches section later in the chapter.

### Summary of Strategies for Selecting a Channel

Once a diagnosis is established and the channels are selected, the next phase in the treatment of emotional trauma is deciding on the most effective points to use on the channels for the pattern at hand. Generally, begin with treating an excess condition before addressing any deficiencies. Understanding the various designations of points along a channel is crucial to a quick resolution of trauma.

Each acupuncture point has unique attributes, and the comprehension of these facilitates an ease to untying even the most complicated knot of trauma. Once the overall shock and frequent triggering caused by the trauma is ameliorated, it is time to begin detailed work on treating the channel(s) affected. The trauma initially scatters the qi and eventually affects certain organ systems. These organ systems are identified, the channel is selected, and the specific point combination is chosen. In some cases, a channel might first need to be opened to allow for smoother regulation of qi and blood. In another scenario, tonification is required. Using the diagnostic methods described in Chapter 2, the practitioner determines the quickest approach to resolve the trauma.

## The Five Transport Points

The five transport points are frequently used in acupuncture, especially by those practitioners who primarily rely on distal point selection, since they powerfully affect the channel system. The following will focus on how each transport point is used in treating emotional trauma.

**THE FIVE TRANSPORT POINTS**

| Channel | Jing-Well | Ying-Spring | Shu-Stream | Jing-River | He-Sea |
|---------|-----------|-------------|------------|------------|--------|
| Lung | LU-11 | LU-10 | LU-9 | LU-8 | LU-5 |
| Spleen | SP-1 | SP-2 | SP-3 | SP-5 | SP-9 |
| Heart | HT-9 | HT-8 | HT-7 | HT-4 | HT-3 |
| Kidney | KD-1 | KD-2 | KD-3 | KD-7 | KD-10 |
| Pericardium | PC-9 | PC-8 | PC-7 | PC-5 | PC-3 |
| Liver | LV-1 | LV-2 | LV-3 | LV-4 | LV-8 |

| Large Intestine | LI-1 | LI-2 | LI-3 | LI-5 | LI-11 |
|---|---|---|---|---|---|
| Stomach | ST-45 | ST-44 | ST-43 | ST-41 | ST-36 |
| Small Intestine | SI-1 | SI-2 | SI-3 | SI-5 | SI-8 |
| Urinary Bladder | UB-67 | UB-66 | UB-65 | UB-60 | UB-40 |
| San Jiao | SJ-1 | SJ-2 | SJ-3 | SJ-6 | SJ-10 |
| Gallbladder | GB-44 | GB-43 | GB-41 | GB-38 | GB-34 |

## Jing-Well Points
### OPENING THE ENTIRE CHANNEL AND RELIEVING FULLNESS
Stimulating the jing-well points treats fullness below the heart, according to Chapter 68 of the *Classic of Difficulties* (*Nan Jing*), and is used to drain excess, dispel stagnation, and clear obstruction (Wang and Robertson 2008, p.447). The points can be used as a way to first open a channel when starting treatment to remove blockages before other points are activated. Emotional trauma affecting a particular channel can lock up the channel flow and create stagnation. The obstructions are cleared by using the jing-well points. When a patient suffers an emotional trauma, frequently there is fullness below the heart. The jing-well points are appropriate to clear this fullness. These points are used in acute conditions to remove blocks from physical trauma and to restore consciousness.

### RESTORING CONSCIOUSNESS
The restoring consciousness function of the jing-well points supports the use of the Emotional Freedom Technique (EFT) to treat emotional imbalance. Patients reliving the old trauma are caught in the past and, by activating the jing-well points included in EFT, the patient returns to the present moment. (For a detailed description of EFT refer to "Secondary Treatment Methods" later in this chapter.)

## Ying-Spring Points
### NOURISHING YIN TO CLEAR HEAT
The ying-spring points clear heat caused by deficiency and generate yin-blood. Ying-spring points treat chronic inflammation that includes deficiency (Wang and Robertson 2008, pp.454–455). Emotional trauma creates heat which eventually depletes yin and the organ energy in general. Using the ying-spring points clears heat created by trauma and supports the organ affected by generating fluids.

## TREATING EMOTIONAL TRAUMA WITH YING-SPRING POINTS

| Ying-Spring Point | Function |
| --- | --- |
| LR-2 | Clears liver heat most effectively when liver blood deficiency is involved (Wang and Robertson 2008, p.455). Emotional traumas deplete the blood due to shock, therefore disturbing the liver's ability to regulate the blood. Reliving the trauma causes heat and irregular movement of the blood that damages the yin and leads to a chronic, inflammatory condition. |
| KD-2 | Indicated for feelings of foreboding or a feeling of alarm and fright (common emotions from trauma) (Deadman and Al-Khafaji 1998, p.339). The fear associated with reliving the trauma memory creates kidney yin and yang deficiency. KD-2 clears heat and nourishes yin in addition to bolstering yang (Deadman and Al-Khafaji 1998, p.339). Strengthening the ming men (gate of vitality) at KD-2 restores kidney function to transform fear into inner wisdom and allow the patient to thrive in the world. |
| HT-8 | Emotional trauma shocks the heart qi, leading to fright, sadness, worry, anxiety, fear of people, and agitation. HT-8 regulates the heart and calms the spirit by moving channel qi and clearing heat (Deadman and Al-Khafaji 1998, p.221). |
| PC-8 | Trapped liver fire generated by the trauma is transmitted to the heart via the pericardium channel. This fire manifests itself in the heart as manic-depression and a propensity toward anger. The fire depletes the heart and pericardium yin, leading to deficiency, fright, sadness, and apprehension. PC-8 clears heart heat, benefits the pericardium, treats yin deficiency, and calms the spirit (Deadman and Al-Khafaji 1998, p.381). |
| ST-44 | Clears yang ming heat from emotional trauma patterns of pure fire in the yang ming channel. Because of the same movement closing channel pairing, ST-44 can also drain excess heat or stagnation that impairs the pericardium. |

### PALPATING THE YING-SPRING POINTS TO REFINE DIAGNOSIS

The presence of nodules at the ying-spring points effectively determines a pattern of heat and yin deficiency. Heat is further confirmed by feeling the pulse qualities blood heat or blood unclear and observing redness on the face and tongue. A patient with these signs benefits from the use of ying-spring points.

### Shu-Stream Points

#### TRANSFORMING DAMP

Shu-stream points treat pain conditions by strengthening the qi, warming the yang, and transforming damp. Joints require yang to circulate qi and fluids, and pain results if dampness and stagnation accumulates (Wang and Robertson 2008, pp.456–458). An emotional trauma blocks the qi in the channels, thus disturbing the fluid circulation, causing dampness. After a trauma, patients frequently report feeling numb and a lack of interest—symptoms signifying the heavy nature of dampness. Deep-seated trauma commonly depletes yang, accumulates dampness, and creates stagnation.

FREEING CHANNEL FLOW

Activating the shu-stream points re-establishes the movement in the channels. These are the yuan-source points in the yin channels and they generate yang, increasing the movement along the channels (Wang and Robertson 2008, p.458). The yin channel shu-stream points will be discussed in detail in the yuan-source section.

The yang channel shu-stream points stop pain and free stagnation in the channel. These are helpful when a trauma is locked in a channel and the patient is experiencing pain. Stimulating LI-3, SJ-3, SI-3, ST-43, GB-41, or UB-65 effectively opens their respective channel.

## *Jing-River Points*

REMOVING PATHOGENS

Jing-river points establish proper movement of qi in the channel and by doing so strongly force pathogens out of the body (Wang and Robertson 2008, p.461). Therefore, they effectively clear the pathogenic nature of emotional traumas. The points are indicated when a trauma is relived and the emotion(s) is/are triggered. Using jing-river points also frees blockages of expression.

TREATING CHANGES IN SOUNDS

Activating the jing-river points treats conditions related to sound, including vocal irregularities. Cough is a classic indication, but other sounds such as hiccuping, belching, and crying are indications. The jing-river points on the yin channels correspond with the metal element, associated with sound. In Wei-Chieh Young's book *The Five Transport Points*, he explains that the *Ling Shu* indicates the jing-river points for treating diseases involving sounds (Young 2013, p.45). This can apply to expressing the inner voice.

IMPROVING EXPRESSION

After an emotional trauma, a person is often unable to move forward in life and find their voice. The trauma can create hopelessness and the avoidance of life. Many patients find themselves shrinking within, going back to the inner child state, and are afraid to speak up. The jing-river points successfully unlock this blockage and free the voice. Once the channel(s) involved is/are identified, stimulating the appropriate jing-river point yields effective results.

**KD-7 and UB-60:** Fear is a common emotion experienced in trauma and, as noted earlier, freezes the qi flow. The kidney channel has an internal pathway passing through the throat and ending at the tongue. The voice is hindered by fear, and using KD-7 enables the patient to "find their voice." Clinically, UB-60 helps open the voice.

The urinary bladder does not have a direct pathway to the throat; the connection with the kidney channel supports this use.

---

## Case Study: Finding the Voice

A 52-year-old man having difficulty expressing his creativity and attempting to improve his singing came in for treatment of chronic neck pain. He had been harshly criticized as a child and this trauma was reactivated in recent months. After using UB-60 his neck pain resolved and he found his voice, reporting that his singing had reached a new level.

---

**GB-38:** Anger can suspend the voice and render a person "choked up." This emotion is generally due to qi stagnation, a liver excess condition. Utilizing channel theory and the idea of treating the yang channel for yin excess, stimulating GB-38 clears stagnant qi and opens the voice.

Further experimentation is needed to explore the use of jing-river points to treat conditions involving the inability of expression. Points such as LU-8 for sadness affecting the voice in trauma or HT-4 for sudden loss of voice in trauma have potential.

### He-Sea Points
#### TREATING COUNTER-FLOW

Observation of the tides is an art practiced by countless fishermen and sea captains for millennia. The flow of water proves powerful in a variety of situations, and resisting its current requires a great deal of energy. Trauma disturbs the rhythm in the body, causing counter-flow. Human bodies, being primarily water, are affected by this counter-flow and become depleted. Emotional trauma scatters the qi, affects the fluids, and disturbs the transformation and transportation of nutrition to the organs. The he-sea points address the counter-flow and regulate the qi transformation by the organs (Wang and Robertson 2008, p.463).

**UTILIZING HE-SEA POINTS TO GATHER THE QI**

| | |
|---|---|
| **LU-5 and SP-9** | Depending on the seasonal flow of energy, LU-5 and SP-9 might be substituted for PC-6 and SP-6 in the "Gathering the Qi" treatment to address scattered qi. SP-9 can be paired with SP-6 as a Dao Ma (Serial Needles) technique, developed by Master Tung, to have a powerful effect on re-ordering the body (Young 2005, pp.xvii–xviii). |
| **ST-36 substituted for SP-6** | During the months when the stomach organ is active (April and October), ST-36 is stronger than SP-6 in "Gathering the Qi." In these months, it has a powerful effect on centering a person's energy and re-establishing harmonious flow. Because of the same movement closing channel pairing with the pericardium, stimulating ST-36 builds blood and qi to protect the heart. |

## Treating Fear with KD-10

Generally, use the he-sea points once the qi is gathered and individual channel treatments are the focus. The he-sea points are frequently combined with the "Soothing the Trauma Memory" protocol when the trauma memory is relived and the qi is disordered. KD-10 is useful when fear is the predominant emotion triggered in a trauma memory. A person who is so scared that they "pee their pants" is a perfect candidate for KD-10. Activating KD-10 re-establishes the flow in the kidney channel and settles the spirit.

KD-10 treats urinary disorders associated with damp heat (Deadman and Al-Khafaji 1998, pp.350–351). Reliving the fear from trauma depletes the kidney yin and can give rise to heat and damp accumulation. Using KD-10 clears the damp heat and in turn benefits the kidney energy. Once the damp heat is cleared, using KD-3, KD-6, or KD-7 is appropriate to tonify the kidneys.

## Regulating Channel Flow

Commonly channels have a combination of excess and deficiency after an emotional trauma. He-sea points regulate the channel and resolve excess by moving the qi in the channels and the organs (Wang and Robertson 2008, p.465). When a channel has an excess condition, the premature use of a tonic point contributes to additional blockages. Activating he-sea points for a few treatments effectively opens the channels to receive tonification.

**LI-11:** LI-11 is helpful in situations when a patient cannot "let go" of a situation or circumstance. Heat brewing in the channels frequently results from holding on to the trauma memory, which can block the lung qi. LI-11 opens the channel flow, removes the lung excess condition, and clears heat.

**GB-34 and HT-3:** He-sea points are crucial in regulating the channel flow after emotional trauma or when reliving the memory. Use GB-34 to regulate the liver and gallbladder. It circulates qi for liver qi stagnation conditions and has a connection with the heart, due to the same movement pivot channel pairing. This relationship gives it an ability to improve blood circulation. This can be paired with HT-3 to work synergistically to re-establish proper circulation.

## Case Study: Regulating with He-Sea Points

A 44-year-old woman, "Monique," sought treatment for leg pain and swelling. She suffered from multiple sclerosis and heartbreak from not being around her family. Facial diagnosis revealed a change in her nose tip, the area representing the heart. Monique's nose was pinched, showing tightness in her heart. Her condition stemmed from a disharmony of heart circulation. The initial treatment included HT-3 with KD-7, but since the result was minimal, HT-3 was combined with SJ-10, KD-10, and UB-62, which quickly re-established circulation and the patient's leg pain resolved (GB-34 would have also been an effective point in her case had she been treated during a different month). Monique's nose went from looking pinched and tight to being full and round. Her heart had opened and her nose reflected the expansion of circulation. The he-sea point on her heart channel regulated the qi flow and removed blockages from past trauma.

## Yuan-Source, Xi-Cleft, and Luo-Collateral Points

Another classification of points, in addition to the transport points, is the yuan-source, xi-cleft, and luo-collateral points. These points, like the five transport points, effectively resolve emotional trauma. The yuan-source points tonify the organ and gently regulate channel flow, the luo-collateral points remove blockages and support their paired channel connection, and the xi-cleft points strongly free the channel. A deep understanding of the mechanism of each point classification enables the best point selection and the quickest untangling of trauma.

**THE YUAN, XI, AND LUO POINTS**

| Channel | Yuan-Source Point | Xi-Cleft Point | Luo-Collateral Point |
|---|---|---|---|
| Lung | LU-9 | LU-6 | LU-7 |
| Spleen | SP-3 | SP-8 | SP-4 |
| Heart | HT-7 | HT-6 | HT-5 |
| Kidney | KD-3 | KD-5 | KD-4 |
| Pericardium | PC-7 | PC-4 | PC-6 |
| Liver | LV-3 | LV-6 | LV-5 |
| Large Intestine | LI-4 | LI-7 | LI-6 |
| Stomach | ST-42 | ST-34 | ST-40 |
| Small Intestine | SI-4 | SI-6 | SI-7 |
| Urinary Bladder | UB-64 | UB-63 | UB-58 |
| San Jiao | SJ-4 | SJ-7 | SJ-5 |
| Gallbladder | GB-40 | GB-36 | GB-37 |

### *Yuan-Source Points*
#### TONIFYING THE BODY AND PROVIDING GENTLE MOVEMENT

Yuan-source points tonify the organ systems by supplementing the qi and warming the yang. Stimulating the yang channel yuan-source points promotes circulation and unblocks the channels (Wang and Robertson 2008, p.497). Clinically, the yuan-source points are used when tonification and gentle movement are needed. Address general weakness by activating all the yuan-source points on the three leg yin channels (SP-3, LV-3, and KD-3) to bring nourishment to the channel system and breathe life into the metabolism of the organs. This point combination is effective for patients who are reliving a trauma memory and experiencing channel exhaustion.

#### UTILIZING YUAN-SOURCE POINTS AFTER THE EXCESS CONDITION IS CLEARED

**LU-9:** In cases where one organ system is deficient, yuan-source points are wonderful at bringing the system back into balance. A patient suffering grief from reliving a trauma memory can develop lung deficiency, and activating LU-9 can tonify and restore proper lung function. Lung deficiency can cause pathogens to invade or create blockages in the lung channel. It is crucial to first clear the excess condition(s) before tonification is addressed. Commonly, a patient will have a weak cough, asthma, fatigue, sadness, and so on following the death of a loved one. A practitioner may be tempted to tonify lung qi. In such a case, using the xi-cleft or luo-collateral point is recommended before using the yuan-source point.

## Case Study: Clearing Excess Before Tonifying

A 75-year-old man, "Nester," reported a lingering cold, asthma, and a recent diagnosis of pulmonary fibrosis after the loss of his wife. He suffered from extreme fatigue and sadness. Examination of Nester's pulse revealed a reduced substance quality in the lung position; however, his superficial lung position was floating, rapid, and tense. The pulse reading confirmed a strong pathogen in his lungs and LU-6 was stimulated along with the bleeding of his ear apex. Just days after the treatment, Nester's cold reduced significantly and his wheezing subsided. Once the external excess was resolved, LU-9 was used. Nester stabilized and moved forward, emotionally secure after several treatments of lung and Zheng qi tonification.

#### STIMULATING THE YANG-SOURCE POINTS TO TREAT EXCESS AND DEFICIENCY

**UB-64:** Channels that have a mix of deficiency and excess can be challenging to treat. Since the yang yuan-source points have the ability to move and open the channel flow, these are helpful in mixed deficiency and excess cases.

## Case Study: Combined Excess and Deficiency

A 52-year-old woman, "Julia," experiencing fear and grief, along with pain in the lower back, was diagnosed with kidney and lung deficiency in addition to qi and blood stagnation in the tai yang channel. UB-64, the yuan-source point of the leg tai yang channel, has the function to open the tai yang channel and remove the stagnation. It also tonifies both the kidney channel (through the yin-yang paired channel connection) and lung channel (through the same movement opening channel pairing). Needling UB-64 resolved her back pain quickly and the fear and grief were reduced.

**SI-4:** Patients with chronic neck pain, gastroparesis (slow digestion), and who ruminate on a trauma benefit greatly from manipulation of SI-4. It opens the arm tai yang channel to reduce neck pain and strengthens the channel to benefit the neck. Most people with chronic neck pain have some element of deficiency in the musculoskeletal channels. SI-4 connects with the spleen because of the same movement opening channel pairing to treat gastroparesis and the rumination on trauma. It connects with the heart from the yin-yang paired connection and helps the patient perceive reality clearly.

**GB-40:** The heart is commonly affected by most traumas since it holds the spirit. Each time the trauma memory is relived, the circulation is impeded and the heart channel becomes deficient. GB-40 is a suitable point to enliven the blood flow because of its connection to the heart from the same moving pivot channel pairing relationship. Stimulating it can powerfully restore the heart energy, bringing stillness to the heart mirror and insight to the patient regarding the trauma, ultimately enabling a patient to process the trauma. Since the shao yang channel clears the space between the external and internal, GB-40 can help remove an entrenched trauma causing cycling in the patient. However, for those acute or tenacious blockages, the channel needs to first be opened using the xi-cleft or luo-collateral points.

### Xi-Cleft Points
#### DETECTING CHANNEL PALPATION CHANGES AT XI-CLEFT POINTS

Xi-cleft points are found at the narrowest part of the channel, akin to the narrowest part of a river gorge, and, when stimulated, strongly open the channel flow (Wang and Robertson 2008, pp.498–500). Emotional trauma shocks the body, creating blockages in channels palpated at the xi-cleft points. A nodule in the area around PC-4 and LU-6 is frequently felt after a patient experiences trauma or relives its memory. When a trauma invades the heart, a nodule at HT-6 is typically detected. Xi-cleft points are a good starting point when addressing the specific channels affected by the trauma.

**PC-4:** It is commonly used for its connection to the heart and the jue yin channel. Clinically, the area around this point develops nodules after trauma. Needling distal to the nodule(s) facilitates the calming of the heart/spirit and regulates the blood flow throughout the body. As noted earlier, the pericardium channel responds quickly to treatment, and the palpatory changes on the channel resolve faster than other channels. It is common for nodules at PC-4 to resolve after just a few treatments.

**LU-6:** It releases deep grief blocking the arm tai yin channel. Often, tenderness and/or nodules will be found here after the loss of a loved one or after a divorce. Opening the channel first with the xi-cleft point establishes flow before tonification is addressed. LU-6 can be used when a person relives a grief memory. The memory could be from several years past, yet it could still trigger the trauma, causing a blockage of the lung channel. Using LU-6 along with the "Soothing the Trauma Memory" protocol is effective in this scenario.

**HT-6:** Activating HT-6 settles acute fright (Deadman and Al-Khafaji 1998, p.219), such as the panic felt when reliving a trauma memory. Nodules in the HT-6 area are common and can be quite subtle. Finding these nodules clue the practitioner to ask the patient about feeling scared, since many patients will not admit this acute fright response. When asked if they are experiencing acute fright, patients can have a release of tears, which opens the heart channel. There are cases when the trauma memory is affecting the paired channel due to blocks in the microcirculation. These situations are better treated by stimulating a luo-collateral point.

## Luo-Collateral Points

### OPENING THE CHANNELS WITH LUO-COLLATERAL POINTS

The initial scattering of qi and blockages throughout the channels can be resolved by using the "Gathering the Qi" and the "Soothing the Trauma Memory" protocols. However, the subtler blockages require a fine-tuned approach, and the luo-collateral points can be utilized to re-establish channel flow. The trauma frequently blocks both the main channel and its paired yin-yang channel. Each channel has its main pathway, its pathway connection between the yin and yang channel, and all the smaller branches off the channel. Trauma can affect the channel microcirculation, hindering the free flow of the spirit. The luo-collateral points are used to access the microcirculation, facilitating the movement in even the smallest of spaces in the body, thus enabling the spirit to flow freely.

### TREATING THE EMOTIONS WITH LUO-COLLATERAL POINTS

The yin luo-collateral points are known for having the function to treat psycho-emotional disorders (Deadman and Al-Khafaji 1998, p.85). Clinically, both the yin and yang luo-collateral points resolve emotional issues created in trauma. There are a few luo-collateral points to highlight.

**LU-7:** Trauma frequently affects the lung first because it is the most external zang organ and causes chest pain, difficult breathing, and body aches. Opening the lung channel via LU-7 resolves blockages and facilitates the qi regulation. Grief or fixations on the trauma memory are also released due to LU-7's connection with both the lung and large intestine. The LU-7 connection with the eight extraordinary channels is discussed below.

**ST-40:** Emotional trauma disrupts the earth element and damages the spleen, resulting in phlegm. ST-40, the luo-collateral point, stimulates the spleen's transformative ability and dispels the phlegm. It also treats phlegm misting the heart because of its connection to the heart via the stomach divergent channel (Deadman and Al-Khafaji 1998, p.166). Trauma is frequently stored in phlegm and in the pericardium. Activating ST-40 circulates fluid and qi in the pericardium channel due to its same moving pivot channel pairing relationship.

---

## Case Study: Bleeding ST-40 to Unlock Potential

A 50-year-old woman, "Jenny," had severe abdominal pain and was diagnosed by her Western medical physician with diverticulitis. She came to the Chinese medical clinic scared about her pain and about her diagnosis. Bleeding the ST-40 area resolved the pain—her fear and panic were abated. The phlegm (another aspect of her condition) reduced, which gave her mind the clarity to realize that she was stuck in her life. Jenny used to be a nationally recognized poker player, but in the last few years she had stopped playing cards. After a few treatments, she "woke up" and returned to playing cards and connecting with her friends. Checking in with the patient years later, she reported that her diverticulitis never returned. It is common for trauma to dampen insight and cause the patient to become stagnant and depressed. Opening the heart and freeing joy is crucial in clearing trauma.

---

**HT-5:** Emotional trauma typically blocks the heart qi and blood. Until the stagnation is addressed, it weakens the heart. The "Gathering the Qi" protocol utilizes PC-6, to free channel circulation. Some cases require additional attention to address the microcirculation in the vessels. The following signs confirm this diagnosis: nodules palpated at HT-5, vessels present in the nose tip, and a choppy pulse quality in the heart position. Activating HT-5 unblocks the collaterals of the heart and the brain to treat stroke and other brain trauma (Wang, personal communication; Wang and Robertson 2008, p.513).

Emotional trauma disrupts the brain communication per Western medicine. Pairing HT-5 with the "Soothing the Trauma Memory" protocol releases stagnation and re-establishes communication between the lobes of the brain. Trauma can cause a patient to shut down and lose their voice and ability to speak openly. Stimulating HT-5 opens the collaterals of the tongue.

**LV-5:** Plum pit qi frequently results from trauma. Commonly patients freeze up, finding it difficult to speak about their past trauma. The trauma creates stagnant qi and generates phlegm, causing the patient to feel choked up. The liver channel is responsible for the free flow of qi in the channels and has a pathway to the throat. Stimulating LV-5 frees the collaterals and opens the throat. Tenderness and/or nodules are often found at LV-5 on palpation in these cases.

## Case Study Revisited: "George" with the Lingering Cough due to Emotional Upset

George's case of a lingering cough and voice loss after a cold demonstrated the effectiveness of needling LV-5. His intense argument with a chamber of commerce member caused liver qi stagnation affecting his expression. After LV-5 was used, the cough abated and his voice returned to normal.

Many of the opening points of the eight extraordinary vessels are luo-collateral points. PC-6, SP-4, and SJ-5 will be discussed in the next section, on the eight extraordinary vessel points.

### *The Eight Extraordinary Vessel Points*
UNIQUELY NATURED FROM THE 12 REGULAR CHANNELS

The eight extraordinary vessels are different in nature from the 12 regular channels and comprise a network to handle/contain/address the overflow of qi and blood from the regular channel system (Wang and Robertson 2008, pp.273 and 276). The eight extraordinary vessels store genetic information and influence the qi on all levels, from the wei qi to the yuan qi (Farrell 2016, p.42). During times of transition, especially of an evolutionary nature, they assist the body with processing stressful events and adapting to change (Farrell 2016, p.42). These functions are essential when a patient is faced with an emotional trauma.

## REMOVING SYSTEMIC BLOCKAGES

The eight extraordinary vessels act as reservoirs for the 12 regular channels. Emotional trauma affects these reservoirs and disrupts the harmonious flow. Trauma is systemic, causing blockages in multiple organ systems and affecting the body on a global level. Using the eight extraordinary vessels removes these blocks and brings nourishment to the organs. The eight extraordinary points are starting places for treating trauma with which to "clean the slate." Once the overall channel circulation is treated, the specific organ/channel systems affected for the individual come to the forefront.

## PROCESSING GENERATIONAL TRAUMA

Most patients' previous generations experienced traumatic events. The lessons learned from these events are inherited. These gifts give the patient their "tools" to manage their emotions during a crisis and allow for their consciousness to choose a different path from their ancestral lineage (Farrell 2016, pp.42–43). However, a patient inherits any unprocessed emotional responses which present as traumas stuck in the body. Activating the extraordinary vessels aids in freeing these deep wounds. Western medical genetic research has proven that trauma can be inherited from a person's ancestors up to at least three generations (Wolynn 2016, p.17). (For more details on generational trauma refer to Chapter 5.)

## UTILIZING THE EIGHT EXTRAORDINARY VESSELS FOR TREATING TRAUMA

Each vessel plays an integral role in untangling trauma. Based on the emotional trauma treatment protocol, there is general flow in determining which channel to select at each stage of treatment. Typically, the patient is first "mothered" ("Gathering the Qi" protocol) to build self-love and then "fathered" ("Soothing the Trauma Memory" protocol) to bolster the courage and determination needed to move forward in the world. They can integrate what they have learned from the trauma and choose a different emotional reaction to the trauma, and ultimately a different path. The patient releases old blockages from traumas in their formative years and from those passed down through their family lineage.

## *Ren Mai (Conception Vessel)*
### MOTHERING THE BODY

The Ren vessel represents the feminine archetype and the archetypal mother. It provides the self-love and nourishment necessary to make one's way in the world (Farrell 2016, p.80). When a person receives love and support from birth into the formative years, they have the resources with which to emerge on their own and manage life's challenges. However, many patients experienced birth trauma, abandonment, and other issues, wherein they lacked mothering. These patients require the activation of the Ren vessel (included in the "Gathering the Qi" protocol). After a traumatic experience, all patients can benefit from mothering to soothe and stabilize them.

## NOURISHING YIN AND BLOOD

The Ren vessel has a deep connection with the yin and blood of the body. Utilizing the Ren vessel resolves blockages, re-establishing nourishment to the body after a trauma. As noted in the "Gathering the Qi" treatment, R-12 is a keystone point used to center the body and support the nourishment of the organs. Activating LU-7, discussed above in the luo-collateral section of this chapter, opens the Ren vessel and increases the effectiveness of the treatment. For example, R-22 and R-23 are used with LU-7 to resolve deep-seated trauma involving expression.

### COMPARISON OF R-4 AND R-6

| Guan Yuan R-4 | R-4 is better to treat cases of blood and yin deficiency (Deadman and Al-Khafaji 1998, p.505). Combined with SI-4 and SP-6 it nourishes and generates blood (Wang, personal communication). For female patients who have been "over-treated," select R-4 and combine it with LI-4, LV-3, and SP-6. |
| --- | --- |
| Qi Hai R-6 | R-6 is the sea of qi, located at the lower Dantian, and is more effective to tonify qi. It is frequently combined with ST-36 to nourish and tonify yin, yang, qi, and blood. For male patients who have been "over-treated," select R-6 and combine it with LI-4, LV-3, and SP-6. |

**R-12:** The Ren vessel connects with the stomach. This connection, through R-12, aids in nourishment and digesting thoughts (Farrell 2016, p.87). Needling R-12, and the Ren vessel in general, helps a person feel supported and able to let go of what no longer serves them (Farrell 2016, p.85). Many patients suffer from addiction (ranging from food or drugs to self-destructive behavior or thoughts) after a traumatic experience as they try to numb the pain and escape. Once they have the resources to feel love and connect with themselves and others, they can break free of their addiction (Farrell 2016, p.86).

**R-17:** Emotional trauma tightens the pericardium and disrupts the qi flow in the chest. Shanzhong (R-17) is the front mu of the pericardium, the meeting point of the qi, and the meeting point of the Ren vessel with the spleen, kidney, small intestine, and san jiao channels. It treats chest tightness and pain by regulating the qi and opening the chest. Activating R-17 treats breathlessness and the inability to speak (Deadman and Al-Khafaji 1998, pp.517–518).

**R-22 and R-23:** Trauma frequently inhibits expression. Tiantu R-22 treats rising qi and opens the voice (Deadman and Al-Khafaji 1998, p.522). It benefits patients who are rendered speechless from rebellious qi moving upward. Trauma can also impede the musculature function of the tongue, and needling Lianquan R-23 is appropriate in these cases (Wang, personal communication).

## Du Mai (Governing Vessel)

### FATHERING THE BODY

Having the courage to venture out into the world is a sign of a healthy Du vessel (Farrell 2016, p.89). The Du vessel represents the masculine archetype and the fathering of the body. Fathers instill strength and confidence in children and show them how to interact with their environment (Farrell 2016, p.89). With each success, the person grows in confidence to attempt more activities on their own. They eventually break free from needing mothering, able to nurture themselves (Farrell 2016, p.90). Stimulating points on the Du vessel encourages the ability to stand tall and walk upright into new experiences (Farrell 2016, p.89).

### CONNECTING TO THE HEART AND THE BRAIN

The Du vessel connects to the heart and the brain. Because of this connection, the "Soothing the Trauma Memory" protocol relies on DU-20 and DU-24 to reduce the physiological disruption caused by emotions. Both points directly connect with the "mud ball palace" and treat spirit disorders. As noted in the *Manual of Acupuncture*, "there are many references to the idea that the spirit concentrates in the head and brain, for example the *Essential Questions* says 'the head is the residence of the intelligence,' the *Ten Works on Practice Toward the Attainment of Truth* says, 'The brain is the ancestor of the body's form and the meeting place of the hundred spirits'" (Deadman and Al-Khafaji 1998, p.532). Reliving the trauma can cause patients to "check out" and not be fully present. Stimulating DU-26 can powerfully restore consciousness and, when appropriate, is a helpful point. Simply tapping this point can effectively anchor oneself in the body and change patterns of dissociation. (EFT draws on this principle. For a detailed description of EFT refer to "Secondary Treatment Methods" later in this chapter.)

### FREEING BLOCKAGES IN THE CHANNELS

The trauma memory blocks the flow in all channels, and the Du vessel effectively distributes the yang qi in the channels. Since the channel travels along the spine, it enables the practitioner to locate which organ(s) are affected. As noted in "Channel Palpation" in Chapter 2, nodules on the Du vessel indicate which organ(s) are out of balance. Needling the Du point associated with the affected organ will unblock the pathways to the organ and bring nourishment.

## Case Study: Treating Physical Symptoms
## Caused by Trauma with the Du Vessel

A 43-year-old patient, "Archibald," experiencing anxiety from the memory of his father's and brother's deaths, reported chest heaviness and tightness each time the memory was triggered. Needling DU-11 brought relief from the chest pains. After a few treatments, Archibald reported less anxiety and reduced emotions around the memory of the deaths. This idea can be applied to other cases involving certain emotions disrupting other organs, for example using DU-4 to treat fear that creates low back pain or activating DU-8 for reducing anger causing hypochondriac pain.

### CLEARING HELD TRAUMA

The documentary movie *Happy* features a case about a middle-aged woman who suffered injuries to her back and subsequently processed an old trauma. The woman's spine, the Du vessel, was run over by a car, requiring her to have several operations and resulting in a slow recovery. The injury and trauma brought up memories that had been in her subconscious prior to her accident. She remembered serious sexual abuse and through trauma counseling could process and move forward. The woman said the injury freed her and she developed a sense of empowerment. This story displays the strength of the human spirit and how trauma can be a gift. It shows how the Du vessel can store hidden memories and, when the channel is stimulated, old memories can be unlocked and processed.

### RESOLVING TRAUMA *IN UTERO*

Patients who experienced trauma *in utero* can benefit from the use of the Du vessel. The Du and Ren vessels are the first to form and connect with the primal channel energy. The Du vessel aids in individuation and the Ren vessel mothers, as all children are mothered *in utero*. The ability to feel, build confidence, and emerge into the world at birth is compromised if there is trauma *in utero*. Treating both the Ren and Du vessels addresses attachment and lack of independence issues that surround this type of trauma. SI-3, the command point of the Du vessel, can be used in conjunction with the "Soothing the Trauma Memory" protocol to activate the Du vessel and bolster confidence.

### *Yin Wei Mai (Yin Linking Vessel)*
### MANAGING LIFE WITH EASE

The Wei vessels help patients "hold it together in the face of change" (Farrell 2016, p.103). The patient does not get stuck in the old trauma or feel discontent with what is (Farrell 2016, pp.106 and 109). One reason PC-6 is included in the "Gathering the Qi" protocol is to activate the Yin Wei vessel and provide support for their navigation through trauma. It facilitates the circulation of blood to the organs and spaces, giving them the foundation to resolve their traumatic experience. The patient can feel content without falling into anxiety, depression, and frustration—emotions that consume the blood (Farrell 2016, p.109).

**CLEARING TOXINS WITH ZHUBIN KD-9**

| Zhubin KD-9 | Function | Common Diagnostic Findings |
|---|---|---|
| Xi-cleft point on the Yin Wei vessel | Trauma creates blockages leading to phlegm and heat, ultimately manifesting itself with toxins that can be tenacious and become hidden between channels and the recesses deep in the body. Stimulating KD-9 clears toxins related to cancer (Wang, personal communication) and clears toxins held in the body from trauma and its memories. | The point is tender upon palpation. A blood unclear pulse quality and a red/dusky tongue with a greasy coat are frequently observed. Select this point after the patient is centered. |

## Yang Wei Mai (Yang Linking Vessel)
### MAINTAINING COMPOSURE WHEN RELIVING A TRAUMATIC MEMORY

Reliving a trauma memory stirs heat and can create aggression. This often results in stagnation in several channels and in the areas outside the 12 regular channels. The patient frequently feels out of control and defenseless. Stimulating SJ-5 (the command point of the Yang Wei vessel) re-establishes circulation in areas outside the 12 regular channels (Wang and Robertson 2008, p.298) and clears heat. Therefore, activating SJ-5 calms the patient and provides them with a sense of security, so as to not react inappropriately, nor cause conflict or burn up resources.

**SJ-5 combined with PC-6:** SJ-5 can be combined with PC-6 using the through and through technique to link the Yin and Yang Wei vessels when a patient is feeling unstable or unconnected (Wang and Robertson 2008, p.298). This technique produces two distinct qi sensations and requires a 2 cun needle. First gently activate the qi at SJ-5, pause for a second, and then continue deeper to PC-6. The qi sensation at SJ-5 is typically a heavy pressure feeling, whereas the feeling at PC-6 is electric. Obtaining these two sensations confirms that both points have been stimulated. Depending on the level of destabilization—and in which month the patient is being treated—this technique can be substituted for simply using PC-6 in the "Gathering the Qi" protocol. The Yang Wei releases trapped heat stemming from trauma, but to clear trauma from the deeper levels, the Chong vessel is needed.

## Chong Mai (Penetrating Vessel)

HOLDING THE FAMILY LINEAGE GENETIC INFORMATION

The Chong vessel, also known as "the sea of blood," provides blood to the 12 regular channels (Wang and Robertson 2008, p.296). Genetic information is transmitted from this vessel to the next generation (including unresolved trauma) (Farrell 2016, pp.61 and 67); thus, treating the Chong vessel can resolve generational trauma (Farrell 2016, p.68). When the Chong vessel is strong, a person feels complete, having all they need to be successful in life (Farrell 2016, pp.64–65). The processing and resolving of past trauma can feel attainable and they sense they have the resources needed.

**Gongsun SP-4:**

- The command point of the Chong vessel, it restores circulation to the organs and centers the patient, since the Chong vessel supplies blood to the organs of the abdomen (Wang and Robertson 2008, p.512).

- The luo-collateral point on the leg tai yin channel, it clears heat from the yang ming channel (Wang and Robertson 2008, p.512), resolving heat created by the trauma.

- The Chong vessel is involved with problems of improper qi movement in the deep internal environment (Wang and Robertson 2008, p.304), thus is effective to treat trauma trapped at a deep level.

- The Chong vessel treats trauma stemming from sexual abuse. (However, starting with the Dai vessel is recommended to first open the channel flow in the abdomen and not overwhelm the patient.)

STIMULATING HUANGSHU KD-16 TO INSTILL STRENGTH

| Huangshu KD-16 | Function | Indication |
|---|---|---|
| A point on the Chong vessel | Located on the abdomen and guides energy and blood flow to the abdomen to center a patient. | Effective for patients suffering from low back pain with fear caused by trauma. |

## Yin Qiao Mai (Yin Motility Vessel)

STEPPING INTO THE PRESENT MOMENT AND SEEING WITH CLARITY

How a patient views and interacts with their environment is managed by the Qiao vessels (Farrell 2016, p.119). The Yin Qiao vessel allows a person to see themselves clearly in the present moment (Farrell 2016, p.120). Activating this vessel enables a person to step out of the past and be in the present moment.

**KD-6:** During an emotional trauma, the communication between the heart and kidney is disturbed. Stimulating KD-6, the command point of the Yin Qiao vessel, restores communication—especially conditions stemming from heat due to kidney deficiency disturbing the spirit (Deadman and Al-Khafaji 1998, p.345). Patients suffering from the miscommunication between the heart and kidney will experience sadness, fright, insomnia, and nightmares. Activating KD-6 and benefiting the Yin Qiao vessel provides a feeling of stability and alignment in the present moment. When present and feeling self-assured, fear dissolves. (*Note:* KD-6 is located below the medial malleolus and talas bone in the fleshy area.)

## Addressing the Cyclical Nature of Trauma

The Yin Qiao vessel has the function to facilitate the timing of channel flow (Wang and Robertson 2008, p.304). Patients frequently complain of reliving trauma at certain times of the day or night. The Yin Qiao vessel addresses the cyclical nature of trauma. The cycle can be daily, hourly, weekly, monthly, or yearly. As noted in the facial diagnosis section on Jing, a certain trauma has a belief system attached to it. This belief system repeats through a person's life. For example, a patient at the age of three feels suppressed by her father, at age nine by her sister, at age 15 by a high school teacher, and so on. This cycle occurs roughly every six years. Until this belief system is addressed, the cycle will continue.

## Seeing the Truth of the Present Moment

Establishing a regular rhythm, the Yin Qiao vessel unlocks the body's ability to awaken and see the pattern of the trauma memory. The patient frees themselves from the trauma cycle and walks freely into the future transformed. The Yin Qiao vessel coordinates the motor movement of the lower body and the opening of the eyes. It could be intuited that the channel assists with the patient's ability to literally move forward and open their eyes to reality. They stride on the path unobstructed by beliefs that are hindering the spirit.

### FOSTERING HARMONIOUS COMMUNICATION IN THE BRAIN

| KD-6 and HT-5 | Western View of Trauma | Treating Trauma |
| --- | --- | --- |
| KD-6 (opening point of the Yin Qiao vessel) HT-5 (luo-collateral point on the heart channel) | Western medicine explains that trauma causes a communication issue with the lobes of the brain; the neurochemicals are imbalanced. | The point combination treats microcirculation issues affecting blood flow to the brain (Wang and Robertson 2008, pp.570–571), thus improving communication in the brain. |

## FEAR SHUTTING DOWN EXPRESSION

The mud ball palace, or brain, is affected in a trauma, and each time the trauma memory is relived the spirit is disrupted. When experiencing a trauma or its memory, the ability to express can become hindered. Patients will often feel tension in their throat or simply be rendered speechless. Stimulating the Yin Qiao vessel can free their voices and resolve the fear (Farrell 2016, p.125). Improving the microcirculation in the brain replenishes the spirit and soothes the effects of the trauma. As the brain is repaired, the ability for clear thought and expression is possible. The consciousness is restored.

### *Yang Qiao Mai (Yang Motility Vessel)*
#### MOVING THROUGH LIFE IN THE PRESENT

The Yang Qiao vessel governs the distribution of the yang qi in the superficial tissues and, when clear, allows for confident physical movement in the present moment (Farrell 2016, p.131). A person can step forward unencumbered. This has powerful implications when treating trauma since patients are frequently caught in the past, not moving through life in the present. Strengthening the Yang Qiao enables a person to progress in processing trauma.

**UB-62:** The command point of the Yang Qiao vessel has great potential in the use of treating trauma. It is one of the 13 Sun Si Miao ghost points and is indicated for mania and depression. Using this point treats rhythmic conditions, benefiting patients who suffer severe mood swings. Activating it also assists patients with moving forward, stepping out of the cycle of reliving the trauma memory. (*Note:* UB-62 is located below the lateral malleolus and the talas bone in the fleshy area.)

---

## Case Studies: Activating UB-62 to Reduce Trauma

An 81-year-old woman, "Silvia," had suffered from Trigeminal Neuralgia for years until Chinese medicine ameliorated her facial pain. She was doing well but had a flash of pain while eating breakfast. Silvia came in for treatment that day, and although the pain was short-lived it triggered the trauma memory of being unable to eat solid food and having to rely on high levels of medication. She was having a PTSD event. One of the main points used was UB-62. The change after treatment was remarkable. Her Shen was glowing and Silvia moved out of the loop of the memory.

Another patient, the 44-year-old woman "Monique" (mentioned earlier in the chapter in the "He-Sea Points" section), was treated successfully needling UB-62. It was after using UB-62 and he-sea points that she felt like she could move forward in life with a joyful heart. Her initial treatment did not include UB-62, but the results after using the point yielded dramatic results. Her Shen increased, her nose changed from being pinched to full, and her face relaxed and rounded. Monique "woke up" from numbness to life and chose to engage.

## Dai Mai (Girdling Vessel)
### REGULATING THE OTHER VESSELS

The Dai vessel is the only vessel to traverse the body horizontally. The horizontal pathway acts as a gateway to regulate the flow of energy between the upper and lower body. A traumatized person is commonly not present in their body, and their ability to be grounded or of sound mind is altered. When this happens, the energy balance is off, resulting in the majority of their energy being trapped in either the upper or lower body. They can feel unsupported in the world. Benefiting the Dai vessel helps coordinate the channel system for the body to function properly (Farrell 2016, p.137).

### TREATING SUPPRESSED TRAUMA

Many emotional traumas have a sexual component, whether from abuse or suppression of personal power. The trauma can be trapped in the genital area, and the Dai vessel effectively clears blocked energy created from such types of trauma. The Dai vessel can act like a reservoir for early trauma, including sexual abuse (Farrell 2016, p.147). People energetically push old trauma away to the Dai vessel (Farrell 2016, pp.141–142). The stored trauma stagnates, causing dampness that can eventually weaken the ming men (the gate of vitality). This decreases the ability to move forward in life and transform old trauma (Farrell 2016, p.142).

**GB-41:** Stimulating GB-41, the command point of the Dai vessel, opens the circulation around the genital area and spreads liver qi. Women who have experienced sexual trauma will frequently have blockages in the Dai vessel that cause menstrual irregularities, back pain, or heaviness in the lower abdomen, for example. Activating GB-41 can powerfully unlock this stagnation. First use the "Soothing the Trauma Memory" protocol before activating the Dai vessel to mitigate any strong emotional reaction from the patient.

Yvonne Farrell, an acupuncture practitioner, mentions in her book *Psycho-Emotional Pain and the Eight Extraordinary Vessels* that, to mitigate the potential strong reaction of opening the Dai mai, she uses LU-7 with GB-41. She says adding LU-7, the command point of the Ren vessel, helps establish a connection to the self and self-love. The Ren vessel also helps with closure, so the patient can let go of the trauma (Farrell 2016, p.146). The author finds Farrel's protocol effective and utilizes this in the beginning stages of resolving trauma after the "Gathering the Qi" and "Soothing the Trauma Memory" protocols.

## The Auricular Points

Activating specific auricular acupuncture points calms the spirit and treats emotional trauma. There are several effective points, some of the most famously known of which are the ones used in the treatment of addictions in the National Acupuncture Detox Association (NADA) protocol. A study, published in 2011, analyzed the NADA protocol and found it to be effective in the treatment of emotional trauma (Raben 2011). Researchers found that applying the protocol in the treatment of PTSD and emotional trauma unblocked the various stages of processing trauma and treated the emotional reactions caused by trauma. Another study conducted on trauma survivors of the 2010 earthquake in Haiti found the NADA protocol a great success in treating residents for PTSD (Cole and Yarberry 2011).

**NADA PROTOCOL**

| |
| --- |
| Shen Men |
| Sympathetic |
| Kidney |
| Liver |
| Lower Lung |

*Source:* Adapted from Raben 2011

## Using Auricular Points to Address Emotions

Auricular points are effective when stimulated by themselves, and can supplement the body acupuncture points in treating the trauma. Insert a needle at each point just under the skin, making sure not to penetrate the cartilage. Alternatively, ear seeds can be placed on each point and retained for up to seven days, given no irritation develops. The following points are helpful in the treatment of trauma and are combined based on the mixture of emotions present (Figure 3.4).

**TREATING SPECIFIC EMOTIONS RELATED TO TRAUMA**

| Emotional/Physical Symptom | Auricular Point(s) |
| --- | --- |
| Restless spirit, general need to calm | Shen Men, Sympathetic, and Heart |
| Anxiety and nervousness | Anxiety |
| Irritation and anger | Point Zero and Liver |
| Fear | Kidney |
| Grief | Upper or Lower Lung |
| Insomnia | Neurologic Point and Neurologic Area |

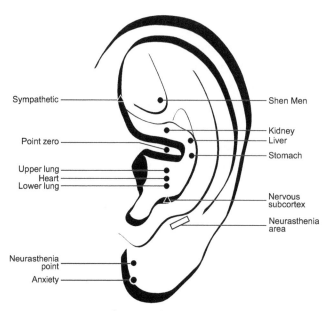

*Figure 3.4 Auricular Points for Treating Emotional Trauma*
*Source:* Kirsteen Wright

**CONTROLLING CRAVINGS AND ADDICTION TO TRAUMA**

| Craving | Point Combination |
|---|---|
| Food | Stomach and Shen Men |
| Alcohol | Liver and Sub-Cortex |
| General Addictions | NADA Protocol |
| Triggering of the Trauma Memory | Shen Men, Point Zero, Heart, and Kidney |

*Summary of the Auricular Points*

Creativity and flexibility play an essential role when treating emotional trauma. Many auricular point combinations exist for each diagnostic pattern, and often trial and error will help guide the practitioner. As the trauma clears, emotions can shift, and utilizing ear acupuncture manages the variety of emotions effectively.

## Heavenly Stems and Earthly Branches

Time and space are the basis of moving through life. Observing the proper timing of things has been the keystone of Chinese culture. The Shaman King, Fu Xi, knew of the importance of timing and flowing with changes and created the *Yi Jing, Book of Change* (Wu 2016, p.64). The one constant in life is that all life is subject to change; these changes influence how the body functions. Just as a gardener would not plant tomatoes in the dead of winter in the Northern hemisphere, so a practitioner employs the energies of those channels and organs in patients that are most active in the time of year in which they are treating.

The channels and organ systems relate to the seasons, the 12-year cycle, the year, the month, the day, and the hour. The heavenly stems and earthly branches clearly indicate what time the different channels and organ systems are active. *Tian Gan Di Zhi* (Wu and Wu 2016) delineates these changes and explains the importance of observing the changes in the body over time periods. (The scope of this text will focus on the basic concepts of stems and branches and how they can be applied to selecting acupuncture points. For a detailed description of the heavenly stems and earthy branches study *Tian Gan Di Zhi*. Master Wu has a certification training program for those interested in heavenly stems and earthly branches.)

Some practitioners select points based on the 12-hour cycle. Every two hours a different channel is open. For example, between 11 am and 1 pm the heart channel is open. Practitioners following this system choose to use a heart point at this time. The five transport points can be selected based on the hourly cycle. Practitioners would choose a ying-spring point early in the day and a he-sea point in the afternoon. However, treatment based on the hourly cycle is logistically difficult and it would be cumbersome for patients to come in for treatment of the liver channel at 2 am.

Master Wu teaches about the stems and branches and discusses the associations with each month throughout the year. This is quite effective in the use of acupuncture points and other Chinese treatment modalities. A year is divided into 12 segments, roughly relating to calendar months, and is associated with a heavenly stem and an earthly branch. The stems relate to the organs, and the branches relate to both an organ and a channel (Wu and Wu 2016, p.93). There is a weather pattern associated with each branch providing clues to the body physiology during that month. Understanding which organs and channels are active during the month of treatment helps the practitioner balance the body's energy. As the seasons change, the body physiology responds to the universal flow; thus, treatments in harmony with this flow improve the speed of recovery in the patient. The following provides a basic overview of the use of heavenly stems and earthly branches (in the Northern hemisphere) in the treatment of emotional trauma. The case studies in Chapter 7 demonstrate the clinical use of this information.

### *Heavenly Stems / Tian Gan*

Each of the five elements has a yin and yang heavenly stem symbolizing the connection to the cosmos; for example, the wood element has Jia/yang wood and Yi/yin wood. The year is broken up into four seasons representing the four directions, east, south, west, and north. There is also the "center" of all the directions, considered earth (Figure 3.5). This "center" represents the time the energy returns to the earth before it emerges into another direction/season. Spring is associated with the eastern direction and relates to most of February to early April. It has both a yang and yin heavenly stem.

Every season begins with the yang heavenly stem and is followed by the yin heavenly stem. In early spring—most of February and early March—the stem is Jia/yang wood relating to the gallbladder organ (Wu and Wu 2016, p.93). The stem changes to the yin heavenly stem in early March until early April (Wu and Wu 2016, p.48). In early April, the energy returns to the center before emerging into summer. The center is earth and relates to the spleen and stomach organs. The energy always returns to the spleen and stomach between seasons.

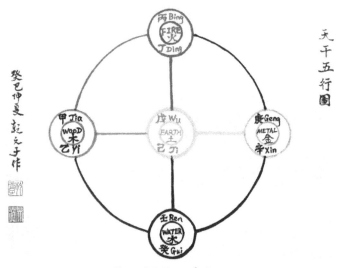

*Figure 3.5 Heavenly Stems*
*Source:* Wu and Wu 2016

The earth element is active during all seasons; however, the spleen and stomach have months when they are the strongest (Wu and Wu 2016, p.68). The stomach is most active during the months of April and October (Wu and Wu 2016, p.55). The spleen is strongest during January and July (Wu and Wu 2016, p.72).

The heavenly stems have many symbols, one of which is an organ. Roughly every 30 days, a different organ is open and active; this is one layer of symbolism for a month.

### Earthly Branches/Di Zhi

The earthly branches have many symbols associated with each branch. Each branch relates to one of the 12 lunar mansion spirit animals—rat, ox, tiger, rabbit, and so on (Figure 3.6)—and has an associated weather pattern. The weather pattern relates to a channel system; for example, in March the weather pattern is Yang Brightness

Dry Metal/Yang Ming, the stomach and large intestine channels (Wu and Wu 2016, p.116). Understanding the quality of that weather pattern gives the practitioner information about the type of pathogens that can be present and which channels require attention. The "dry metal" weather pattern clues the practitioner that the yang ming channel is active and dryness can invade the body. Shoring up the energy of, or clearing of, the represented channel can improve the health of the channel system at large and the body in general.

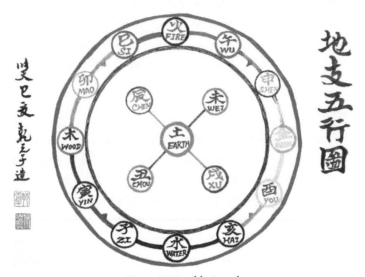

*Figure 3.6 Earthly Branches*
*Source:* Wu and Wu 2016

The earthly branch also links each month to the two-hour circadian rhythm of the 12 channels. Each month has a channel that is open, based on this two-hour delineation; for example, in the month of March the time is 5:00–6:59 am, associated with the large intestine channel (Wu and Wu 2016, p.116). This information is in addition to the weather pattern. Coincidentally, March happens to be associated with the yang ming weather pattern and the large intestine channel. However, in the month of April the weather pattern is Major Yang Cold Water/Tai Yang and the channel by the circadian rhythm is stomach (Wu and Wu 2016, pp.122–123).

Each branch is associated with an organ. These are the same as the organs of the heavenly stems; in April the organ is stomach. Gathering all this information allows the practitioner to deeply understand how the universal energy flow is affecting the body's physiology.

### The Three Months of a Season Grouped as a Triad

The months in each season can be grouped in a "triad." (*Note:* This is a term introduced by the author to help with organization.) The "spring triad" is comprised of February,

March, and April. The first two months of the triad represent the seasonal energy, that is, February and March, the wood element. The last month of the triad is when the energy returns to the earth element.

In addition to the last month of the triad representing earth element energy, it has a reservoir of energy remaining from the previous season. For example, July, the last month of the summer triad relating to the earth element, has a reservoir of wood from the spring season. Understanding the excess of the element in reserve during these four different months can guide treatment. For example, the month of October has a reservoir of fire (it holds the excess energy from the previous season, summer, representing the fire element). Treatments for clearing fire can be utilized in October to remove any extra fire lingering in the body accumulated in summer.

### *The Four Directions*

Each section below is arranged by a triad representing a season, one of the four directions. The earth element is present in all seasons and is strongest at the end of each season, as noted above. At the end of each season, the energy returns to the center (Figure 3.7). The earth element is the last of each triad and represents the center of the four directions. The triads of each season/direction are approximately divided into 30-day segments. The symbolism is rich and is beyond what this text can cover. Basic information about the stems and branches is presented, along with how to use the information to formulate a Chinese medicine treatment.

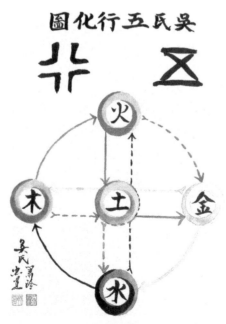

*Figure 3.7 Wu Family Five Elements Transformation*
Source: Wu and Wu 2016

## Northern Triad

Just as Samuel Clemens navigated his steamship, the *Natchez*, by reading the subtle currents below the mighty Mississippi River, the practitioner reads the powerful emotions under the surface. The water element begins the rhythm of the qi flow and life; all life stems from this awesome power. The three months in the northern direction/winter triad, November, December, and January, mark the dawning of life and the development of the human being.

**EARLY NOVEMBER TO EARLY DECEMBER = FLOW**

| Heavenly Stem | Ren (yang water) = urinary bladder organ (Wu and Wu 2016, pp.83–84) |
|---|---|
| Earthly Branch | Hai = pig<br>Reverse Yin Wind Wood weather pattern = jue yin<br>21:00–22:59 = san jiao channel<br>Organ = urinary bladder (Wu and Wu 2016, pp.163–165) |
| Helpful Treatment Hints | Benefit the water element by using the urinary bladder organ and san jiao channel. He-sea points on these channels return the energy to the sea of the body and guide the flow of qi into the storing time of the season. The weather pattern jue yin is characterized by winds and transformation; use of the liver and pericardium channels manages strong fire or wind. |

**EARLY DECEMBER TO EARLY JANUARY = EXTREME YIN**

| Heavenly Stem | Gui (yin water) = kidney organ (Wu and Wu 2016, pp.87–88) |
|---|---|
| Earthly Branch | Zi = rat<br>Minor Yin Imperial Fire weather pattern = shao yin<br>23:00–00:59 = gallbladder channel<br>Organ = kidney (Wu and Wu 2016, pp.97–100) |
| Helpful Treatment Hints | At this time energy is the deepest in the body and has the power to shift and transform into powerful yang. Focusing on the kidney, heart, and gallbladder channels will balance water and fire and benefit heart and kidney communication. This time is helpful to build kidney yang and tonify the heart. |

**EARLY JANUARY TO EARLY FEBRUARY = YIN EARTH**

| Heavenly Stem | Ji (yin earth) = spleen organ (Wu and Wu 2016, pp.71–72) |
|---|---|
| Earthly Branch | Chou = ox<br>Major Yin Damp Earth weather pattern = tai yin<br>01:00–02:59 = liver channel<br>Organ = spleen (Wu and Wu 2016, pp.103–104) |
| Helpful Treatment Hints | This is a time of damp penetrating cold and energy being stored at the deepest level. Since the liver and spleen channels are activated, the condition of liver overacting on spleen commonly occurs in many patients, with both channels being active. Nourishing the earth and giving the wood strong soil to root in sets the stage for the emergence of spring. The reservoir of metal energy left over from the previous season can be used to benefit the lungs (Wu and Wu 2016, pp.103–104). |

## Eastern Triad

As the Big Dipper or Plough asterism (Ursa Major) points in an easterly direction and the seedlings emerge, the human is born. The spring season is represented by the wood element, the baby-to-adolescence time of a person's life. The budding energy during early February through early May expands and brings change.

**EARLY FEBRUARY TO EARLY MARCH = NEW LIFE**

| | |
|---|---|
| **Heavenly Stem** | Jia (yang wood) = gallbladder organ (Wu and Wu 2016, pp.47–49) |
| **Earthly Branch** | Yin = tiger (not the same as the White Tiger of the west/fall season)<br>Minor Yang Ministerial Fire weather pattern = shao yang<br>03:00–04:59 = lung channel<br>Organ = gallbladder (Wu and Wu 2016, pp.109–111) |
| **Helpful Treatment Hints** | It is important to regulate the gallbladder and its effects on the other organ systems. Patients frequently present with grief and anger during this time of year and require harmonization of the metal and wood elements. |

**EARLY MARCH TO EARLY APRIL = YANG ENERGY ADVANCING**

| | |
|---|---|
| **Heavenly Stem** | Yi (yin wood) = liver organ (Wu and Wu 2016, pp.55–57) |
| **Earthly Branch** | Mao = rabbit<br>Yang Brightness Dry Metal weather pattern = yang ming<br>05:00–06:59 = large intestine channel<br>Organ = liver (Wu and Wu 2016, pp.109–111) |
| **Helpful Treatment Hints** | Using the liver and large intestine channels, paired by the closing movement resonant channel pairing relationship, will improve the circulation of qi and benefit the immune system (Wu and Wu 2016, pp.115–118). The blockages created by emotional trauma can swiftly be eliminated using these channels. |

**EARLY APRIL TO EARLY MAY = RETURN TO CENTER**

| | |
|---|---|
| **Heavenly Stem** | Wu (yang earth) = stomach organ (Wu and Wu 2016, pp.67–68) |
| **Earthly Branch** | Chen = dragon<br>Major Yang Cold Water weather pattern = tai yang<br>07:00–08:59 = stomach channel<br>Organ = stomach (Wu and Wu 2016, pp.121–123) |
| **Helpful Treatment Hints** | The digestive system can be easily accessed and, following the five element transformation cycle, earth gives birth to metal; the lung and large intestine channels can be used to benefit earth. Using the stomach channel during this month can benefit the digestion. Water (left over from the winter) is the reservoir for this month with the weather pattern being cold water. The urinary bladder and small intestine channels can access the water element (Wu and Wu 2016, pp.121–123). Managing water during this time aids in the transition to the fire season, summer. |

## Southern Triad

During this period a person is reaching full growth and stepping into maturity. The Big Dipper points in the southern direction and the element of fire is present. The time from early May to early August represents the southern triad and brings passion, excitement, warmth, freedom, and joy.

### EARLY MAY TO EARLY JUNE = BRIGHTNESS

| | |
|---|---|
| **Heavenly Stem** | Bing (yang fire) = small intestine organ (Wu and Wu 2016, pp.59–60) |
| **Earthly Branch** | Si = snake<br>Reverse Yin Wind Wood weather pattern = jue yin<br>09:00–10:59 = spleen channel<br>Organ = small intestine (Wu and Wu 2016, pp.127–128) |
| **Helpful Treatment Hints** | Heat and many warm sunny days allow for life to take hold in the earth and mature. Dampness found in the spleen channel balances the fire of the small intestine. Using the spleen and small intestine channels during this time is fruitful for the powerful growth that is occurring. The weather pattern of jue yin commonly generates wind in this month; therefore attention to the liver and pericardium channels is needed (Wu and Wu 2016, pp.127–128). Balance the wood, fire, and earth channels to soothe the trauma memory and clear any blazing fire during this month. |

### EARLY JUNE TO EARLY JULY = UPLIFTING ENERGY

| | |
|---|---|
| **Heavenly Stem** | Ding (yin fire) = heart organ (Wu and Wu 2016, pp.63–64) |
| **Earthly Branch** | Wu = horse<br>Minor Yin Imperial Fire weather pattern = shao yin<br>11:00–12:59 = heart channel<br>Organ = heart (Wu and Wu 2016, pp.133–134) |
| **Helpful Treatment Hints** | Fire flares during this period, and treatments which balance the fire are used. Treatments utilizing kidney yin balance this fire (Wu and Wu 2016, pp.133–134). Reliving a trauma memory creates fire, and balancing it with the water element is crucial during this month. |

### EARLY JULY TO EARLY AUGUST = YIN EARTH

| | |
|---|---|
| **Heavenly Stem** | Wei (yin earth) = spleen organ (Wu and Wu 2016, pp.71–72) |
| **Earthly Branch** | Wei = goat<br>Major Yin Damp Earth weather pattern = tai yin<br>01:00–02:59 = small intestine channel<br>Organ = spleen (Wu and Wu 2016, pp.139–141) |
| **Helpful Treatment Hints** | The three elements for longevity—earth, water, and fire—are all present during this month. In Daoist alchemy, balancing these brings enlightenment, longevity, and good health. Since this segment is the last of the triad, there is a reserve of wood energy from the spring season (Wu and Wu 2016, pp.139–141). The point combination SP-3 and SI-4 effectively benefits the earth element and brings stability to a patient reliving trauma. Both yuan-source points activate the earth and increase a patient's ability to remain centered when a trauma memory is triggered. |

## Western Triad

The fall symbolizes reaping the benefits of the labors of summer. The Big Dipper points to the west, the heat begins to cool, and the energy declines. The wisdom gained from the maturing of life can be enjoyed during early August through early November, offering a mellowing of life.

**EARLY AUGUST TO EARLY SEPTEMBER = SHARP**

| | |
|---|---|
| Heavenly Stem | Geng (yang metal) = large intestine organ (Wu and Wu 2016, pp.75–77) |
| Earthly Branch | Shen = monkey<br>Minor Yang Ministerial Fire weather pattern = shao yang<br>03:00–04:59 = urinary bladder channel<br>Organ = large intestine (Wu and Wu 2016, pp.145–146) |
| Helpful Treatment Hints | Benefiting the large intestine improves the urinary bladder channel (metal generating water) (Wu and Wu 2016, pp.145–146). The water energy balances the fire of the shao yang heat. Fire can blaze and patients can experience surges of heat with the trauma memories. Clearing heat using the large intestine, gallbladder, and san jiao channels is effective during this month. |

**EARLY SEPTEMBER TO EARLY OCTOBER = CLEAR**

| | |
|---|---|
| Heavenly Stem | Xin (yin metal) = lung organ (Wu and Wu 2016, pp.79–80) |
| Earthly Branch | You = rooster<br>Yang Brightness Dry Metal weather pattern = yang ming<br>05:00–06:59 = kidney channel<br>Organ = lung (Wu and Wu 2016, pp.151–152) |
| Helpful Treatment Hints | It is important to protect patients from dryness (Wu and Wu 2016, pp.151–152). Reliving the trauma memory creates heat and wind, both of which dry the fluids. This month can be particularly problematic for patients with yin deficiency; nourishing fluids is essential, and the point combination LU-5 and KD-7 is effective. This is also an ideal time to address deep grief to protect the lung qi. |

**EARLY OCTOBER TO EARLY NOVEMBER = RETURN TO CENTER**

| | |
|---|---|
| Heavenly Stem | Wu (yang earth) = stomach organ (Wu and Wu 2016, pp.67–69) |
| Earthly Branch | Xu = dog<br>Major Yang Cold Water weather pattern = tai yang<br>07:00–08:59 = pericardium channel<br>Organ = stomach (Wu and Wu 2016, pp.157–159) |
| Helpful Treatment Hints | Being the last segment in the triad, it has a reservoir of fire. The climate pattern can be cold (Wu and Wu 2016, pp.157–159). This cold energy can be used to clear the excess fire left over from the summer months and any fire generated by the trauma memory. |

## *Using the Four Directions to Diagnose the Origin of Trauma*

Emotional trauma can occur at any time in a person's life. Knowing when the trauma happened can improve the accuracy of the diagnosis, and treatment can be based on what organ and channel energies were involved at the time of trauma. The four directions symbolize the flow of a person's lifetime. Therefore, if a person had trauma *in utero*, this could point to issues in the water element or kidney and urinary bladder. If they had trauma around age 40, the heart and small intestine could be affected.

THE TIME A TRAUMA OCCURS AFFECTS CERTAIN ORGANS

| Time Trauma Occurred | Element/Organ System Affected |
|---|---|
| Time *in utero* | Water/Kidney |
| Childhood through the teen years | Wood/Liver |
| Maturity | Fire/Heart |
| Later years of life | Metal/Lung |

## *Summary of Heavenly Stems and Earthly Branches*

The use of heavenly stems and earthly branches has been practiced for millennia. In the last several years, the availability of this knowledge and how to apply this system is sparse and often miscommunicated. The author has found that staying true to the system described above yields better results than not observing the universal changes. Practitioners who follow the flow of energy and apply the teachings of the ancients discover great benefit from this information. However, the above merely scratches the surface of the depth of the symbolism and interconnections. The universe is always in flux. Seeing the human body, the organ systems, and the channels as a mini-universe in tune with the heavenly and earthly energy is core to Chinese medicine.

Use the energy that is present and in accordance with the universal energy flow at the time when treating a patient. This conserves the practitioner's energy. This is likened to picking low-hanging fruit. The apple at the top of the tree might be the best-looking apple, but to get that apple requires obtaining a ladder, climbing to the top, and bringing it down. There might be a wonderful treatment that has worked in the past, but if it is not in harmony with the current universal energy flow, it requires a lot of energy from the body to meet the needs of the channels. Why not simply use the energy available and save both the patient's and practitioner's energy? A person practicing the water qigong form during the winter solstice will harvest greater amounts of energy for the kidneys than practicing the form during the middle of spring—just like a gardener would not plant corn seeds at the end of fall in the Northern hemisphere. The ancient shamans acknowledged this concept and conserved essence by using what energy was accessible.

## Moxibustion

Moxibustion (commonly called "moxa") is another treatment for emotional trauma, and is a powerful and effective modality. However, the author has limited experience using moxa and so its use will be discussed only minimally in this book. Infrared heat is generally used in place of moxa, which will be mentioned in the treatment protocols in Chapter 4. The reader is encouraged to seek other references for the use of moxa in treating emotional trauma.

## Bloodletting

Bloodletting produces quick and miraculous results in the clinic. The modality, rarely used in many modern clinics, is a safe and elegant technique for releasing pressure and blockages in the channels. When hearing the term "bloodletting," many people think of the bleeding done in the Middle Ages for removing "humors" from the body. People can therefore be hesitant to consider bloodletting a viable therapy. The history of priests, barbers, and others performing bleeding for several different conditions from epilepsy to gout (Cohen 2012) can cause confusion about bloodletting in Chinese medicine.

### Emotional Trauma Disturbing the Spirit and Causing Pressure

Emotional trauma creates blockages, pressure, and heat in the channels. When used appropriately and when indicated, bloodletting is essential in restoring balance in the channels. Shamans bled to clear evil spirits from the body since the blood holds the spirit. Releasing some drops of blood at specific sites helps to clear emotional disturbance. A "few drops of blood" is the key phrase for this type of bloodletting—this procedure is not about draining pints of blood from an artery. Only a vein is pricked to remove a minimal amount of blood that is not in circulation. Like a steam valve in a pressurized system, bloodletting releases pressure and heat to keep the channels flowing.

The bloodletting technique was mentioned in the classics. In the *Su Wen*, translated by Paul Unschuld (2003), Chapter 26 includes:

> When heaven is warm and when the sun is bright,
> then the blood in man is rich in liquid
> and the protective qi is at the surface
> Hence the blood can be drained easily, and the
> qi can be made to move on easily.
>
> (UNSCHULD 2003, P.271)

The technique eliminates stagnation created from chronic conditions. In Chapter 54 of the *Su Wen*, the author explains:

> As for "what is densely compacted and old, eliminate
> it," [that is to say:] let the bad blood.
>
> (UNSCHULD 2003, P.270)

When a patient is traumatized, the channels can become blocked; thus the channel inter-network of communication is inhibited. Chapter 20 of the *Su Wen* includes:

> Squeeze [the vessels] and follow them [with the fingers],
> Search for their knotted network vessels,
> Pierce them, and let their blood flow out
> To make them passable [again].
>
> (UNSCHULD 2003, P.270)

There are many subtleties to the technique of bloodletting; thus personal training by a specialist in bloodletting is imperative. (The bloodletting technique presented herein was taught to the author by Dr. Wei-Chieh Young and Susan Johnson, L.Ac.) These techniques are presented for those who already utilize the technique or who are interested in further pursuing their education in bleeding therapy.

## Protocols

### Educating the Patient

Most patients have neither heard of nor experienced bloodletting, and the education of the patient is crucial in achieving acceptance and approval of this technique. Explaining the mechanism of bloodletting is necessary for them to understand why such a procedure is needed and to calm their fears. Educate the patient about pricking the skin to release pressure built up in the channels and to restore proper circulation. A few seconds of time to educate the patient will make a world of difference and help them to relax. As always, the patient must approve of the technique and then it is up to the practitioner to follow protocols for a successful experience.

### Safety

- The practitioner must always wear gloves.

- An ample supply of cotton and paper towels must be available and placed near the area to be bled.

- The practitioner should keep their face at a safe distance from the puncture site since the pressure in the vessels can be strong and blood may potentially spurt out.

- Ask the patient to take a breath in and then cough as the site is punctured. (This reduces the pain of the needle prick.)

- The appropriate needle or lancet should be used to release the amount of blood determined. (A three-edged needle must be used for the points on the arms, legs, temples, and back.)

- It is important for the patient to not look at the blood, to prevent fainting.

- Cover the area with a self-adhesive bandage after bloodletting the limbs or back.

### Contraindications

- Pregnancy

- Having recently lost blood

- Patients with clotting issues

- During menses

- Intoxication

- Overly tired or hungry

- Patients taking blood thinners.

There can be exceptions to these but, in general, the contraindications hold true.

### Best Time to Bleed

- During the summer and spring

- In the afternoon.

### Locating the Correct Site

Points are always bled on the same side of the body that is affected. If the issue is systemic, then both sides are bled. The location of the bleeding site is not always directly on the acupuncture point but in the vicinity. For example, when bleeding UB-40, look for where the vessel is engorged—this can be a few inches above or below UB-40. The practitioner must look for the vessel and bleed the aspect of the vessel most engorged. Often, a vessel is bled at two or three sites.

Typically bleed the most proximal point first and then move to a distal position on the vessel. The amount of blood released varies, depending on the condition and the location of the bleeding site. It is always important to let the point bleed completely and not try to stop it, as this will create a large bruise. Bruising can still result even with the best technique. A patient should be made aware of this before bleeding. The vessels bled are veins. If an artery is pricked, it must be stopped immediately by applying direct, firm pressure.

## Patterns

Acute and chronic patterns, when indicated, both respond well to bleeding. Emotional trauma can result from physical injury, and patients experiencing bruising or swelling from a physical trauma can greatly benefit. For example, a patient fracturing the ankle in an accident will benefit from bleeding the jing-well points on the affected channels at the trauma site. Releasing the blood stagnation from a physical injury helps release the emotions blocked in the channels.

Chronic conditions respond well to bleeding. Heat created by trauma can present as migraine headaches, and bleeding the acupuncture point tai yang clears the heat and pressure and resolves the headache. Certain conditions of heat and blood stagnation respond better and faster to bloodletting than acupuncture.

## Commonly Bled Points

**Jing-Well Points:** These are some of the most commonly bled points, and a lancet is ample to release enough blood to restore balance in the channels. Commonly used in cases of heat and blood stagnation in the channels, the jing-well points are the location of yin and yang transformation. Bleeding the jing-well points can quickly relieve acute conditions such as high fever and physical trauma.

Reliving an emotional trauma provokes a miscommunication between the lobes in the brain that sends a rush of hormones to the body, causing it to behave as if it is a fight-or-flight situation. A patient frequently experiences heat and/or chest fullness, both of which can be cleared by bleeding the jing-well points. Research on the jing-well points has proven their effectiveness for neuroprotection in stroke patients (Fu *et al.* 2016) and for helping protect the brain in a severe traumatic brain injury (Tu *et al.* 2016). Both of these studies support the use of jing-well points to address the brain and improve communication between lobes.

**Erjian (M-HN-10) or Ear Apex:** Inflammation due to heat from trauma can be resolved with bleeding the ear apex. Hold the ear firmly with one hand and bleed the vessel at the top of the ear. (If a vessel is not apparent, simply bleed the uppermost point of the ear.) This reduces the heat and pressure caused by reliving the trauma memory.

A study published in the *Chinese Journal of Integrated Medicine* found that patients with Gan (liver)-type depression benefited from bleeding the ear apex (Shi *et al.* 2016). In this pattern, heat is typically generated due to pressure caused by liver qi stagnation. The heat rises and needs to be released. Research has proven auricular stimulation, including the bleeding of the ear, "to have a close relationship with the autonomic nervous system, the neuroendocrine system, neuroimmunological factors, neuroinflammation, and neural reflex, as well as antioxidation" (Hou *et al.* 2015). The ear apex, like the jing-well points, has an ability to affect the communication between the "logical brain" and the "emotional brain." (For the Western medical mechanism of emotional trauma refer to Chapter 6.)

**Tai Yang (M-HN-9):** Tai yang clears heat moving upwards. For migraine headaches, bleeding tai yang is effective and often resolves the migraine within minutes. As noted earlier, headaches can be a physical symptom of trauma locked in the body. The blockages created by reliving the trauma memory cause heat, which rises. Bleeding tai yang relieves this heat and pressure. This technique is advanced and consists of having the patient tilt the head to the side, which can be done sitting up or lying supine. A three-edged needle is inserted and twisted clockwise as the needle deeply penetrates the point and then is quickly removed. Generally, several drops of blood are released and the patient will usually feel relief immediately. This technique, when performed accurately, elicits little pain and rarely bruises.

**BLEEDING HE-SEA POINTS**

| Point | Action and Indication(s) | Helpful Hints |
|---|---|---|
| LU-5 | Releases heat and pressure in the lungs and restores the lung circulation. For patients holding onto grief that has caused stagnation and fire, creating a deep cough. | The cubital vein is not bled; the small vessels in the area are pricked to release a few drops of blood. |
| UB-40 | Resolves pressure caused by fear affecting the urinary bladder channel. Many patients with this pattern present with low back pain. | UB-40 is a broad area for bleeding; the vessel can be found high on the leg at the level of UB-38 or low at the level of UB-56. |
| ST-36, ST-37, and ST-39 | Clear heat that is disturbing the circulatory system. Trapped fire from an old trauma commonly causes hypertension, and bleeding this area is effective. | In many cases the blood pressure will be reduced by 20 points. |

**Rangu KD-2:** Stimulation of KD-2 treats distended feelings in the head, headache, dizziness, and blurred vision (Young 2005, p.81). Bleeding KD-2 resolves the symptoms of a concussion and effectively treats acute and chronic head injuries. Bleed the vessel found near the KD-2 area on the same side of the injury. Once bled, the patient can experience immediate relief, even for a head injury suffered years prior. A patient with any serious physical trauma should always first seek medical evaluation and advice from a Western medical doctor.

---

## Case Studies: Bleeding KD-2

A 58-year-old male, "Johnny," was under a great deal of stress and, while in a hurry, hit his head on a car door. He suffered a concussion. After seeing his physician and being examined, he came to the clinic (one week after the injury) for treatment of dizziness, disorientation, fatigue, uneasiness, and slight headache. Johnny reported feeling embarrassed about the injury and having a sense of vulnerability. His feelings were associated with fear, the emotion of the kidney system. Two vessels in the KD-2 area on the right foot (the side of the injury) were bled. Dark blood was expelled, and the patient reported immediate clarity. Upon returning the next week, he stated that his symptoms resolved within a few days (including the emotions associated with the trauma) and was pleased at the rate of recovery. Fear is linked with physical injury. Once someone has been injured there is fear of re-injury or of being vulnerable. These fears commonly affect the physiology of the shao yin channel and can generate changes along the channel pathway.

A 67-year-old man, "Duane," had worked in construction for over 40 years and suffered several head injuries. He sought Chinese medicine treatment for low back pain and was always treated in the prone position. During the course of treatment, other points were selected that involved having the patient in the supine position. Duane said that since one particular head injury, 20 years ago, he had been unable to lie on his back without getting extremely nauseous and dizzy for hours afterward. Duane's foot channels were examined and several vessels were found at KD-2. The point was bled bilaterally. Duane could lie on his back during the treatment without issues. When he returned a week later, he said he had been able to lie on his back all week without any problems. Bleeding KD-2 released pressure in Duane's head that was causing dizziness and nausea.

## OTHER CLINICALLY EFFECTIVE POINTS TO BLEED

| Point | Action and Indication(s) | Helpful Hints |
|---|---|---|
| ST-43 | Relieves the pain and clears the emotional trauma of oral surgery. | Bleeding the vessel around ST-43 is usually painful, but the results are impressive. |
| DU-16 | Eliminates wind and calms the spirit (Deadman and Al-Khafaji 1998, p.548). The triggering of old trauma generates internal wind, causing dizziness, nausea, and vomiting. | A vessel is generally found in the area and a significant number of drops are commonly released. Very effective to resolve dizziness and vomiting due to wind. |
| Zhiwu 11.26 Master Tung Point | Restores the earth energy and astringes fluids. Long-term colds and flu, non-healing sores, re-occurring viruses, and uncontrolled bleeding are symptoms of a weak earth element exhausted by trauma and its memory. | Zhiwu can be translated as "control dirt," hinting at its ability to benefit the spleen. The finger is pinched first to engorge the thumb with blood. |

**Points on the Inner Cheek:** A patient under great emotional distress whose channels become weak and susceptible to an external invasion can suffer from Bell's palsy (an invasion of external wind). Bleeding the inner cheek will clear the wind from the channels. To bleed this point, the practitioner presses the outside of the cheek gently for the inside of the cheek to rest between the upper and lower teeth. The other hand enters the mouth and bleeds two to three points (with a lancet) on the inside of the cheek at the level where the teeth would meet. This technique prevents the patient from biting the practitioner's hand and secures the area to bleed.

## Case Study: Bleeding the Points on the Inner Cheek to Resolve Bell's Palsy

A 44-year-old man, "Bernie," under stress from work, recently divorced, and in the middle of a home remodel, woke one morning with Bell's palsy. He went to his Western doctor for treatment and was given Prednisone. A week later the left side facial pain and drooping remained and worsened with stress. The trauma of his divorce, paired with the other life stresses, allowed wind to enter the yang ming channel. Bernie sought acupuncture treatment. Since his condition was acute and the drooping was significant, bleeding the inner cheek (on the affected side) was added to the "Gathering the Qi" treatment. After one treatment with this bleeding technique, his condition reduced by 80 percent. Without the use of this technique, his condition would have required several visits.

## Summary of Bloodletting

Utilized for many patterns caused by emotional trauma, one bloodletting treatment is equal to four to five acupuncture treatments, quickly assisting in the resolution of symptoms. The technique is an under-used art in Chinese medicine, but its presence is expanding into clinics around the world as books and seminars on bloodletting are becoming popular.

# Cupping Therapy

The ancient art of cupping is practiced all over the world and has existed in many cultures for centuries (Mehta and Dhapte 2015). The technique involves using rubber, glass, bamboo, or plastic cups, creating suction with a vacuum technique. The shamans in ancient China used cupping to clear evil spirits from the body and cleanse the soul (Samovar, Porter, and McDaniel 2012). Cupping therapy removes blockages in the body created by emotional trauma. (There are many styles of cupping and what is presented below comes from the teaching of Susan Johnson; the reader is encouraged to complete one of her comprehensive cupping seminars.)

## Treating the Body and Spirit

Cupping affects the physical and emotional body. Physically, cupping relaxes the muscles by pulling on the tissue to release tension. The suction draws the blood in the muscles to the surface, creating a vacuum, forcing fresh blood into the muscle tissue (Mehta and Dhapte 2015). The blood exchange clears toxins from the tight muscle tissue and rehydrates the muscles. On a spirit level, this process of cleansing the blood can be thought of as cleansing the spirit and freeing emotions trapped in the channels.

Typically, cupping is administered to the large muscle groups (cupping below the elbows and knees is not recommended due to the delicate nature of the tissue in these areas). The cupping techniques on the upper/mid-back, on the umbilicus, and on DU-10 are effective in treating emotional trauma. As with bloodletting, cupping has important protocols to ensure success. Training is essential before anyone performs cupping.

## Protocols

### Educating the Patient

Before starting the procedure, educate the patient about cupping. Many patients are completely ignorant of cupping, and taking the time to explain the treatment improves the success of the experience. Patients suffering from trauma might have experienced physical abuse, and seeing the marks left by cupping may trigger a trauma memory;

the discoloration may also trigger psychological trauma in their loved ones. Inform the patient prior to the procedure about the possibility of sensitivity and ache after cupping. Let them know that the resulting marks can last for over a week.

The marks are often thought of as bruises—this is a misconception. Bruising is caused by impact trauma resulting in the breakage of capillaries and a rush of fluids to the injured tissue. There is no compression or impact in properly performed cupping. Bruises are tender to the touch; cupping marks are not. Bruises take up to two weeks to resolve; cupping marks last on average four to seven days. For those practitioners who use fire cupping, educate the patient about the safety of the procedure. Each patient must be evaluated on a case-by-case basis as not everyone is a candidate for cupping.

*Safety*

- Avoid drafts and cold air on the cupping site for two days.

- Refrain from swimming or using an outdoor hot-tub for two days after the procedure.

- Use a gentler approach for children, the sensitive, and elderly patients.

- Proceed with caution for patients who are over-tired or have fragile skin.

- Always stay with the patient during the cupping process to observe for any skin irritation or if the patient becomes uncomfortable.

- Sterilize the cups properly after each use.

- Abundant hair growth in the area needs to be shaved if the patient is amenable (otherwise the suction is compromised).

- Perform cupping over the same area (if needed) at least ten days after the previous session to prevent tissue damage.

- Increase water intake 24 hours after cupping therapy, due to the release of toxins.

*Procedure*

- Use a strong suction to the patient's comfort level.

- Leave cups on the skin for one to three minutes before they are shifted to the next area.

- Cup the entire area being addressed, for example the whole upper back.

- Only cup the upper back/mid-back *or* the lower back in a session to avoid releasing too many toxins.

- Cupping the back: the cups must be placed bilaterally next to the spine to avoid misalignment of any vertebrae.

- Cupping on the shoulders or hips is performed unilaterally or bilaterally.

*Diagnosing from the Marks Left from the Cups*

Cupping is used as a diagnostic tool, that is, the darker the marks, the greater the toxins and blockages there are in the channels. This diagnostic helps with emotional trauma. Patients who have darker marks at the level of the third thoracic vertebra may have issues of trapped grief, compared with a patient who has trapped anger—indicated by darker marking at the ninth thoracic vertebra.

Typically, the cup marks lighten with each session. However, if the marks continue to discolor darkly with each session, there is an issue of toxins not being properly processed by the body. The area lateral to SI-11 is considered the toxin area, and observing the discoloration in this area reveals the quantity of toxins—including trapped emotions—in the body.

## Cupping Upper/Mid-Back

The old saying "monkey on your back" reflects the idea of emotions, old beliefs, traumas, hardships, and so on trapped in the upper back, a common place of tension weighing a person down, until released and cleared. Cupping lifts this emotion and tension off the back and lightens the spirit.

*The Technique*

The broad stimulation of qi and blood offers a powerful supplemental treatment in clearing trauma. Cup the area from the top of the shoulders down to the level of the seventh thoracic vertebra while the patient is lying in the prone position with the head straight—preferably in a head rest.

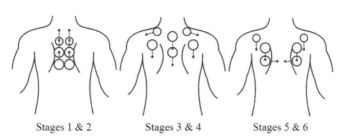

Stages 1 & 2          Stages 3 & 4          Stages 5 & 6

*Figure 3.8 Cupping Procedure for the Upper Back*
*Source:* Julian Holman

Perform the cupping bilaterally to maintain the alignment of the spine. Place three cups on either side of the vertebra (one medium and two large). Refer to Figure 3.8 for the order of the cup placement. First attach the two medium-sized cups bilateral to the second thoracic vertebra with the four large cups closely inferior to them. Leave the cups on the skin for one to three minutes and then move them superiorly a few inches, with the large cups filling in the gaps. After one to two minutes, move the cups again, continuing until the entire upper/mid-back, from GB-21 to UB-17 and across, is filled in with cup marks.

### Calming the Spirit

The upper/mid-back and shoulders have many acupuncture points relating to the spirit. The back shu of the lung, pericardium, and heart are located here along with UB-42 (Door to the Corporeal Soul), UB-44 (Hall of the Spirit), and UB-46 (Diaphragm Gate). The "toxin area," found laterally to the scapula (a segment of the small intestine channel), is part of the upper back involved in the cupping procedure. The small intestine separates the clear from the turbid, and activating this area helps the organ fully clear out trapped toxins. Cupping the upper back frees up old trauma on several levels. Therefore, monitor patients during and after the procedure for emotional changes.

### Freeing Trapped Emotions

Releasing tension from UB-46 and softening tightness in the diaphragm allows for deeper breaths to be taken and frees any trapped trauma held there. Some patients who have had heartbreak also possess an inflated quality in the diaphragm pulse position (Hammer 2001, p.579). This pulse position is part of the Shen-Hammer pulse system and is found on patients who have suppressed trauma. After cupping the area around the seventh thoracic vertebra, where UB-17 and UB-46 are located, the diaphragm pulse position can return to normal.

## Cupping Shen Que R-8

Cupping R-8 can awaken the digestion. It also establishes proper flow and counteracts rebellious stomach qi (chronic hiccups, gastroparesis, acid reflux, etc.). The technique effectively gathers qi and stabilizes a patient suffering from digestive disorders due to emotional trauma.

A single medium cup is placed over the umbilicus for up to five minutes. The sensation is unique and the practitioner is encouraged to personally experience the technique. Patients with abdominal sensitivity and a history of sexual abuse are generally not candidates for this technique.

## Cupping Ling Tai (Spirit Tower) DU-10 with Bloodletting

Stimulating DU-10 (Spirit Tower) clears toxins and heat, primarily in dermatological conditions. An ancient term for the heart, the point name refers to the Spirit Tower built by emperor Wen Wang to provide a vantage point to see all that lay around him. Located medial to UB-15 (the heart back shu point), the name Spirit Tower alludes to the heart's reasoning ability (Deadman and Al-Khafaji 1998, pp.541–542). Heat and toxin accumulation unsettles the spirit and hinders the heart's function to accurately perceive.

Trauma, when left unresolved, generates heat, blockages, and ultimately toxins. Bleeding DU-10 releases toxins built up from trapped emotional trauma. Toxins in the skin reflect toxic heat internally. Acne, furuncles, and carbuncles can be treated with this point (Deadman and Al-Khafaji 1998, p.542). Bleeding DU-10 should only be used when there are significant heat toxins in the skin. This can be coupled when there are skin toxins and chemical sensitivities. Releasing the heat trapped in the skin clears the lungs and stabilizes the Po, therefore reducing chemical sensitivities.

### The Technique

The patient can be seated or lying prone for this procedure. First, prick DU-10 with a three-edged needle. (Follow the bleeding protocols listed above in "Bloodletting.") Immediately afterward, place a small or medium cup over the point. Leave the cup on the skin for one to two minutes, depending on the constitution of the patient. Typically, the cup draws several drops of blood from the point, requiring an abundance of cotton to clean the site when the cup is removed. Cover the area with a self-adhesive bandage afterwards.

## Summary of Cupping Therapy

Cupping therapy can stir the energy and overwhelm a patient if performed prior to the qi being settled. Once the qi is gathered and the trauma memory is soothed, use this therapy to help the patient process the blocked trauma. Cupping resolves the emotional and physical symptoms of trauma and can speed the recovery. To assist the body with processing trauma, Chinese herbal formulas are commonly used.

# Chinese Herbal Formulas

Chinese herbal formulas affect the body systemically and access deep-seated emotional trauma. The formulas follow a staged approach similar to the acupuncture protocols. Begin with gathering the qi and calming the spirit, followed by addressing excess and/ or deficiency in the organ systems. Individual formulas are presented in Chapter 4. A formula frequently used to initiate treatment of emotional trauma is described below.

## "Gathering the Qi" and "Soothing the Trauma Memory"

The chief of the psychological department of the Beijing Chinese Medicine Hospital in 2002 taught the modification of Gan Mai Da Zao Tang (Licorice, Wheat, and Jujube Decoction) to treat a variety of emotional conditions.[3] Unfortunately, his name is not mentioned here due to the author having lost contact with the department.

The base formula calms the spirit, harmonizes the middle jiao, and strengthens the spleen (Chen and Chen 2009, p.731). Modifying the formula adds the ability to soothe the trauma memory and powerfully gather the qi and calm the spirit.

**GAN MAI DA ZAO TANG MODIFIED (LICORICE, WHEAT, AND JUJUBE DECOCTION MODIFIED)**

- Gan Cao (Radix et Rhizoma Glycyrrhizae) 9g
- Fu Xiao Mai (Fructus Tritici) 9–15g
- Da Zao (Fructus Jujubae) 5–7 pieces
- *Hu Po (Succinum) 6g*
- *Long Gu (Os Draconis) 6g*
- *Bai He (Bulbus Lilii) 6–9g*

**ACTIONS OF THE MODIFICATIONS OF GAN MAI DA ZAO TANG**

| Chinese Herb(s) | Action |
| --- | --- |
| Hu Po (Succinum) and Long Gu (Os Draconis) | They stabilize and calm the spirit (Chen and Chen 2009, pp.758–760). They reduce the intensity of the trauma memory, allowing the patient to be present. |
| Bai He (Bulbus Lilii) | It tonifies the qi and nourishes fluids, and most importantly, it tonifies the heart and calms the spirit (Chen and Chen 2009, p.955). It stabilizes the Shen so that the patient can accurately perceive the environment. |

This incredibly effective formula can be further modified based on each patient's specific presentation. It is not appropriate for all patients. Once the patient is grounded and the trauma memory is soothed, utilize other formulas to address the patient's specific channel and organ imbalances.

## Shamanic Qigong, Visualizations, and Meditations

Viewed as rungs on a ladder, treatment methods in Chinese medicine comprise a hierarchy based on the level of intervention performed by the practitioner on the patient. The higher up the ladder, the less the intervention by the practitioner. Qigong (cultivation of vital energy) rests on the top rung of the ladder; thus, the patient

---

3   Lecture by Head of the Psychiatric Department of the Beijing TCM Hospital, 2002.

performs their own healing through visualizations, breathing techniques, and physical movement. The bottom rung consists of herbal formulas where the patient plays a passive role and the practitioner's treatment literally gets into the patient's bloodstream. The rungs between involve nutrition, exercise, feng shui, astrology, massage, and acupuncture. (For details about this concept refer to Appendix 1.)

As the patient climbs the ladder, their sense of empowerment increases—ultimately bringing healing to a new level. This concept is especially pertinent when treating emotional trauma. Damage to the psyche through trauma renders a patient lacking in self-worth. Qigong provides them with healing exercises they can practice daily to fully engage in the healing process. The word qigong is a modern one encompassing physical forms such as tai ji, sitting meditations, basic/complex movements, visualizations, and other self-cultivation techniques. A few forms presented below serve as an introduction to the wealth of information available. As with any physical form, it is recommended to learn these movements from a teacher.

## Shamanic Qigong

Many powerful and effective forms of qigong exist. The qigong presented below is taught by Master Zhongxian Wu, who is the eighteenth generation lineage holder of the Mt. Wudang Dragon Gate style of qigong and eighth generation lineage holder of the Mt. Emei Sage/Shaman style of qigong (Wu 2016, pp.119–120). (Master Wu teaches internationally and has written several books on multiple forms. For the best description and presentation about the type of qigong he teaches, it is encouraged to personally study with Master Wu and read his wonderfully crafted texts.)

### Standing Qigong Form

The Standing Qigong Form offers powerful healing, but it appears as though a "person is just standing there." However, strong healing is occurring internally. Many of the forms of qigong taught by Master Wu begin with this stance. When doing this standing form, the person connects to heaven and earth, feeling empowered and calm (Figure 3.9). This form brings them into the present moment and allows access to the available energies. Standing still enables the person to ground themselves and gather their qi. They connect to the cosmic qi and receive a qi shower coming down from the heavens into DU-20, which softens the intensity of the trauma memory. This simple form is powerful, and just a few minutes of daily practice yields wonderful results.

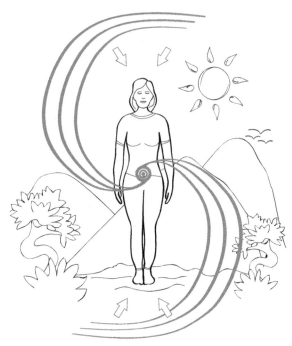

*Figure 3.9 Standing Qigong Form*
*Source:* Kirsteen Wright

1.  Stand with the feet together, toes clutching the ground, and legs straight.

2.  The hands are relaxed a few inches from the outer thighs, arms straight, with fingers together and pointing at the ground. The arms are not stiff (as a soldier standing at attention), yet not limp like a wet noodle either. They are in between these extremes, similar to a "needle in cotton."

3.  The back is straight, head upright, imagining a string is attached to the top of the head, lifting it upright. The vertebrae are like pearls on a string.

4.  The shoulders are relaxed.

5.  The eyelids are relaxed, "closing the curtain." The lids gently cover most of the eyes, with the nose tip slightly visible.

6.  The mouth is closed, the teeth touching gently, and the tongue is touching the skin above the back of the front teeth.

7.  The earthly door (the anus) is closed, the perineum is lifted, and the lower belly is tucked and held.

8.  DU-20 (Hundred Meetings), located on the top of the head, is open.

9.  The breathing imagery is *Mi Mi Mian Mian*. This is a breath like "spun silk"— slow, smooth, deep, and even.

10. Imagine being surrounded by sunlight. With each inhalation, the golden universal light is taken in by the lungs and into all the pores of the body. With each exhalation, the energy condenses in the lower belly—the lower Dantian.

Standing and connecting to the universal energy aids in treating multiple pathologies, including emotional trauma. Feeling the rooting and grounding ability of the earth provides patients with a sense of safety and calmness. When practiced as part of a daily routine, the intensity of the trauma reduces and the patho-mechanism of the trauma clears.

Scientists trained schoolchildren in a standing form that concentrated on posture and breathing. They found it reduced anxiety and improved circulation. The study included thermagrams showing the stark contrast of circulation before and after qigong. Researchers found that, several weeks after doing the form, the subjects still experienced increased circulation. This demonstrated the lasting effects of qigong (Matos *et al.* 2015). The Standing Qigong Form significantly improves emotional states and the flow of energy in the body. Patients can practice moving forms to remove old energy, memories, and patterns. The Shaking Qigong Form is one such effective form.

*Shaking Qigong Form*

Shaking comes from the Chinese shamanic tradition and opens the spiritual gates (joints) and wakes up the energy of the body. This special movement allows patients to connect with the spiritual energy and enables them to enliven their rhythmic vibration. In ancient times, shamans melded with the spiritual energy through drumming and dancing. This is a ritual of the heart—feeling the rhythm of the earth to awaken the spirit.

Practicing the Shaking Qigong Form moves energy within the body. Visualize letting go of old energy to create space for the new energy to enter. As the old energy and patterns release, the person's energy field unites with the universal qi. The person must always stay mindful of the present moment and where they are, avoiding the urge to "leave the body," and venture into space.

The following provides a description of the Shaking Qigong Form. To best incorporate the practice, train with Master Wu or one of his lifelong qigong students.

1. Begin with the Standing Qigong Form (described above).

2. Connect with heaven and earth.

3. Take in a breath and, with the exhalation, step out with the right foot. The feet should be pointing straight ahead and slightly wider than shoulder-width apart.

4. Take in a breath and, with the exhalation, rotate the palms facing outward. Take in another breath and lift the arms up, keeping them straight and relaxed, making a "V" shape. Imagine touching the heavens. If possible, roll up onto the balls of the feet and keep the heels off the ground. This enhances the posture.

5. Imagine all the joints opening—the toes, feet, ankles, knees, hips, vertebrae, jaw, shoulders, elbows, wrists, hands, and fingers. The joints are the gates to the spiritual energy, and opening these spaces allows for the spiritual energy to energize the body.

6. Hold this posture for several slow, deep, and even breaths, feeling the body's qi expanding.

7. After a few minutes, take in a deep breath, hold the breath, and lower oneself into a squat. Then leap into the air. As your feet reconnect with the earth, breathe out and say the Chinese word *heng* (pronounced "hung"), keeping the mouth closed.

8. Begin "shaking."

Shaking is bouncing on the ground, alternating between each foot. Shaking should be done at a pace and rhythm that feels comfortable. If there are joint problems, simply standing in place and imagining your body shaking is powerful on its own. Shaking is bringing in new qi and getting rid of the old energy. Periodic stomping is encouraged. Remember to say the word *heng* with each exhalation, keeping the mouth closed. Feel the sensation of the word *heng* resonate in the lower belly—the lower Dantian. The resonation should not irritate the throat. If it does, the technique is incorrect. The mouth is closed and teeth are kept together, with the tongue touching the upper tooth ridge behind the front teeth, unless otherwise noted.

1. Imagine a red golden ball bouncing up and down in the lower Dantian. Throughout the shaking, keep the earthly door closed and the heavenly gate open. Imagine feeling the qi shower.

2. After a few minutes of shaking the whole body, begin to shake the various parts of the body:

   i. Head: Heaven Level. The head represents the "Heaven Level" of the body. This is the connection to the Father Sky energy, and to the lineages and spiritual leaders that relate to each person. Continue to bounce from foot to foot making the *heng* sound. Spend a few minutes with each part of the body, starting with the eyes and working down to the neck.

    a.   Eyes: Rotate the eyes clockwise and counter-clockwise.

    b.   Nose: Rub and shake the nose.

    c.   Lips: Keeping the lips together, breathe out while vibrating the lips.

    d.   Tongue: Open the mouth and make whatever noise you wish as the tongue is moved. Whatever comes naturally is fine.

    e.   Teeth: Click the teeth together gently while keeping your mouth closed and the tongue touching the upper tooth ridge behind the front teeth.

    f.   Ears: Gently massage and rub the ears.

    g.   Neck: Gently massage your neck with one or both hands. For those without neck injuries or issues, gently rotate and extend the neck.

ii.   Upper Limbs: Human Level. The upper limbs and torso represent the human level and the connection to the human family. Continue to bounce from foot to foot making the *heng* sound. Spend a few minutes with each part of the body, starting with the shoulders and working down to the fingers.

    a.   Shoulders: Gently open and rotate the shoulders.

    b.   Elbows: Shake and move the elbows.

    c.   Wrists: Gently rotate and stretch the wrists.

    d.   Fingers: Shake the fingers.

iii.  The Torso: Human Level. Continue to bounce from foot to foot making the *heng* sound. Spend a few minutes with each part of the body, starting with the back and finishing with the kidneys.

    a.   Back: Visualize your back being as strong as a mountain while shaking.

    b.   Vertebrae: Imagine shaking the spine, starting from the low back up to the neck. Those with disk problems need only stand still and simply visualize the spine shaking.

    c.   Chest: Lift the arms up to shoulder level with your palms facing upward and imagine the heart and lungs bouncing in your chest. Tapping the chest as you shake is an option.

    d.   Abdomen: Pat down the abdomen and visualize shaking the internal organs.

e.  Kidneys: Place the palms in the small of the back and say the Chinese words *hai hei* (pronounced "hi hey"). Keep the mouth closed. The sound of *hai hei* should resonate in the kidneys.

iv.  Lower Limbs: Earth Level. The lower limbs represent the connection to the earth and its energies: the water, fire, and wind. This is the connection to Mother Earth energy. Continue to bounce from foot to foot making the *heng* sound. Spend a few minutes with each part of the body, starting with the hips and working down to the feet.

a.  Hips: Rotate and shake the hips gently.

b.  Knees: Temporarily stop shaking/bouncing and place the feet shoulder-width apart. Bend the knees and grasp the knee caps with the fingertips. Slowly rotate the knees, bringing them together and then moving them apart in a circular motion. As the knees come together inhale, and as they move away from each other exhale. Do both clockwise and counter-clockwise rotations. For patients with knee problems, simply stand with the fingertips on the knee caps and imagine rotating the knees.

c.  Ankles: Begin bouncing again and rotate and shake the ankles, alternating from one to the other.

d.  Feet: Stomp and shake the feet for a few minutes while imagining all the old energy draining out into the earth.

3.  Finish: Imagine the golden red ball bouncing in the lower Dantian. Focus on the red golden ball for a few minutes while bouncing.

4.  Take a deep breath and leap into the air; land firmly on the ground, exhaling. Say the word *heng* and then stand still silently. The feet are shoulder-width apart with the feet and toes clutching the ground. The back is straight and the head is upright. The earthly door is closed, the heavenly gate is open. The hands and arms are next to the sides of the body with fingers pointing at the ground. The mouth is closed, and the eyelids are relaxed. Feel the tingling, warmth, and movement in the body. Take several gentle breaths, returning to the *Mi Mi Mian Mian* style breathing (smooth, slow, deep, and even).

5.  After a few minutes, take a deep breath and on the exhalation slowly turn the palms of the hands outward. Inhale, lifting the arms up over the head and bringing the palms together. At the same time bring the right foot to the left foot so they are touching again. Exhale and make the sound *heng*, placing the

hands on the lower Dantian. The hands form the "Tai Ji Mudra." The Tai Ji Mudra is interlocking the hands with the thumbs—with the one palm touching the lower abdomen. For women, the right palm touches the abdomen, and for men it is the left palm.

6. Focus on the lower Dantian for a few minutes and then close the form by exhaling three times making the *heng* sound. This seals the energy in the lower Dantian.

This Shaking Qigong Form incorporates all the aspects of the body. It moves the qi, frees blockages, and brings nourishment to the organs. Each element is equally cleansed and recharged. If a patient has a specific element needing attention, additional time may be spent on those areas of the body relating to that element. Practicing this form daily rekindles joy, brings peace within, and resolves the emotional trauma. Master Wu recommends practicing any qigong form 49 days in a row to determine if the form is effective for the individual.

**RESEARCH STUDIES OF QIGONG TREATING EMOTIONAL SYMPTOMS**

| Medical Journal (Date) | Research Finding |
| --- | --- |
| *Journal of Health Psychology* (2009) | After one month of qigong practice, depression and anxiety were reduced, and the quality of sleep was improved (Manzaneque *et al.* 2009). |
| *BMC Journal* (2014) | Researchers reviewed several random control trials and concluded that qigong reduces stress and anxiety after one month of practice, and, in many cases, immediately after practicing qigong one time (Wang *et al.* 2014). |

Both the Standing Qigong Form and the Shaking Qigong Form gather the qi, center the patient, and soothe the trauma memory. The forms bring the patient to the present moment and help "trash out" old energy. Specific forms to benefit the brain and improve the communication system of the body are described below.

## *Qigong to Benefit the Brain*
### HAIR WASHING FORM

This form can be practiced either while seated or standing. Place the fingertips where the hairline begins and inhale as the head gently tilts back. Firmly move the fingertips across the scalp to the crown of the head. Exhale and slowly move the fingertips down the back of the head, while the neck relaxes and the chin drops to touch the chest. With the exhalation say *heng*, keeping your mouth closed, teeth closed, and your tongue touching your upper tooth ridge behind the front teeth. Repeat this technique nine times. This form activates the acupuncture points used in the "Soothing the Trauma Memory" protocol.

### Brain Rotation

Gently rotate the head eight times clockwise and eight times counter-clockwise, visualizing your brain, that is, see the brain rotating in space. Keep the mouth closed and the teeth together, with the tongue touching the upper tooth ridge behind the front teeth. This exercise powerfully calms the mind and opens the flow of energy from the head to the body.

---

## Case Study: The Remarkable Benefit of the Brain Rotation Exercise

A 61-year-old male, "Burt," presented with Lou Gehrig's disease and was being treated with Western medicine. He was skeptical about Chinese medicine, but decided to try it. Burt came in for a Chinese medicine treatment wearing a neck brace to support his head. His neck muscles no longer had the strength to keep his head upright.

The brain rotation exercise was given to the patient and he practiced it diligently twice a day. He rotated his head eight times each direction and then added eight times for each lobe of the brain. After two weeks of practice, he only wore the neck brace at the end of the day or when he was tired. In four weeks, he no longer required the brace. A year later, the last few weeks of his life, when his energy was very weak, he once more relied on the brace.

---

### *Summary of Shamanic Qigong*

A door hinge gets rusty if the door is not used. This saying applies to the body in general. Moving the body clears blockages created by trauma and assists the patient in connecting with the body and the present moment. The charge of the trauma memory reduces when the patient remains present and in their body. Their sense of empowerment and ability to move forward improves. Qigong is a valuable tool for patients to use to step beyond the old trauma and experience a different perspective.

Some patients could find the Shaking Qigong Form too stimulating at first and would benefit from beginning with just the Standing Form to gather their qi. They could progress to the Hair Washing Form to soothe the trauma memory and then, when they feel ready, incorporate the Shaking Qigong Form (starting with a few minutes and increasing the time each day). The physical body function and strength increases with practicing qigong, providing a healthy vessel for the patient. The patient successfully climbs the ladder of Chinese medicine, utilizing qigong when faced with rising emotions from an emotional trauma.

## Visualizations

Visualizations activate the spirit and the power of intention. Qigong, and Chinese medicine in general, incorporates the three treasures Jing, Qi, and Shen. People engaged in exercise move their bodies, but if thoughts run wild they leave the present moment. Caught up in the past or future, the full potential to incorporate all the activity going on inside the body is not realized. The following two visualization exercises focus on the Shen level, or intention, and when practiced regularly reduce the triggering of emotional trauma.

Reliving emotional trauma causes a person to experience multiple emotions and body sensations. A person generally responds by mentally running away from these feelings. They attempt to distract themselves with outside stimuli, deny their feelings, or hate themselves for having their feelings. Running from the feelings rising from the trauma memory amplifies the charge of the trauma—the patient gets caught in a vicious circle. If a patient focuses on their breath and feels the sensations, they activate the body's ability to naturally cleanse itself of the trauma.

### Transforming the Emotional Surge

The focus of the "Transforming the Emotional Surge" visualization is to feel the sensations in the body.[4] Experiencing the sensations and letting go of the energy/emotions/body feelings becomes easier with each practice. This powerful visualization can yield effective results in clearing trauma held in the body. Ideally, work with a counselor/therapist to guide the practice.

- When there is a strong surge of emotion, sit with the sensation and experience it.

- Mentally describe the body sensation(s) in terms of its location in the body, the color(s), the shape, the texture, the weight, and if it is moving or still. (Avoid labeling the sensation as anxiety, fear, anger, etc.)

- Focus on the feeling and refrain from thinking of something else, suppressing the feeling, or attempting to mentally run from it (a common reaction). Put all the attention on the feeling to allow for transformation of the trauma.

- Sense the hands and feet and note the feeling—tingling, warmth, vibration, and so on.

- During the practice, the body inherently shifts the emotional surge, reducing the feelings brought on by the emotions.

---

4    Personal communication with Karen Davis, a counselor and astrologer, living in Bend, Oregon, who taught this technique to the author.

- Visualize the feeling moving out of the body and into the earth. (The earth receives old energy and can transform it, like compost.)

- With practice and focus, this exercise becomes easier.

- For those open to the idea of calling on helpers, guides, or angels, for example, this can assist with the practice.

## *Meditations*

Meditations enhance the body's ability to settle and bring about healing from within. After a trauma, patients can hyper-focus on the event and lose sight of the present moment. Intentions and phrases shift the mental focus away from the trauma and improve energy, presence, and strength.[5]

### VERSES FOR LOVING-KINDNESS, COMPASSION, AND SYMPATHETIC JOY

> May all beings be happy and peaceful.
>
> May all beings be healthy and strong.
>
> May all beings be safe and free.
>
> May all beings be able to care for themselves with ease and joy.

### COMPASSION FOR THOSE WHO SUFFER

> I care about this pain; I care about the pain in the world.
>
> May all beings be free of suffering and all the causes of suffering.
>
> May all beings be comforted, supported, cared for, and healed.
>
> May all suffering sentient beings be surrounded with loving-kindness.
>
> May all beings be surrounded with kindness.

### FORGIVENESS REFLECTION

> If I have hurt or harmed anyone knowingly
> or unknowingly, I ask forgiveness.
>
> If anyone has hurt or harmed me knowingly or unknowingly, to the
> extent that I am able to do so at this time, I extend forgiveness.

---

5   Jude Rosen of Tacoma, Washington, taught these meditations to the author at the Cloud Mountain Retreat Center in 2009. The reader is encouraged to study with Ms. Rosen. She teaches Vipassana and Metta meditation retreats and holds meditation groups in Washington state.

I extend forgiveness to myself.

APPRECIATIVE JOY/SYMPATHETIC JOY

May all those experiencing success and happiness continue to experience it.

May it grow for them, and may their joy always be with them.

## Variety of Meditations

The different meditations release the trauma and bring positivity. Growing the love and positivity for oneself and others shifts the hurt and charge of the trauma. The shift creates positive space in the body. These short and simple phrases bring about significant change.

**RESEARCH STUDIES OF MEDITATION TREATING EMOTIONAL SYMPTOMS**

| Medical Journal (Date) | Research Finding |
|---|---|
| *Current Opinion in Psychiatry* (2016) | Mindfulness-based cognitive therapy (MBCT) practices are on par with antidepressant therapy. MBCT increased brain activity in the pre-frontal cortex and insula—regions responsible for regulating emotions (Segal and Walsh 2016). |
| *Medical Care* (2014) | Metta meditation improved environmental mastery, personal growth, purpose in life, and self-acceptance in veterans with PTSD. The triggered emotions from the trauma were reduced and positive emotions increased (Kearney *et al.* 2014). |
| *Military Medicine* (2016) | After one month, 83 percent of soldiers with PTSD who added transcendental meditation (TM) to their treatment regimen stabilized, reduced, or stopped their medication, and over a six-month period experienced fewer psychological symptoms (Barnes *et al.* 2016). |
| *Brain Connectivity* (2015) | Daoist meditators' brains scanned during resting and meditative states revealed reduced activity in the sensory cortex areas, an increase in the thalamus regions, and increased connections in the brain during meditation (Jao *et al.* 2016). |

## Summary of Meditations

Meditation enables the patient to take charge of their healing process and transform the emotional and physical effects of emotional trauma. As with any practice, the patient determines which meditation works for them through trial-and-error. The above is a small offering of the multiple loving-kindness meditations available and serves as a starting point for patients to feel the power of meditation.

## Chinese Medicine Nutrition

Two millennia ago Qi Bo, in the *Huang Di Nei Jing* (*The Yellow Emperor's Classic*), stressed the importance of good nutrition and restful sleep for sound mind, health, and longevity. By simply following general Chinese nutritional recommendations, one's health improves greatly and emotions are balanced.

RESEARCH STUDIES OF NUTRITION TREATING EMOTIONAL SYMPTOMS

| Medical Journal (Date) | Research Finding |
| --- | --- |
| *Metabolism* (2015) | People who consumed trans-fatty acids and who slept less were more likely to suffer from PTSD (Gavrieli *et al.* 2015). |
| *Psychiatry Clinical Neuroscience* (2014) | Healthy eating habits increased the resilience of the survivors of the massive earthquake and tsunami that struck the northeastern coast of Japan and reduced the intensity of PTSD symptoms (Kukihara 2014). |

### *General Nutritional Guidelines*

#### *A Balanced Diet*

Maintaining the middle, or earth, element is essential for post-natal qi production. Mindful dietary choices with room for flexibility and fun preserve the spleen and stomach qi and produce abundant energy for the body. Increased energy in the body promotes resilience to stress and less reactivity to trauma. Li Dong Yuan, author of the *Pi Wei Lun* (*Treatise on the Spleen and Stomach*), emphasized the concept that all pathogens stem from the digestion, and if the digestion is healthy, all other organ systems will improve. He centered his practice on digestion, first and foremost. In an article about Dr. Li, Rosenberg noted:

> Dr. Li pointed out that with the extreme stress and grief of war, loss of life, impure water, and inadequate food or shelter, that the epidemics were caused by depletion, and that people needed supplementation to overcome the epidemic evils. (Rosenberg n.d.)

Li indicated the importance of good nutrition to ward off pathogens and affirmed the impact of emotional trauma on the body and its immune system. Good nutrition is what you eat and how much of it. The Chinese dietary approach varies considerably as opposed to a typical American diet (a large piece of meat, a large portion of carbohydrates and maybe a small amount of vegetables).

**THE CHINESE MEDICINE BALANCED DIET**

| | |
|---|---|
| 50% | Whole grains (an equal mix of rice, millet, rye, and barley) |
| 20–30% | Seasonal vegetables and fruits |
| 10% | Protein (variety of meats and fish, tofu, tempeh, and legumes) |
| 5–10% | Soups (one to two cups per day) (refer to Appendix 2 for recipes) |

The first formula listed in the *Huang Di Nei Jing* is white rice porridge. This treats digestive upset and wasting disorder since white rice is easy to digest and benefits the earth element. It can be eaten several times per week to improve overall digestion. Brown rice may be substituted, but must be soaked overnight to break the hulls on the rice. If it is not soaked for the proper time, the hulls will not open, irritating the digestion system, and ultimately will go undigested.

**ESTABLISHING STABILITY WITH GENERAL NUTRITIONAL GUIDELINES**

| Recommendation | Explanation |
|---|---|
| *Regular Mealtimes* | The earth follows natural rhythms. To bring clear thoughts and proper nourishment, the mind of the spleen—the Yi/intent—processes and flows at a steady pace. Eating at similar times each day reduces the body from going into a "starvation mode" and allows the metabolism to function optimally. |
| *Warm Cooked Foods* | Warm cooked food is recommended since cold/raw food tends to deplete the energy of the body. When a person eats raw food, the spleen has the additional task of "cooking" the food and breaking down the cellulose structure before transporting the nutrition throughout the body. In warm climates or during late spring and summer, eating salads and other raw vegetables in moderation is appropriate. Eating organic food is recommended. Organic meats are most important since the accumulation of pesticides is greater in non-organic meats. |
| *Chewing Food* | Chew food 40 times per bite to provide the necessary time needed for saliva to break down the food for smooth digestion (Dawes *et al.* 2015). The proper amount of chewing slows down eating, allowing the body to register when it is full, preventing over-eating (Vázquez *et al.* 2016). |
| *Eating While in a Calm State of Mind* | Stress inhibits the digestive function (Dehghanizade *et al.* 2015); thus, encourage patients to eat in a relaxed, calm environment. When eating, avoid stressful conversations, reading, watching television, or surfing on the internet. |

| Recommendation | Explanation |
|---|---|
| *Enjoying Food* | Foods that bring the spark of lightness (fire and joy) generate earth—a digestive environment hungry to absorb the nutrients. Patients who explore different foods, and eat fresh seasonal foods, tend to enjoy food more. |
| *Fluids and Digestion* | Fluids are an important part of digestion and, depending on the patient's level of activity and constitution, about eight glasses of room-temperature fluids (primarily highly pure water) a day should be consumed. This refers to all fluids, including those in foods and soups. Clear broth soup provides easy absorption of nutrients and is gentle on the spleen and pancreas. |

## *Additional Nutritional Information*

### *Exercise and Nutrition*

Physical movement is a vital part of maintaining a healthy metabolism and assimilating nutrients. The earth element governs the muscles; therefore, when the muscles are activated, so is the digestive process. Chinese medicine recommends "1000 steps" (a leisurely stroll, not speed walking) after eating to promote digestion and activate the metabolism.

### *Eating Disorders*

PTSD or emotional trauma can be the root cause of eating disorders, and often eating habits change when the trauma memory is triggered. In 2014, subjects suffering from an eating disorder were studied over a six-month period. Researchers found that the subjects with PTSD had a higher prevalence of eating disorders, and were prone to insecurity, interpersonal distrust, and impulsivity. They had a decrease of interceptive awareness (Vierling *et al.* 2015).

Resolving the emotional trauma frequently treats the eating disorder. Due to the impulsivity created by an emotional trauma, maintaining a healthy diet can be challenging. However, as the intensity of the trauma memory reduces, healthy choices are achievable.

ADDITIONAL NUTRITIONAL INFORMATION

| Recommendation | Explanation |
|---|---|
| *Food Combining* | Typically, fruit and vegetables are not mixed; however, apples mixed with vegetables are easy to digest. Fruits require different enzymes and a longer time to be digested compared with vegetables. Fruits are best eaten in the morning; if consumed at night they will ferment, causing gas and poor digestion. |
| *Supplements and Nutrition* | Stress and toxins deplete the body of essential nutrients and are present in most environments. Adding whole food nutritional supplements to the basic diet regimen is essential, especially when treating trauma. Finding the balance between correct and incorrect amounts of supplements can be challenging and is best guided by a licensed practitioner. |
| *Juicing* | Over the last few decades juicing has become quite popular; however, it is not part of the typical Chinese medicine recommended diet. Incorporating herbs (such as ginger) with juices aids digestion. |
| *The Human Biome and Mental Clarity* | The bacteria balance in one's gut has been linked to the mental state of the individual. Further work and study is being conducted on the human biome (bacterial levels in the gut). Overuse of antibiotics has upset this balance in many people's digestive systems. Organic kombucha drinks and other fermented foods, in addition to probiotic supplements, create a healthy human biome and bring clarity of thought. |
| *The Macrobiotic Diet* | Selecting foods and observing cooking methods based on the flow of seasons (macrobiotic diet) brings a person in sync with the harmony of the universe. Scientific studies on the macrobiotic diet show its benefit in helping patients with diabetes and cancer (Soare *et al.* 2015). Studies have proven that the macrobiotic diet reduces inflammation (Harmon *et al.* 2015), such as the heat created by emotional trauma and its memory. |

## *Observing the Universal Energy Flow*

### *Eating with the Seasons*

The ancient Chinese shamans and doctors recognized the importance of following nature in all ways of life—including nutrition—to prevent disease and promote well-being. Cooking methods, the flavors of foods, and the quantity of foods to eat are chosen by differentiating the qi in each season. Different organs are active each season and thrive when eating/cooking is selected based on the seasonal energy. Certain types of cooking methods add heat to foods and change with each season, as does the amount of food consumed.[6]

---

6    Nam Singh, a Chinese herbalist and Daoist priest in San Francisco, taught Chinese dietetics to the author, including the way of eating with seasons. The reader is encouraged to study with Mr. Singh at his Culinary Arts School.

Eating foods correlated to the seasonal energy balances the specific emotional tendencies associated with that time of year. People suffering from emotional trauma build up resilience to reliving trauma by following such practices. The foods recommended below by Nam Singh are to be incorporated into the overall diet and are not the only things consumed in that season.

**Spring** is when the wood element thrives and the energy is reborn. This is an appropriate time to cleanse any heat or toxins remaining in the body from winter. Anger and irritation commonly flare in the spring, and the trauma memory can trigger such emotions.

- Eating small amounts of foods is recommended along with abstention from rich foods.

- Consume less meat and increase vegetables and fruits.

- Utilize flash cooking, steaming, and stir fry methods.

- Augment the diet with bean sprouts, chicken, citrus fruits, lentils, greens, and barley (foods in harmony with spring), in addition to seasonal foods.

- Enjoy a tea of Gou Qi Zi (goji berries) and Ju Hua (chrysanthemum) to soothe the liver and remove toxins. This simple tea, taken daily, calms the spirit and flushes built-up toxins. Take care to steep chrysanthemum for only one minute to prevent the tea from being too bitter and causing diarrhea.

**Summer** signals the peak of yang energy and heat in the body. Following the spring diet idea of less food and flash cooking continues. During summer, heart fire easily depletes yin (the fluids). The summer heat triggers emotional reactivity that can accentuate a trauma memory.

- Avoid consuming sugar, chocolate, alcohol, greasy fried foods, and heavy foods (cheeses, sauces, etc.).

- Enjoy a tea of Xi Yang Shen (American ginseng) to calm the spirit, increase fluids, and benefit the kidney energy.

**Late summer** is the transition from summer to fall. The energy returns to the center direction (the earth element). Dampness can be generated in the body, and patients can obsess about past trauma.

- Use aromatic seasonings such as mint, basil, and cilantro to reduce dampness.

- Add millet, eggs, tuna, sweet potatoes, and apples to the diet.

- Bake apples with honey, Da Zao (jujubes), and cinnamon to benefit the earth element and reduce overthinking.

**Fall** is the time of harvest and the metal element—the energy turns inward. Eating pungent foods (the taste associated with the metal element) is recommended. Utilizing slower cooking methods is advised to draw out the essence of the food, increasing the nutrient concentration. Patients typically experience an increased sense of grief around the trauma (grief and sadness are the emotions of fall); thus shoring up energy and building substance stabilizes the Po to root the spirit in the body.

- Prepare stews, casseroles, baked dishes, roasts, and slow grilled food.

- Add soybeans, wild rice, cauliflower, pumpkin, water chestnuts, and pears to the diet.

- Consume the "Nourishing the Fluids Cocktail" (dryness commonly invades in the fall): ¾ teaspoon sea salt (Celtic is preferred), 1 teaspoon maple syrup (Grade A), ½ squeezed lemon, and 1½ cups warm water.

**Winter** signifies the most inward and storing time of the year; it is associated with the water element and cold. As with fall suggestions, similar cooking methods are used to draw out the essence of food and infuse heat into the food. Just as the plants are returning to the root, so is the body, and it needs extra nourishment for this period. Fear is the emotion associated with the winter season. Sustenance grounds the spirit and provides stability; earth controls water/fear.

- Augment the diet with almonds, walnuts, celery, mushrooms, avocados, and winter pears.

- Utilize baking, stewing, roasting, and slow grilling methods.

- Avoid eating raw or cold foods.

### Summary of Chinese Medicine Nutrition

*Let food be thy medicine, and medicine be thy food.*

*Hippocrates*

A stable foundation is achieved with whole cooked foods along with routine mealtimes, adequate fluid consumption, seasonally appropriate choices, supplementation with vitamins/minerals, and enjoyment of food. These contribute to the patient's inner strength, and when the earth element is cared for, post-natal qi production is optimal. Emotions are regulated and the intensity of the trauma memory reduces until the trauma no longer affects the patient's organs and channels. This provides patients with the ability to navigate the resolution of emotional trauma.

## Sleep Hygiene

Eat, sleep, be happy, repeat. Sleeping is one of the best forms of medicine and plays an important role in successful treatment of emotional trauma. Allowing the body to replenish itself and store energy creates a stable environment to process and resolve trauma.

### Chinese Medicine and Sleep

Lying down increases a person's wisdom/inner knowing, the aspects of the water element. Well-rested people can tap into their inner knowing; wisdom aids in the processing and transformation of emotional trauma. The classic phrase "sleep on it" speaks to this idea. Each time the body rests, water increases. A healthy water element supports the wood element.

Water gives birth to wood. In Chinese medicine, all the blood returns to the liver to be cleansed and replenished during the night. The spirit resides in the blood and is cleansed with a restful sleep. The wood element is associated with action and, if healthy, increases the patient's ability to transform the old trauma.

*When sleeping women wake, mountains move.*

*Chinese proverb*

It is important for patients to sleep, rest, or meditate between 11 pm and 3 am (when the qi surges in the wood channels) to allow the liver to efficiently process and cleanse the blood. Patients who are stressed commonly wake during this time. A vicious cycle ensues when waking between these hours, and stressing when unable to fall back to sleep. Practicing deep breathing and meditation calms the mind and body, aiding the liver in processing the blood. Sleep and deep meditation recharge the body's energy, ultimately reducing stress and allowing for the resolution of trauma. As night falls, yin strengthens and yang declines. Following these activities helps the body flow with this rhythm.

*Deep Sleep Helpful Hints*

- Maintain a regular bedtime (making sure to sleep between 11 pm and 3 am).

- Avoid caffeine in the afternoon/evening.

- Avoid eating large meals one to two hours before bed.

- Discontinue screen use (cell phones, TV, computers, etc.) one hour before bed.

- Drink a small cup of herbal tea, such as chamomile, to settle the body and mind.

- Gently stretch or read to relax the body and allow the yin energy to build.

- Dim the lights one hour before bed and sleep in a darkened, cool room.

- Take flower essences and diffuse essential oils with calming properties.

- Keep a notepad near the bed to write down and release thoughts arising during the night.

- Meditate before bedtime.

## Napping

Napping is not just for grandparents and toddlers. The "siesta" and other such routines have been practiced in cultures all over the planet for centuries to replenish reserves. Western culture, in its desire for productivity, does not observe naptime; however, regular napping after lunch improves energy and brain function (Lovato and Lack 2010). In Chinese medicine, the horary clock time from 1 pm to 3 pm is associated with the heart; thus resting during this time replenishes the heart, benefits the circulation, and roots the spirit.

*Napping Helpful Hints*

- Nap for 20 minutes *or* 90 minutes to allow for a full REM cycle (Ketcham 2015; Soong n.d.) and prevent waking from the nap groggy.

- Maintain a daily napping routine to train the body, allowing for deep sleep at night.

- Nap between 1 pm and 3 pm (napping later in the day causes restless sleep at night).

## Summary of Sleep Hygiene

A calm mind allows for harmonious organ systems and ultimately a happy body. A refreshed body improves the ability to process the old trauma, let go of the old toxins, and enjoy life. Having fun is an essential aspect of life: "A good laugh and a long sleep are the two best cures for anything" (Irish proverb).

# Shamanic Drumming

> *Music and rhythm find their way into*
> *the secret places of our soul.*
>
> *Plato*

The first sound a human hears is the heartbeat of the mother. A simple, steady drumbeat soothes a person and connects them with this first sound of existence. For centuries, shamans used the drum to shift energy and transform illness. A resurgence of vibrational treatments with tuning forks, chimes, singing bowls, and chanting is occurring in Chinese medicine clinics and is proving effective in the treatment of emotional trauma.

## Drum Vibrations Create a Free-Flowing Environment

The importance of establishing a healing space for a patient to heal is essential for treatment, and the drumbeat is one way to create a calming, nurturing environment. The trauma memory initiates an emotional loop and the drumbeat shifts the energy, which births a new perspective in the patient. The drum becomes a vehicle for the spirit to manifest itself and shine. Performing a simple yet powerful beat over the patient, or near them, shakes up the old pattern and clears out stuck energy. The vibration of the drum massages the cells, moves fluid through the lymph system, improves the cardiovascular system, calms emotional reactivity, enhances the immune system, moves qi, and clears out toxins.

**WESTERN MEDICAL JOURNAL ARTICLES SUPPORTING DRUM HEALING**

| Medical Journal (Date) | Research Finding |
| --- | --- |
| *American Journal of Public Health* (2003) | "Difficult patients," who were not helped by counseling, responded positively to drumming and stopped using drugs (Winkelman 2003). |
| *American Journal of Drug and Alcohol Abuse* (2012) | Drumming links people with their culture. Native Americans reconnected with their heritage through drumming, giving them purpose, resulting in less substance abuse (Dickerson *et al.* 2012). |
| *Journal of Cardiovascular Medicine* (2014) | Drumming benefits the cardiovascular system (reduces blood pressure, blood lactate levels, stress levels, and anxiety levels) and provides low-to-medium-intensity exercise; therefore it is less likely to cause the risks associated with high-intensity exercise (Smith, Viljoen, and McGeachie 2014). |
| *Alternative Therapies in Health and Medicine* (2001) | The immune system improves with drumming. Researchers studied group drumming in adult populations and concluded the following: "Group drumming resulted in increased dehydroepiandrosterone-to-cortisol ratios, increased natural killer cell activity, and increased lymphokine-activated killer cell activity..." (Bittman *et al.* 2001). |
| *Evidence-Based Complementary and Alternative Medicine* (2011) | Drumming proved effective at treating anxiety, attention deficit problems, internalizing issues, hyperactivity, and traumatic stress problems in children from low-income homes in Los Angeles (Ho *et al.* 2011). |

## *Drumming and Acupuncture*

The Chinese character for medicinal substances is 藥 *yào*. The character is composed of components that include one meaning grass 草 (herbal medicine) resting on top of the character for happiness/joy: 樂 *lè*. The part of the character indicating joy can also be pronounced *yuè*, to mean "music." Therefore, the character for Chinese medicinals can be understood as "a healthy body creates joyful and harmonious music."[7] Similarly, the medicinal effects of drum vibrations generate harmony and restore balance after emotional trauma. Drumming, like all music, is a form of medicine. The combination of drumbeats with acupuncture results in a synergistic treatment.

### *Choosing a Drum for Healing*

All types of drums can be used in treating patients. Clinically, the hoop drum (a drum common in many indigenous cultures) is convenient to play over a patient after

---

7    Teaching to the author by Master Zhongxian Wu.

the needles are inserted (Figure 3.10). Other drums such as djembes, congas, tama (referred to as a "talking drum"), djun djun, and others can be used. These other types of drums are logistically challenging to play over the patient while receiving acupuncture treatment. However, played near the patient, the vibrations of the drum still activate the needles.

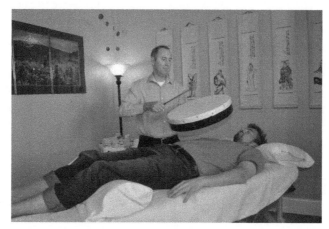

*Figure 3.10 Drumming over a Patient Receiving Acupuncture*
Source: Dean Holman

### Shamanic Journey Beat Technique

Many drumbeats can be used in healing. A steady drumbeat, commonly referred to as the "trance beat" or the "Shamanic Journey Drumbeat," produces relaxation and movement in the channels. Begin the drumbeat once the needles are placed in the patient. Play the steady rhythm for a few minutes over the patient, moving the drum from their head to their feet several times up and down the body. After drumming for a few minutes, the patient is left to rest for approximately 30 minutes. Before removing the needles, perform the closing drumbeat (described below).

#### DRUMMING WITH ACUPUNCTURE PROTOCOL

1. Insert needles.
2. Perform the Shamanic Journey Drumbeat (one to five minutes).
3. Let patient rest with needles.
4. Close treatment with slow, seven-stroke drumbeat.

### Focusing on Areas with the Drum

The Shamanic Journey Drumbeat is generally played equally over the body. Playing the drum gently and softly gathers the qi and soothes the trauma memory. Once the qi is centered, the patient can handle louder and more powerful drumming. The vigorous drumming clears blockages and releases the toxic element of the trauma. Each patient must be assessed individually—there is not a mechanical approach. Depending on the chief complaint, extra time can be spent on specific areas of the body. Longer drumming over the knee of a patient who reports knee pain helps to release the pain and improve circulation. For someone with liver qi stagnation, lengthen the drumming time over the rib area. If a patient has a diagnosis of heart and kidney miscommunication, the drumming can be emphasized over the chest and lower abdomen.

### Closing the Treatment

Before the needles are removed, a slow drumbeat of seven strokes is played three times over the body. This seven-stroke beat grounds the patient and roots the spirit in the body. The seven beats are played while moving the drum over the body from the head to the lower abdomen. This activates the different levels of the body. The first set of seven beats is played holding the drum over the top of the head at acupuncture point DU-20 (Hundred Meetings), moving down the torso, finishing at the lower abdomen, the lower Dantian. The second set is played holding the drum over the lower Dantian and moving back up the torso, finishing at the level of DU-20. The third set is repeated, the same as the first set. This drumbeat is important to help center the patient and return them to the present moment.

## Case Study: Stabilizing the Shen with Drumming

An 85-year-old woman, "Sasha," had been receiving monthly treatments to maintain her health and called to come in sooner, due to a severe emotional trauma. She reported that her husband had been killed in a car accident one week earlier, and was experiencing great sadness and acute insomnia. They had been married for over 50 years and the blow of her husband's sudden death was intense. She was sleeping minimal hours and was disoriented. Her stomach was upset and she had intestinal cramping. Surrounded by tremendous family support, she felt love amongst the devastation. She was legally blind and her husband had been her source of transportation and way to engage with the world through volunteering at their church's "meals on wheels" program. He had been a wonderful companion and they had frequently gone out to dinner and visited friends. Besides grieving her husband, she was faced with a great fear of how she would now get around and interact with the community. She felt let down by life and was feeling a sense of hopelessness.

Her diagnosis was Scattered Qi. Treatment focused on gathering the qi and grounding the Shen. The acupuncture treatment "Gathering the Qi" was used in conjunction with the Shamanic Journey Drumbeat. The drumming was performed gently and focused on her chest and abdominal areas. Hendrik Kappen, a fellow acupuncturist visiting from Germany, was observing in the clinic. Once the drumming commenced, Kappen reported noticing an incredible softening and relaxing of her Shen. He explained that Sasha's energy field had become significantly peaceful and grounded. The closing seven beats were played and the patient was prescribed Gan Mai Da Zao Tang (Licorice, Wheat, and Jujube Decoction) Modified.

Four days later Sasha returned and stated she had slept well the first two nights after treatment. Her stomach ache had reduced and her energy was improving. Weekly acupuncture and drumming treatments continued for a month. Sasha recovered and continued to be an active member in the community. A year after the accident, she was still volunteering, going out to dinner with friends, and still sporting her sparkling smile.

The shamanic drumming helped her connect and settle, and brought her Shen to the present moment. At her age, this trauma could have been devastating and resulted in a severe decline in health. Chinese medicine stepped up and brought her energy back to center. The drum played an incredible role in helping Sasha regain her energy and spirit.

### *Summary of Shamanic Drumming*

Combining this effective technique with acupuncture helps to focus treatment on specific organ systems and resolve stubborn blocked energy. Old toxic emotions associated with a trauma are released, which increases the space in the body for the spirit to comfortably reside. The sounds of the drum soothe the mind, regulate the emotions, and establish harmony of the organ and channel systems. Drumming over a patient for the first and second visit after experiencing an emotional trauma is recommended. Then, the drum healing can be revisited on subsequent treatments as needed, especially when a trauma memory has been triggered.

## SECONDARY TREATMENT METHODS
### Emotional Freedom Technique

The Emotional Freedom Technique (EFT)[8] is used throughout the world to help balance emotions. EFT regulates emotions and releases old trauma via the stimulation of acupuncture points (Figure 3.11). This easy-to-learn, zero cost, convenient self-care technique serves as an effective supplement to the primary Chinese medicine treatment methods.

---

8    See www.emofree.com.

**EFT POINTS**

| Head Points | Torso Points | Hand Points |
|---|---|---|
| • DU-20 | • KD-27 | • LU-11 |
| • UB-2 | • R-17 | • LI-1 |
| • Tai Yang | • R-12 | • HT-9 |
| • ST-2 | • SP-21 | • SI-3 |
| • DU-26 | • LV-13 | • SJ-4 |
| • R-24 | | |

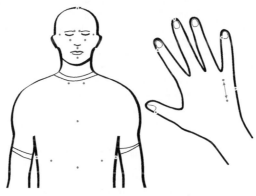

*Figure 3.11 EFT Protocol*
*Source:* Kirsteen Wright

## Procedure

- Tap the points gently with the fingertips for five to ten seconds.

- Utilize EFT at any time, especially when emotions surface with the trauma memory.

- Begin with the points on the head and face, then move to the torso points, and finally finishing with the points on the fingers and hands. (This comprises one cycle of stimulating the points.)

- Typically, complete two or three cycles to settle the emotions and stabilize the spirit.

- Repeat the following phrase silently as the points are tapped: "Even though I feel _____, I deeply and completely love and accept myself." (Fill in the blank with the emotion(s) felt at the time.)

- Daily practice improves the ability to implement the technique when emotions surge and the trauma memory activates.

### The Chinese Medicine Theory of Treating Emotional Trauma with EFT

The EFT points treat emotional trauma and calm the spirit. The jing-well points HT-9, LU-11, LI-1, and DU-26 restore consciousness. Tapping the EFT points anchors the body in the present moment, releasing emotions related to the past or future. Numerous studies have shown that PTSD, anxiety, depression, and fear are reduced with EFT.

RESEARCH STUDIES OF EFT TREATING EMOTIONAL SYMPTOMS

| Medical Journal (Date) | Research Finding |
| --- | --- |
| *Explore (NY)* (2014) | Fifty-nine combat veterans received six sessions of EFT. It reduced their PTSD, anxiety, depression, and pain. At a six-month follow-up, their PTSD, anxiety, depression, and pain was still reduced (Church 2014). |
| *Journal of Nervous and Mental Disease* (2013) | A treatment group received six one-hour trainings in EFT (compared with the control group that did not) and, when measured afterwards, 90 percent of the group no longer met the clinical criteria for PTSD. The results were so positive that the control group was then taught EFT. After six months, 80 percent of the entire population that learned EFT still no longer met the clinical criteria for PTSD (Church *et al.* 2013). |
| *Journal of Clinical Psychology* (2012) | EFT effectively treats couples with PTSD and releases fear associated with trauma (Greenman and Johnson 2012). |

### Children and EFT

Adults with children who suffer from emotional trauma can tap on their own bodies for their child. Since there is a connection between parent and child, EFT works for the child without having to tap on the child's points. If the children are open to trying EFT they can tap on themselves, or use a stuffed animal instead. Children respond well to EFT. The technique is approachable and is a great substitute for acupuncture for children—or even adults who have needle phobia. Once the child feels the results of EFT, they gain confidence in the practitioner and become open to acupuncture treatment. EFT can be a great way to simply help settle a patient's fear regarding needling before treatment.

## Case Study: The Accessibility of EFT

A six-year-old girl, "Dora," complained of anxiety and sought treatment with Chinese medicine. She was hesitant to get acupuncture, and instead of needling she was taught EFT. Dora practiced the technique in the clinic and, after one cycle of tapping the points, her Shen changed and became lighter, relaxed, and open. Leaving the clinic smiling and calm, she practiced the technique daily. Upon returning to the clinic she said her anxiety had been reduced by 75 percent. Dora liked the technique so much she taught EFT to her fellow students and kindergarten teacher.

EFT is practiced in schools, and many teachers across the U.S. have students begin each day with it. Teachers find EFT an effective way to improve classroom behavior and mental focus and reduce emotional outbursts.

### Summary of Emotional Freedom Technique

Counselors achieve great success using EFT and cognitive therapy to resolve behavioral patterns and emotional blocks in their patients. Rooted in Chinese medicine, the technique empowers the patient and gives them a useful way to treat themselves. Since it is cost-effective, this technique can be applied in several situations.

## Affirmations

> *You, yourself, as much as anybody in the entire*
> *universe, deserve your love and affection.*
>
> *Buddha*

The internal dialogue of the brain is powerful and can create heaven or hell on earth. The words people say internally play a major role in the emotional environment of the body. Positive affirmations benefit health, education, and relationships (Cohen and Sherman 2014). Reducing emotional trauma by shifting the internal dialogue with positive affirmations is profound. In a study of Vietnam war veterans, researchers concluded that positive affirmations successfully reduced the severity of PTSD (Dohrenwend *et al.* 2004).

Positive affirmations vary, and Louise Hay has contributed significantly in this area. Her book *You Can Heal Your Life* is filled with many variations of affirmations patients can use for creating a positive internal dialogue. Another author, Christiane Beerlandt, shares several positive affirmations in her book *The Key to Self-Liberation* for numerous emotional and physical conditions. Multiple combinations of affirmations are available, and each patient resonates with different words. Allow for flexibility in creating affirmations to foster optimum healing.

### *Examples of Positive Affirmations*

- "I deeply and completely love and accept myself."

- "I am safe and loved and protected by the universe."

- "I am surrounded by love and have all that I need."

- "I am centered and feeling strong and healthy."

- "I am thankful for all the gifts I receive and live in gratitude."

- "I walk confidently forward in life, taking action and making wonderful choices."

- "I have kindness in my heart and my body is flowing freely."

- "I am mentally clear and emotionally calm and live in balance."

- "I calmly approach life and enjoy each moment."

These are just a few examples to guide the creation of affirmations for patients. Affirmations redirect thought patterns and, even though a patient might not feel calm and centered, simply saying these words to the psyche will begin to produce calm and centered feelings.

> *Watch your thoughts. They become words. Watch*
> *your words. They become deeds. Watch your deeds.*
> *They become habits. Watch your habits. They*
> *become character. Character is everything.*
>
> *Lao Zi*

## Flower Essences

Since the dawn of flowers on the planet, perfumes have been sought after for their aromatic healing properties. Distilled flower essences taken internally can transform blockages from difficult emotional patterns. They can be consumed on the go to bring quick relief for emotional symptoms (such as grief, anger, fear, worry, and anxiety) and other symptoms (e.g., insomnia, fatigue, and poor concentration).

Essences are generally taken in a tincture form—simply added to water and sipped throughout the day. They prevent the surging of a trauma memory and can be taken if there is a strong reaction to a trauma memory. With each daily use, the trauma reaction reduces and, in time, the patient can simply take the remedy as needed and serve as an effective supplemental modality to Chinese medicine treatment.

## Essential Oils

Certain essential oils reduce the trauma memory, calm emotional reactions, increase courage, and harmonize the organ systems. The oils can be used topically or internally and work at a deep cellular level to transform emotional states and reduce the triggering of a trauma memory. They are a beneficial addition to a comprehensive treatment of emotional trauma.

## SUMMARY OF THE VARIOUS TREATMENT METHODS

*The body is a community made up of its*
*innumerable cells or inhabitants.*

*Thomas Alva Edison*

For the community of the body to thrive, its systems must function well together. As Henry Ford proved in his business, "Working together is success." Incorporating several treatment modalities increases the speed of healing and provides multiple paths to the top of the mountain. Each person is an individual and resonates with certain treatments. The practitioner can select from a variety of methods to best treat the patient.

### References

Barnes, V.A., Monto, A., Williams, J.J., and Rigg, J.L. (2016) "Impact of transcendental meditation on psychotropic medication use among active duty military service members with anxiety and PTSD." *Mil. Med. 181*, 1, 56–63.

Bittman, B.B., Berk, L.S., Felten, D.L., Westengard, J., *et al.* (2001) "Composite effects of group drumming music therapy on modulation of neuroendocrine-immune parameters in normal subjects." *Altern. Ther. Health Med. 7*, 1, 38–47.

Bremner, J.D. (2006) "Traumatic stress: effects on the brain." *Dialogues in Clinical Neuroscience 8*, 4, 445–461.

Bridges, L. (2012) *Face Reading in Chinese Medicine* (Second Edition). London: Churchill Livingstone Elsevier.

Chen, J., and Chen, T. (2009) *Chinese Herbal Formulas and Applications.* City of Industry, CA: Art of Medicine Press.

Ching, N. (2016) *The Fundamentals of Acupuncture.* London: Singing Dragon.

Church, D. (2014) "Reductions in pain, depression, and anxiety symptoms after PTSD remediation in veterans." *Explore (NY) 10*, 3, 162–169.

Church, D., Hawk, C., Brooks, A.J., Toukolehto, O., *et al.* (2013) "Psychological trauma symptom improvement in veterans using emotional freedom techniques: a randomized controlled trial." *J. Nerv. Ment. Dis. 201*, 2, 153–160.

Cohen, G.L., and Sherman, D.K. (2014) "The psychology of change: self-affirmation and social psychological intervention." *Ann. Rev. Psychol. 65*, 333–371.

Cohen, J. (2012) *A Brief History of Bloodletting.* Available at www.history.com/news/a-brief-history-of-bloodletting, accessed on 24 May 2017.

Cole, B., and Yarberry, M. (2011) "NADA training provides PTSD relief in Haiti." *Deutsche Zeitschrift fur Akupunktur 54*, 1, 21–24.

Dawes, C., Pedersen, A.M., Villa, A., Ekström, J., *et al.* (2015) "The functions of human saliva: a review sponsored by the World Workshop on Oral Medicine VI." *Arch. Oral Biol. 60*, 6, 863–874.

Deadman, P., and Al-Khafaji, M. (1998) *A Manual of Acupuncture.* Hove: Journal of Chinese Medicine Publications.

Dehghanizade, Z., Zargar, Y., Mehrabizadeh Honarmand, M., Kadkhodaie, A., and Eydi Baygi, M. (2015) "The effectiveness of cognitive behavior stress management on functional dyspepsia symptoms." *J. Adv. Med. Educ. Prof. 3*, 2, 45–49.

Dickerson, D., Robichaud, F., Teruya, C., Nagaran, K., and Hser, Y.I. (2012) "Utilizing drumming for American Indians/Alaska Natives with substance use disorders: a focus group study." *Am. J. Drug Alcohol Abuse 38*, 5, 505–510.

Disney, D., and Miller, P.M. (1957) *The Story of Walt Disney.* New York: Dell Publishing Co.

Dohrenwend, B.P., Neria, Y., Turner, J.B., Turse, N., *et al.* (2004) "Positive tertiary appraisals and posttraumatic stress disorder in U.S. male veterans of the war in Vietnam: the roles of positive affirmation, positive reformulation, and defensive denial." *J. Consult. Clin. Psychol. 72*, 3, 417–433.

Dzung, T.V. (2004) *Teaching.* Bastyr University, Washington, DC: VHS video release.

Farrell, Y.R. (2016) *Psycho-Emotional Pain and the Eight Extraordinary Vessels.* London: Singing Dragon.

Fu, Y., Li, Y., Guo, J., Liu, B., *et al.* (2016) "Bloodletting at jing-well points decreases interstitial fluid flow in the thalamus of rats." *J. Tradit. Chin. Med. 36*, 1, 107–112.

Gavrieli, A., Farr, O.M., Davis, C.R., Crowell, J.A., and Mantzoros, C.S. (2015) "Early life adversity and/or posttraumatic stress disorder severity are associated with poor diet quality, including consumption of trans fatty acids, and fewer hours of resting or sleeping in a US middle-aged population: a cross-sectional and prospective study." *Metabolism 64*, 11, 1597–1610.

Greenman, P.S., and Johnson, S.M. (2012) "United we stand: emotionally focused therapy for couples in the treatment of posttraumatic stress disorder." *J. Clin. Psychol. 68*, 5, 561–569.

Hammer, L. (2001) *Chinese Pulse Diagnosis, Revised Edition.* Seattle: Eastland Press.

Hao, J.J., and Hao, L.L. (2011) *Chinese Scalp Acupuncture.* Boulder, CO: Blue Poppy Press.

Harmon, B.E., Carter, M., Hurley, T.G., Shivappa, N., Teas, J., and Hébert, J.R. (2015) "Nutrient composition and anti-inflammatory potential of a prescribed macrobiotic diet." *Nutr. Cancer 67*, 6, 933–940.

Ho, P., Tsao, J.C., Bloch, L., and Zeltzer, L.K. (2011) "The impact of group drumming on social-emotional behavior in low-income children." *Evid. Based Complement. Alternat. Med.*, Epub 2011, Art. 250708.

Hou, P.W., Hsu, H.C., Lin, Y.W., Tang, N.Y., Cheng, C.Y., and Hsieh, C.L. (2015) "The history, mechanism, and clinical application of auricular therapy in Traditional Chinese Medicine." *Evid. Based Complement. Alternat. Med.*, Epub 2015, Art. 495684.

Jao, T., Li, C.W., Vértes, P.E., Wu, C.W., *et al.* (2016) "Large-scale functional brain network reorganization during Taoist meditation." *Brain Connect. 6*, 1, 9–24.

Judith, A. (2015) *Wheels of Life* (Second Edition). Woodbury, MI: Llewellyn Publications.

Kearney, D.J., McManus, C., Malte, C.A., Martinez, M.E., Felleman, B., and Simpson, T.L. (2014) "Loving-kindness meditation and the broaden-and-build theory of positive emotions among veterans with posttraumatic stress disorder." *Med. Care. 52*, 12, Suppl. 5, S32–38.

Ketcham, C. (2015) *How to Power Nap for All-Day Energy.* Available at www.huffingtonpost.com/2014/09/15/power-nap-all-day-energy_n_5798256.html, accessed on 26 May 2017.

Kukihara, H., Yamawaki, N., Uchiyama, K., Arai, S., and Horikawa, E. (2014) "Trauma, depression, and resilience of earthquake/tsunami/nuclear disaster survivors of Hirono, Fukushima, Japan." *Psychiatry Clin. Neurosci. 68*, 7, 524–533.

Lovato, N., and Lack, L. (2010) "The effects of napping on cognitive functioning." *Prog. Brain Res. 185*, 155–166.

Manzaneque, J.M., Vera, F.M., Rodriguez, F.M., Garcia, G.J., Leyva, L., and Blanca, M.J. (2009) "Serum cytokines, mood and sleep after a qigong program: is qigong an effective psychobiological tool?" *J. Health Psychol. 14*, 1, 60–67.

Matos, L.C., Sousa, C.M., Gonçalves, M., Gabriel, J., Machado, J., and Greten, H.J. (2015) "Qigong as a traditional vegetative biofeedback therapy: long-term conditioning of physiological mind-body effects." *Biomed. Res. Int. 2015,* 531789.

Mehta, P., and Dhapte, V. (2015) "Cupping therapy: a prudent remedy for a plethora of medical ailments." *Journal of Traditional and Complementary Medicine 5,* 127–134.

Raben, R. (2011) "Stages of coping with stress: trauma management and acupuncture [Phasen der Stressbewältigung: Traumaverarbeitung und Akupunktur]." *Deutsche Zeitschrift fur Akupunktur 54,* 4, 13–17.

Rosenberg, Z. (n.d.) *Li Dong-Yuan's Treatise on the Spleen and Stomach and Treatment of Autoimmune Disorders.* Available at www.bioethicus.com.br/d_artigos/1182991725.pdf, accessed on 26 May 2017.

Samovar, L., Porter, R., and Edwin McDaniel, E. (2012) *Communication Between Cultures* (Eighth Edition). Boston, MA: Cengage Learning.

Segal, Z.V., and Walsh, K.M. (2016) "Mindfulness-based cognitive therapy for residual depressive symptoms and relapse prophylaxis." *Curr. Opin. Psychiatry 29,* 1, 7–12.

Shi, H.F., Xu, F., Shi, Y., Ren, C.Y., *et al.* (2016) "Effect of ear-acupoint pressing and Ear Apex (HX6,7) bloodletting on haemorheology in chloasma patients with Gan depression pattern." *Chin. J. Integr. Med. 22,* 1, 42–48.

Smith, C., Viljoen, J.T., and McGeachie, L. (2014) "African drumming: a holistic approach to reducing stress and improving health?" *J. Cardiovasc. Med. (Hagerstown) 15,* 6, 441–446.

Soare, A., Del Toro, R., Roncella, E., Khazrai, Y.M., *et al.* (2015) "The effect of macrobiotic Ma-Pi 2 diet on systemic inflammation in patients with type 2 diabetes: a post hoc analysis of the MADIAB trial." *BMJ Open Diabetes Res. Care 3,* 1, e000079.

Soong, J. (n.d.) *The Secret (and Surprising) Power of Naps.* Available at www.webmd.com/balance/features/the-secret-and-surprising-power-of-naps, accessed on 26 May 2017.

Tu, Y., Miao, X.M., Yi, T.L., Chen, X.Y., *et al.* (2016) "Neuroprotective effects of bloodletting at Jing points combined with mild induced hypothermia in acute severe traumatic brain injury." *Neural. Regen. Res. 11,* 6, 931–936.

Unschuld, P.U. (2003) *Huang Di Nei Jing Su Wen: An Annotated Translation of Huang Di's Inner Classic—Basic Questions: 2 Volumes.* Oakland, CA: University of California Press.

Van der Kolk, B. (2014) *The Body Keeps the Score.* London and New York: Penguin.

Vázquez, S., López Gutiérrez, G., Acosta Rosales, K., Cabrales, P., *et al.* (2016) "Control of overweight and obesity in childhood through education in meal time habits: the 'good manners for a healthy future' programme." *Pediatr. Obes. 11,* 6, 484–490.

Vierling, V., Etori, S., Valenti, L., Lesage, M., *et al.* (2015) "Prevalence and impact of post-traumatic stress disorder in a disordered eating population sample." [In French.] *Presse Med. 44,* 11, e341–352.

Wang, C.W., Chan, C.H., Ho, R.T., Chan, J.S., Ng, S.M., and Chan, C.L. (2014) "Managing stress and anxiety through qigong exercise in healthy adults: a systematic review and meta-analysis of randomized controlled trials." *BMC Complement. Altern. Med. 14,* 8.

Wang, J.-Y., and Robertson, J. (2008) *Applied Channel Theory in Chinese Medicine.* Seattle: Eastland Press.

Winkelman, M. (2003) "Complementary therapy for addiction: 'drumming out drugs.'" *Am. J. Public Health 93,* 4, 647–651.

Wolynn, M. (2016) *It Didn't Start with You.* New York: Viking.

Wu, Master Z. (2016) *Seeking the Spirit of the Book of Change.* London: Singing Dragon.

Wu, Master Z., and Wu, K. (2016) *Heavenly Stems and Earthly Branches—TianGan DiZhi: The Heart of Chinese Wisdom Traditions.* London: Singing Dragon.

Young, W.-C. (2005) *Tung's Acupuncture.* Taipei: Chih-Yuan Book Store.

Young, W.-C. (2013) *The Five Transport Points.* Rowland Heights, CA: American Chinese Medicine Cultural Center.

Zheng, Y., Qu, S., Wang, N., Liu, L., *et al.* (2012) "Post-stimulation effect of electroacupuncture at Yintang (EX-HN3) and GV20 on cerebral functional regions in healthy volunteers: a resting functional MRI study." *Acupunct. Med. 30,* 4, 307–315.

# CHAPTER 4

# Differentiation of Symptoms

*A journey of a thousand miles begins with a single step.*

*Lao Zi*

Untangling an emotional trauma requires skill and grace. There are three categories of emotional trauma symptomology: emotional, behavioral, and physical. Symptoms manifest themselves after a person experiences a trauma; the homeostatic balance in the body is disturbed. Until this discord is resolved, the ingrained tissue memory of the trauma continues to be triggered and intensifies the symptoms. The patient develops what can be called PTSD (Mayo Clinic 2017a; National Institute of Mental Health 2016) and typically exhibits several of the symptoms shown in the table below. For ease of organization they are separated into three sections.

**EMOTIONAL TRAUMA SYMPTOMOLOGY**

| Emotional | Behavioral | Physical |
|---|---|---|
| Fear | Avoidance/Disassociation | Insomnia |
| Anger | Negative Thinking | Panic Attacks |
| Depression | Self-Destructive Actions | Fatigue |
| Worry | | Poor Concentration |
| Grief | | Body Pains |
| Mood Swings | | |

A great strength of Chinese medicine lies in its ability to differentiate symptoms and accurately diagnose which system(s) are affected. Once the cause is identified, treatment can be carried out with precision. A correct diagnosis leads to efficient treatment, which resolves even the most complex symptoms as easily as removing a thorn from the skin.

## Treatment Protocol

Before specific symptomology is addressed, the initial shock of the trauma and its intense memory must be treated. The protocol is:

1. Treating the shock of the trauma: "Gathering the Qi."

2. Reducing the intensity of the triggers: "Soothing the Trauma Memory."

3. Treating the individual symptoms.

This chapter focuses primarily on the individual symptoms, though the first two phases of treatment are covered under "Shock and Reliving the Trauma Memory."

### *Diagnostic Signs*

Each symptom section begins with a description of the pathophysiology of each pattern. This guides the practitioner's intent, allowing for a higher rate of success in treatment. Several diagnostic methods are covered: facial changes, channel palpation findings, common pulse changes, tongue diagnostic signs, physical symptoms, and emotional symptoms. A patient will rarely display all the signs and symptoms, but must have several in order to qualify for the diagnosis. Once there is understanding of how the trauma and its memory affect the body, the treatment techniques can be applied easily.

#### *Merging Treatment Patterns and Utilizing Multiple Modalities*

Patients commonly experience a combination of symptoms requiring a combination of treatments. The practitioner must differentiate the main diagnosis and blend the treatments of secondary and tertiary diagnoses. Understanding the diagnostic root and crafting a treatment strategy is truly the skill and art of practicing Chinese medicine.

### *Treatment Methods*

#### *Acupuncture Point Combinations*

The acupuncture treatment protocols list several options for point prescriptions, and practitioners are encouraged to select points based on the open channels designated by the heavenly stems and earthly branches—while remaining mindful of the diagnosis. Several points found to be clinically effective are listed. They are not meant to be the absolute, final list but will hopefully inspire the reader to discover other combinations.

Typically, two or three points are generally sufficient to achieve optimal results, keeping the total number of needles used in a treatment to between four and ten. The adage "less is more" guides the point selection. Using too many points causes the qi to scatter and the message to the body is unclear. Generally, retain the needles for 30–45 minutes.

### Chinese Herbal Formulas

Chinese herbal formulas are listed for most of the patterns but are just a guideline to use for the diagnosis as they do not necessarily apply to every patient. Due to the limitations of the scope of the text, referring to herbal textbooks is encouraged. Flower essences and essential oils are not mentioned in the treatment sections below due to the extensive variety of brands on the market; however, they are successfully used in clinical practice and are a great supplement to successful treatment.

### Affirmations

Examples of affirmations are offered to inspire the creation of personal affirmations that resonate with the patient. The general intention of the affirmation is to transform the trauma pattern.

## General Treatments Applied to All Patterns

### Drum Healing

The Shamanic Journey Drumbeat is recommended for each pattern. The overall beat is consistent, but the volume, intensity, and focused-on areas change based on the diagnosis. Clinically, it can be difficult to apply drumming during every treatment, so, typically, it is used during the first treatment and added to every third or fourth treatment, depending on the patient.

### General Lifestyle Recommendations

Encourage patients to build a daily routine of qigong, meditation, visualization practice, and EFT, to speed the resolution of emotional trauma. Educate them in the basic building blocks of nutrition and recommend specific dietary changes for their individual imbalances. Some patterns indicate particular clear broth soups for treatment (for the recipes refer to Appendix 2).

Patients are advised to be under the care of a Western general family medical practitioner and counselor—an integrated approach yields the best results. Chinese medicine is effective in transforming trauma memories and it is important that patients have an outlet through which they can express the changes and feelings that surface. Counselors, psychologists, and psychiatrists provide a wonderful arena for this.

# TREATMENT PROTOCOLS ONE AND TWO: TREATING THE SHOCK OF THE TRAUMA AND ITS MEMORY

## Shock and Reliving the Trauma Memory

Shock is a unique symptom of trauma since it is associated with just one diagnosis—scattered qi. The natural rhythm of the body is disrupted and requires coordination. A patient experiencing shock should always be evaluated by a Western medical doctor before seeking care with Chinese medicine. The treatment for shock in Chinese medicine is "Gathering the Qi" and applies to unresolved trauma experienced years before the patient seeks treatment.

Once the qi is gathered and the patient's spirit is back in the body, specific symptoms can be addressed. When the patient appears stable, the "Soothing the Trauma Memory" treatment can be administered. It is tempting to incorporate both the "Gathering the Qi" and "Soothing the Trauma Memory" into the initial visit. However, this is not recommended. Sending too much information to the body creates disharmony. After a few treatments of centering the patient, the scalp points can be woven into the treatment.

There are some instances when patients have seen a variety of practitioners and undergone several types of treatments without achieving results. This situation results in exhausted channel energy and is referred to as "over-treatment" of the channels.[1] Similar to "rebooting" one's computer, the channels require a reset before the "Gathering the Qi" treatment is administered.

## *Scattered Qi*

### *Pathophysiology*

Shock disrupts the qi flow, causing a scattering effect, thus hindering the ability of the body to restore homeostasis. The Shen is destabilized. The qi must be gathered and centered for the body to re-establish its innate healing ability. Diagnostic signs are generally obvious, most notably in the patient's Shen.

The acupuncture protocol "Gathering the Qi" is coupled with the patient following regular meal, waking, and sleeping times, to benefit the earth element and establish stability. Patients should avoid stressful situations to prevent further scattering the qi. Once a patient is settled, however, there can be flexibility with schedules.

Transformation after the "Gathering the Qi" treatment is typically profound and patients notice a significant shift in their ability to feel grounded, calm, and mentally focused, and have an improved sense of well-being. Pronounced changes in the Shen

---

1   Personal training with Wang Ju-Yi and conversation with Jason Robertson.

and pulse are typically noticed. The Shen on their face is glowing and the eyes have changed from muddy to translucent. The pulse is smoother and more relaxed. The body has regained its harmonious rhythm. As Bob Marley explained, "I like to see you move with the rhythm; I like to see when you're dancing from within."

## Diagnostic Signs

| Face | Channel Palpation |
|---|---|
| • Shen is muddy | • Nodules in the san jiao channel |
| • Clouded eyes | • Tightness and nodules in the pericardium channel |
| • Vacant, confused look | • Small nodules and/or tightness throughout the lung channel |
| • Pale skin | • Nodules at PC-4 and LU-6 area |
| • A sense of vacancy or disorientation is detected | |

| Pulse | Tongue |
|---|---|
| • Scattered, choppy, muffled, flat, slippery, smooth, and/or rough vibration throughout (*note:* not all pulses are present—these are possible qualities) | • Normal tongue color and shape |
| | • Pale dusky color |
| • Rapid, tight | |
| • Spinning bean in the distal position(s) | |
| • Tight in left distal position | |

| Physical Symptoms | Emotional Symptoms |
|---|---|
| • Numbness | • Confusion |
| • Cold sensations | • Fear |
| • General body ache | • Worry |
| • Fatigue | • Emotionally numb |
| • Foggy headedness | |
| • Poor concentration | |
| • Disconnected feeling | |

## Treatment Principle

Gather the Qi, Stabilize the Shen, and Ground the Hun.

## Acupuncture

| "Gathering the Qi" Protocol |
|---|
| • Yin Tang M-HN-3 |
| • Nei Guan PC-6 |
| • Zhong Wan R-12 |
| • San Yin Jiao SP-6 |

Apply infrared heat on the R-12 area unless the patient has excess heat.

## MODIFICATIONS TO THE "GATHERING THE QI" PROTOCOL

| Point Substitutions | Time of Year | Notes |
|---|---|---|
| SJ-5 for PC-6 | February; August; November | Needling SJ-5 to PC-6 is preferred. |
| ST-36 for SP-6 | March; April; September; October | The stomach channel effectively benefits the earth during these months. |
| LU-5 and SP-9 for PC-6 and SP-6 | January; February; July; September | There are notable changes on the lung channel (the lung's ability to regulate qi is compromised). |
| GB-34 for SP-6 | February; August; December | If the heart is strongly affected, GB-40 can be added to benefit the Shen. |

The next step after the "Gathering the Qi" protocol is to apply the "Soothing the Trauma Memory" protocol followed by treatments for the patient's individual imbalances. When to proceed to the next protocol is determined by whether the patient is centered.

*Herbal Formula*

Gan Mai Da Zao Tang Modified (Licorice, Wheat, and Jujube Decoction Modified)

Add:

>   Hu Po (Succinum) 6g
>
>   Long Gu (Os Draconis) 6g
>
>   Bai He (Bulbus Lilii) 6–9g

*Affirmation*

>   "I am fully present in my body, feeling grounded and calm."

### Reliving the Trauma Memory

*Pathophysiology*

Once the patient is stabilized, the "Soothing the Trauma Memory" protocol will reduce the intensity of the trauma memory. This protocol can be incorporated with aspects of the "Gathering the Qi" protocol until the patient's Shen is sufficiently centered. Then treatments targeting the specific channel and organ changes are added.

Each time the patient relives the trauma there is a chance the qi will scatter and the spirit will be disturbed. Many patients speak of not being "present" or "leaving their body" after a trauma reliving a trauma memory. If a patient relives the trauma memory and the qi is scattered, they will usually respond quickly to the "Gathering the Qi" treatment. They commonly require only one or two treatments to adequately treat the shock of the trauma memory and restore their spirit to the body.

The general diagnostic signs and symptoms are the same as shock since the patient is reliving the trauma. The main goal with this treatment is to calm the spirit and improve the patient's ability to be present.

### Treatment Principle

Soothe the Trauma Memory, Increase Cosmic Water, Benefit the Sea of Marrow, Calm the Spirit, Pacify Wind, and Nourish the Water.

### Acupuncture

| **"Soothing the Trauma Memory" Protocol** |
| --- |
| • Baihui DU-20 |
| • Shenting DU-24 |
| • Ah Shi 2 cun lateral to Shenting DU-24 (*between Chu Chai UB-4 and Tou Lin Qi GB-15*) |

### Herbal Formulas

Due to the variety of ways a trauma memory affects a patient emotionally, specific differentiation of the pattern is needed in order to prescribe a correct Chinese herbal formula. (To determine the patient's individual pattern refer to the symptomatic sections below.)

### Affirmation

"I am safe, I am settled, and I am present."

## Over-Treatment

### Pathophysiology

Patients tend to seek treatment with Chinese medicine after trying several other modalities and finding them unsuccessful. These are cases wherein a patient's qi is scattered from over-treatment.

In the cases of over-treatment, patients have been treated to the point of channel exhaustion (a term used by Dr. Wang Ju-Yi). They have seen many practitioners and have been treated with several types of modalities that depleted their channel energy. The spirit lacks root and the qi becomes disordered.

The symptoms are the same as those listed in the Scattered Qi section above.

*Treatment Principle*

Re-set the Channels, and Improve Qi and Blood Circulation.

*Acupuncture*

| Protocol for Resolving Over-Treatment |
| --- |
| • Hegu LI-4 and Taichong LV-3 (four gates) |
| • Sanyinjiao SP-6 |
| Add: |
| • Guanyuan R-4 for women |
| • Qihai R-6 for men |

*Source:* Lecture from Dr. Wang Ju-Yi and conversation with Jason Robertson

This simple yet powerful treatment re-establishes channel circulation and allows the patient to receive the general protocol for treating emotional trauma. Once the channels are re-set, the "Gathering the Qi" protocol is utilized.

# TREATMENT PROTOCOL THREE: DIFFERENTIATING THE EMOTIONAL, BEHAVIORAL, AND PHYSICAL SYMPTOMS OF TRAUMA

## EMOTIONAL SYMPTOMS

### Fear

Fear is associated with the water element and primarily affects the kidney organ system. However, other elements can be affected. Fear—a common emotion experienced due to trauma—sinks or freezes the qi and causes general qi stagnation; over time it depletes the kidney energy. It is important to first move qi, and then tonify the kidneys. In some cases, the patient is so deficient that the kidneys require tonification prior to addressing the qi stagnation.

Fear drains the water element and leads to kidney yin, yang, or qi deficiency. Deficient water precludes adequate nourishment for the wood element, causing qi stagnation in the channels, since the liver's ability to open the channels is compromised.

The Zhi provides the basis to move through life. When the kidney yin and/or yang is deficient, the patient feels afraid to push forward in life. Anchoring the Zhi by nourishing yin or unfreezing it by warming the yang removes the fear, allowing the continuation down one's life path, motivated and determined.

The kidneys hold the Jing, the link to the ancestors. When trauma is passed down from previous generations, it is transferred via the Jing. Patients suffering from a past generational trauma have some form of kidney deficiency; the trauma is locked in the tissue. The Zhi relates to a patient's connection with the family history (Maclean and Lyttleton 2000, p.99). If a patient has difficulty maintaining momentum on their life path, this could be an indication that there is a trauma that has been passed down. Addressing the kidneys aids in transforming the trauma. (For more details on treating inherited trauma refer to "The Eight Extraordinary Channels" in Chapter 3 and "Unresolved Emotional Trauma Affects Future Generations" in Chapter 5.)

## Qi Stagnation

### Pathophysiology

The water element weakens with long-term fear and lacks the ability to nourish wood. The liver qi congests, creating tension throughout the body. The shao yang, yang ming, jue yin, and shao yin channels can all have nodules and tension due to the blockage. Weakness results, since the channels are not receiving energy and nutrition. The channels are blocked either from the liver's inability to maintain channel flow or to fear freezing the energy. In either case, the qi circulation must be re-established. (*Note:* At this stage, there are no heat signs and/or symptoms.)

### Diagnostic Signs

| Face | Channel Palpation |
|---|---|
| • Chin is wobbly, dimpled, lined, skin texture of an orange | • Overall weak and slippery sensation or tension when palpating the liver, gallbladder, pericardium, san jiao, kidney, heart, stomach, and large intestine channels |
| • Temples are dark | |
| • Skin has a dusky/murky/muddy hue | • Tenderness with or without nodules at LV-2 and LV-3 |
| • Dark circles under the eyes | |
| • Irritation lines in the third-eye area | • Nodules and/or tenderness at GB-20, GB-34, GB-41, and GB-31 |
| • White, frozen Shen | |
| • Eyes appear frozen in fear | • Tenderness at KD-4 |
| | • A stick-like change at KD-3 |

| Pulse | Tongue |
|---|---|
| • Tense, tight, and wiry | • Curled-up sides |
| • Tense/tight in middle left position | |

| Physical Symptoms | Emotional Symptoms |
|---|---|
| • Teeth clenching and/or grinding | • Irritation |
| • Body tension, especially in shoulders and neck | • Fear |
| • Tension headaches | |
| • Premenstrual symptoms | |
| • Constipation | |
| • Insomnia with waking between 1 and 3 am | |
| • Frequent sighing | |
| • Digestive upset | |

## Treatment Principle

Open the Channel Pathways and Relieve Constraint, Dredge the Liver, Benefit the Kidneys, Calm the Shen, Unbind the Hun, and Benefit the Zhi.

## Acupuncture

| | |
|---|---|
| UB-32 and UB-53 | SI-3 and UB-65 |
| UB-23 and UB-52 | LI-6 and UB-57 or UB-58 |
| KD-10 and LV-7 | LI-11 and LV-5 |
| GB-31 deep with 3–4 cun needle | SI-3 and KD-6 |
| SJ-5 and LV-5 | LU-5 and SP-9 |
| LI-4 and LV-3 | Auricular: Shen Men, Point Zero, Kidney, Liver, |
| SJ-6 and GB-34 | Sympathetic |
| SJ-6 and KD-4 or KD-5 | |

Cupping on the upper or mid-back area to establish proper circulation.

## Herbal Formula

Xiao Yao San (Rambling Powder)

**MODIFICATIONS TO XIAO YAO SAN**

| Headaches | Man Jing Zi (Fructus Viticis) 10g |
|---|---|
| | Qing Xiang Zi (Semen Celosiae Argenteae) 10g |
| | Chuan Xiong (Radix Ligustici Wallichii) 10g |
| Lower back pain | Ji Xue Teng (Radix et Caulis Jixueteng) 10g |
| | Chuan Niu Xi (Radix Cyathulae) 10g |
| | Jiang Huang (Rhizoma Curcumae) 10g |
| | Mu Gua (Fructus Chaenomelis Lagenariae) 5g (Yanping 2004) |

## Affirmation

"My body is flowing freely and is well nourished."

## Kidney Qi Deficiency

### Pathophysiology

Fear exhausts the water element and qi of the kidneys. Over time, the yin and yang are affected, but in this case there are no strong signs of temperature change. The primary signs and symptoms involve general weakness of the water element. This pattern tends to respond quickly to treatment compared with when the yin or yang are affected. If the water element is treated promptly after the trauma, the yin and yang are preserved.

### Diagnostic Signs

| Face | Channel Palpation |
|---|---|
| • Chin: wobbly, wrinkled, dimpled; skin like an orange peel | • Weakness, slippery, soft sensation throughout the kidney channel |
| • Under the eyes: white, dusky, hollow | • Visible indentation at KD-3 |
| • Eyes snap open; surprised shocked look; less light in the eyes; dark or gray, murky eyes; three-sided eyes | • Weakness at R-6 |
| | • Nodules and/or tenderness at UB-64 |
| • Raised eyebrows | • Tenderness at SJ-4 |
| • Glazed look; sideways glance(s) | • Tenderness at UB-23 |
| • Murky, muddy, dark skin hue | |
| • White, frozen Shen | |

| Pulse | Tongue |
|---|---|
| • Feeble, slow, deep, and thin in the proximal position | • Dip in the rear of the tongue |

| Physical Symptoms | Emotional Symptoms |
|---|---|
| • Low back and knee pain | • Fear |
| • Night-time urination | • Isolation |
| • Frequent urination | • Phobias |
| • Tinnitus | • Timidity |
| • Fatigue | |
| • Craving salty foods | |

### Treatment Principle

Tonify the Kidney Qi, Calm the Shen, and Benefit the Zhi.

### Acupuncture

| | |
|---|---|
| KD-3 and UB-23 | LU-9 and SP-3 |
| SJ-4 and KD-6 | ST-36 and R-6 |
| HT-7 and KD-7 | Auricular: Kidney, Shen Men, Sympathetic |
| KD-16 and UB-64 | |

Infrared heat on the lower abdomen.

*Affirmation*

"I am safe and strong with a deep reserve of energy."

## Kidney Yin Deficiency with Heat

*Pathophysiology*

Fear drains the water energy and depletes fluids. Reliving the trauma memory exhausts kidney yin and the patient experiences dryness and symptoms of heat. Dr. Yang Jie Bin (杨介宾) emphasized the use of Chinese herbs and good nutrition to nourish yin. Dr. Yang, a Chinese medicine doctor who practiced in Cheng Du, China (known as the "Living Dictionary"), taught that yin needs substance to be renewed; acupuncture alone was insufficient. This pattern is treated primarily by utilizing Chinese herbal formulas and adopting nutritional changes. Sufficient yin anchors the Zhi and allows clear motivation and direction, thus removing the fear. Fortified yin also roots the Shen and the patient's connection with reality.

*Diagnostic Signs*

**Face**

- Chin: wobbly; wrinkled; dimpled; skin resembles an orange peel with redness and dryness
- Redness on lower eyelids and under the eyes; dryness
- Face is red (especially in the cheeks)
- Three-sided eyes
- Raised eyebrows
- Red and dry philtrum
- Thin ear cartilage
- Glazed look; sideways glance(s)
- Dry, withered skin

**Channel Palpation**

- Dryness on the kidney channel
- Thickening, visible indentation, and/or nodules at KD-7
- Tenderness at UB-23
- Weakness at R-4 and/or R-6

**Pulse**

- Thin; deep; tight; wiry; rapid at the proximal positions (more apparent on the left side)

**Tongue**

- Red; cracked; dry; less coat; mirror coat; saliva lines on sides
- Dip in the rear of the tongue

| Physical Symptoms | Emotional Symptoms |
|---|---|
| • Low back and knee pain | • Fear |
| • Night-time urination; frequent urinary tract infections | • Isolation |
| • Tinnitus | • Phobias |
| • Fatigue | • Timidity |
| • Premature aging | • Agitation |
| • Brittle bones | • Anxiety |
| • Five-center heat | |
| • Night sweats | |
| • Excessive thirst and hunger | |
| • Craving salty foods | |

### Treatment Principle

Nourish the Kidney Yin, Clear the Heat, Calm the Shen, and Stabilize the Zhi.

### Acupuncture

| | |
|---|---|
| HT-6 and KD-7 | PC-7 and LV-2 |
| HT-7 and KD-2 | UB-23 and UB-52 |
| KD-3 and UB-23 | LU-10 and SP-9 |
| LU-5 and KD-7 | Yin Tang (M-HN-3) and R-4 |
| SJ-5 and KD-7 | ST-36 and R-6 |
| SJ-4 and GB-39 | Auricular: Kidney, Sympathetic, Shen Men |

### Herbal Formula

Zhi Bai Di Huang Wan (Anemarrhena, Phellodendron, and Rehmannia pill) (Chen and Chen 2009, p.636)

### Affirmation

"I am safe and strong with a deep reserve of energy. I have a harmonious balance between fire and water."

## Kidney Yang Deficiency

### Pathophysiology

Fear, stemming from the initial trauma or reliving its memory, can freeze the kidneys, resulting in yang deficiency. The Zhi is frozen/weakened, and the determination to follow through on goals is compromised. Tonifying the kidney yang returns the Zhi to a healthy state. This pattern is common in older patients since their yang is typically less strong and they are prone to fear. Kidney yang deficiency is primarily differentiated from the other kidney pathologies by signs of cold.

## Diagnostic Signs

### Face

- Chin: wobbly, wrinkled, and dimpled; skin resembling an orange peel with a pale and blue/dusky tint
- Shen is perceived as cold
- Eyes dark or gray; light is lost from the eyes; eyes snap open
- Face is pale with a blue, dusky, murky hue
- Under the eyes: pale; dusky; swollen
- Three-sided eyes
- White philtrum
- Glazed look; sideways glance(s)
- White, frozen Shen

### Channel Palpation

- Kidney channel feels weak
- Visible indentation at KD-3
- Cold sensation in the lower abdomen
- Weakness at R-6

### Pulse

- Deep; slow; thin; empty in the proximal positions (notably on the right side)

### Tongue

- Dip in the rear of the tongue
- Pale and thick coat
- Scalloped and swollen

### Physical Symptoms

- Cold sensations
- Early morning diarrhea
- Low back and knee pain
- Loose sphincter muscles
- Night-time urination
- Frequent urination
- Incontinence
- Tinnitus
- Fatigue
- Craving salty foods
- Impotence; low libido; infertility

### Emotional Symptoms

- Fear
- Isolation
- Withdrawn
- Depression
- Low motivation

## Treatment Principle

Warm the Kidney Yang, Calm the Shen, and Benefit the Zhi.

*Acupuncture*

| | |
|---|---|
| SJ-4 and KD-3 | DU-4 and UB-23 |
| ST-36 and R-6 | 1010.22 Bi Yi (Nasal Wing), right side for female |
| KD-16 and UB-64 | and left side for male |
| KD-6 and UB-23 | Auricular: Kidney, Shen Men |
| UB-23 and UB-52 | Moxa: Salt and moxa at R-8 |
| LU-9 and SP-3 | |

Infrared heat on the lower abdomen.

*Herbal Formula*

Jing Gui Shen Qi Wan (Kidney Qi Pill from the Golden Cabinet)

*Affirmation*

"I am safe and strong with a deep reserve of energy and have a feeling of warmth in my lower abdomen."

# Anger

Anger is typically a shield for deep, hidden emotions. When addressed and reduced, underlying emotions, such as fear and grief, become apparent. Qi and blood stagnation—with or without heat—is the common diagnosis. However, anger can be a result of water deficiency, or simply an overall blood and yin deficiency. Reliving the trauma memory generates wind in the body, which stokes the fire. It is important to discern the amount of heat involved and clear it as necessary.

The Hun, or ethereal soul, provides the body with courage and clear decision making. If the Hun is constrained, angry outbursts become common. These eruptions are fueled by fire generated from the stagnation and give rise to "hot headedness." The yin and blood can be exhausted from trauma and fail to ground the Hun. An ungrounded Hun results in lack of courage or decision making, regularly leading to frustration and defensive outbursts.

## *Liver Qi Stagnation*

### *Pathophysiology*

Emotional trauma, and reliving its memory, scatters the qi and blocks the flow, creating disorder in the liver function. The liver is responsible for maintaining channel flow and "keeping all the options open." It chooses where the blood (housing the spirit) is needed by the body and commands it appropriately. Like a general observing the battlefield and strategizing, all the options are considered before deciding to engage.

If the flow of blood is reduced, pressure results in the channels and anger surfaces. Imagine a general who is confused and unable to give proper orders. His emotional state would quickly turn to irritation and compromise his abilities.

In this pattern, heat is not generated from the qi stagnation, so the main objective is to return the smooth flow of energy through the channels. If signs of heat are detected, this pattern is not applicable for the patient. This condition is about the flow of qi and blood throughout the body and when properly addressed establishes free-flowing movement as the symptoms resolve.

## Diagnostic Signs

| Face | Channel Palpation |
|---|---|
| • Temples are dark | • Overall weak and slippery sensation when palpating the liver, gallbladder, and san jiao channels or a tightness and/or bumpiness along these channels |
| • Skin has a green, dusky hue | |
| • Eyes: mildly red sclera (in chronic cases the sclera can become yellow/green/gray) | |
| • A hard look about the eyes | • Nodules and tightness and/or a bumpy feeling along the large intestine channel |
| • Tight lips and mouth | • Tenderness with or without nodules at LV-3 |
| • Irritation lines in the third-eye area | • Nodules and/or tenderness at GB-34 and GB-31 |
| • Intense glare; hyper-focused gaze | |
| • (In chronic cases the face hardens) | |

| Pulse | Tongue |
|---|---|
| • Tense; tight; wiry | • Curled-up sides |
| • Tense; tight in middle left position | |

| Physical Symptoms | Emotional Symptoms |
|---|---|
| • Teeth clenching and/or grinding | • Irritation |
| • Body tension, especially in shoulders and neck | • Mood swings between anger and fear |
| • Tension headaches | • Depression |
| • Premenstrual symptoms | • Sadness |
| • Constipation | |
| • Insomnia with waking between 1 and 3 am | |
| • Frequent sighing | |
| • Digestive upset | |
| • Hypochondriac pain | |
| • Cough (if Tai Ji circulation is affected, insulting the lungs) | |

## Treatment Principle

Open the Channel Pathways, Soothe and Dredge the Liver, Unbind the Hun, and Calm the Shen.

## Acupuncture

| | |
|---|---|
| SJ-6 and GB-34 | LI-6 and ST-43 |
| 4 gates (LI-4 and LV-3) | SJ-9 and GB-38 |
| LU-5 and SP-9 | UB-13 and UB-18 |
| LI-11 and LV-5 | UB-18 and UB-25 |
| PC-6 and LV-5 | 33.11 Ganmen (Liver Gate) |
| GB-4 to GB-7 using a 1.5 cun needle and GB-31 using a 3–4 cun needle | Auricular: Shen Men, Liver |

Cupping on the upper or mid-back to move the stagnation.

## Herbal Formula

Xiao Yao San (Rambling Powder)

**MODIFICATIONS TO XIAO YAO SAN**

| | |
|---|---|
| Pronounced qi stagnation | Zhi Ke (Fructus Citriseu Ponciri) 10g<br>Xiang Fu (Rhizoma Cyperi Rotundi) 10g |
| Depression and frequent crying | He Huan Pi (Cortex Albizziae Julibrissin) 10g<br>Fo Shou (Fructus Citri Sarcodactylis) 10g<br>Xiang Yuan (Fructus Citri Medicae) 10g |
| Irritability with dizziness and headaches | Tian Ma (Rhizoma Gastrodiae Elatae) 10g<br>Xia Ku Cao (Spica Prunellae Vulgaris) 10g |
| Headaches | Man Jing Zi (Fructus Viticis) 10g<br>Qing Xiang Zi (Semen Celosiae Argenteae) 10g<br>Chuan Xiong (Radix Ligustici Wallichii) 10g (Yanping 2004) |

## Affirmation

"My body is flowing freely and is nourished."

## Liver Heat/Fire

### Pathophysiology

The qi stagnation generates pressure and engenders heat and fire, which produces a flaring, intense quality to the pattern. The diagnostic signs and symptoms are the same as liver qi stagnation but include signs of heat and fire. Reliving the trauma memory fuels the fire and results in reckless behavior and outbursts of anger. Beneficial lifestyle and diet choices significantly reduce the fire.

Liver heat can increase in intensity and give rise to liver and heart fire. Suicidal thoughts, aggressive behavior, violent outbursts, and other severe symptoms indicate fire.

## Diagnostic Signs

(*Note:* The signs and symptoms are the same as liver qi stagnation, plus the following.)

| Face | Channel Palpation |
|---|---|
| • Red, inflamed sclera | • Nodules and tenderness at LV-2, GB-41, SJ-5, and LI-11 |
| • Red in the third-eye area | |
| • Flushed, red face | • Stick-like nodule between ST-44 and ST-43 and between LV-2 and LV-3 |
| • Laser-focused look in the eyes | |
| • Wild, fiery gaze | |

| Pulse | Tongue |
|---|---|
| • Rapid; tense; tight (especially in the middle left position) | • Red body |
| | • Curled red edges |
| • Blood heat; blood unclear; blood thick | • Yellow coat |
| • Tense; hollow; full; overflowing | |
| • Robust | |

| Physical Symptoms | Emotional Symptoms |
|---|---|
| • Heat sensations | • Angry outbursts |
| • Excessive thirst | • Short temper |
| • Restlessness | • Mood swings |
| • Blurred vision | |
| • Migraines | |
| • Hypochondriac pain | |
| • Self-destructive behavior | |

## Treatment Principle

Clear Heat from the Liver, Open the Channel Pathways, Calm the Shen and Hun, and Drain Fire.

## Acupuncture

| | |
|---|---|
| SJ-5 and GB-41 | Auricular: Shen Men, Point Zero, Sympathetic, |
| LI-3 and LV-2 | Liver |
| LI-11 and ST-44 | Bleed ear apex |
| PC-7, PC-8, or HT-8 | Bleed DU-10 and cup the point |
| GB-4 to GB-7 using a 1.5 cun needle | |

## Herbal Formulas

| Diagnosis | Formula | Notes |
|---|---|---|
| Liver Heat | Dan Zhi Xiao Yao San (Moutan and Gardenia Rambling Powder) | *If patient has insomnia add:*<br>Ren Dong Teng (Ramulus Lonicaerae Japonicae) 9g<br>Ye Jiao Teng (Caulis Polygoni Multiflori) 12g<br>Zhen Zhu Mu (Concha Margaritafarae) 15g<br>Geng Mi (Oryzae Semen) 30g [for patients with digestive weakness] (Maclean and Lyttleton 2000, p.835). |
| Liver Fire | Long Dan Xie Gan Tang (Gentiana Decoction to Drain the Liver) | It is only used short term. Many patients will need herbs to warm the spleen afterward to mitigate the cooling effects of the formula (Chen and Chen 2009, p.371). |
| Liver Fire causing Mania | Dang Gui Long Hui Wan (Tangkuei, Gentiana, and Aloe Pill) | The original prescription includes She Xiang (Moschus), which is no longer used due to the ingredient being from an endangered animal (Chen and Chen 2009, p.379). |

## Affirmation

"I am rooted and grounded with my energy flowing and refreshed, as a cool wave of water."

## Yin and Blood Deficiency with or without Heat

### Pathophysiology

Chronic anger exhausts the liver and leads to yin and blood deficiency. This depletion is frequently compounded by heat, a result of qi stagnation, burning the fluids. When the yin and blood are deficient, the Hun is not rooted and the spirit becomes restless and agitated. The signs and symptoms are similar to those in the liver heat/fire category, and include yin and blood deficiency signs. Commonly, the yin deficiency gives rise to heat, and heat signs will be detected. Herbal formulas and nutritional support play a large role in replenishing the yin and blood.

## Diagnostic Signs

### Face

- Dryness in the third-eye area
- Lines in the third-eye area
- Thinning eyebrow hairs
- Intense glare; hyper-focused gaze
- A hardened look about the face

*With heat:*

- Flushed face
- Redness on the lower eyelids
- Redness in the third-eye area

### Channel Palpation

- Dryness along the liver and/or kidney channels
- Nodules, visible indentation, and/or thickening at KD-7

*With heat:*

- Nodules and tenderness at LV-2, GB-41, SJ-5, and LI-11
- Stick-like nodule between ST-44 and ST-43, and between LV-2 and LV-3
- Overall weak and slippery sensation when palpating the liver, gallbladder, and san jiao channels or a tightness and/or bumpiness along these channels
- Nodules and tightness in the large intestine channel or a bumpy feeling along the channel

### Pulse

- Tense, tight, or reduced substance at the middle left position
- Tense, tight, or empty deep in the proximal positions (especially on the left)
- Tight-to-wiry; hollow; full; overflowing

*With heat:*

- Rapid; tense; tight (especially in the middle left position)
- Blood heat; blood unclear; blood thick
- Tense; hollow; full; overflowing
- Robust

### Tongue

- Curled edges
- Rough, lacerated edges
- Pale edges

*With heat:*

- Red body (especially on the edges)
- Cracked and dry
- Less coat
- Mirror coat
- Saliva lines on sides

### Physical Symptoms

- Teeth clenching and/or grinding
- Body tension (especially in shoulders and neck)
- Tension headaches
- Premenstrual symptoms with heat
- Insomnia with waking between 1 and 3 am
- Frequent sighing
- Forgetfulness
- Dizziness
- Hypochondriac pain
- Digestive upset and hunger

*With heat:*

- Thirst
- Five-center heat
- Restlessness with heat sensations and night sweats
- Redness in the third-eye area

### Emotional Symptoms

- Irritation
- Agitation
- Panic sensations
- Depression

*With heat:*

- Angry outbursts
- Quick temper

*Treatment Principle*

Nourish the Liver Yin and Blood, Open the Channel Pathways, Calm the Shen, and Stabilize the Hun.

*If there is heat:* Clear Heat from the Liver.

*Acupuncture*

| | |
|---|---|
| LV-3 and UB-18 | *With heat:* |
| GB-31 deep toward the bone with a 3–4 cun needle | PC-7 and LV-2 |
| | LI-11 and KD-2, KD-6, or KD-7 |
| SP-6 and R-4 or R-6 | |
| DU-4 and UB-23 | |
| DU-20 and DU-24 | |
| GB-4 to GB-7 and GB-39 | |
| HT-7 and GB-40 | |

*Herbal Formula*

Suan Zao Ren Tang (Zizyphus Combination) (Chen and Chen 2009, p.722)

*This is the classically indicated formula for this condition. Clinically, a general formula to build qi and blood, such as Ba Zhen Tang (Eight Treasure Decoction) (Chen and Chen 2009, p.604), is used along with nutritional recommendations.*

*Affirmation*

"My body is restored and harmoniously flowing with life. I regenerate my blood easily and rest with ease."

## Depression

Depression is literally a dampened spirit; the spirit is not shining or flowing. When someone suffers an emotional trauma, the qi and blood are blocked and/or weakened. Each time a patient relives a trauma memory, these patterns are exacerbated, hindering the spirit; depression results. Moving and/or benefiting the qi and blood enliven the spirit and clear the fog of depression.

It is crucial to determine the main underlying factor in depression. Often there is a combination of patterns involved. Balancing treatment approaches requires skill and flexibility as the pathogens can change over the course of treatment. A case might begin as primarily qi and blood stagnation, but when cleared, the deficiency becomes the priority.

The subject of depression is immense, and this section focuses on the five main diagnoses. The other emotions that occur along with depression such as anxiety, worry, fear, and sadness are listed in separate sections. A patient commonly experiences several emotions when reliving the trauma. The disharmony could involve multiple diagnoses addressing several organ systems. For example, qi stagnation in the lungs primarily produces grief, whereas qi stagnation in the kidneys causes fear. The pattern of qi stagnation covered in this section will focus on the liver.

### Addressing Postpartum Depression

Postpartum depression affects many women. The syndrome is mainly due to heart deficiency, resulting in women feeling anxious and depressed. During childbirth, a significant amount of blood is lost, reducing the stability of the Shen because of the special connection between the uterus and the heart. The body naturally rebalances, but in some cases intervention is needed. It is the restless Shen, due to the blood loss, that primarily causes postpartum depression, and in most cases the treatment emphasis is on the heart, not the liver. Liver qi stagnation is rarely the cause of postpartum depression since the woman has experienced a major blood loss. Thus, attention is placed on the blood—either tonifying and/or moving it. The pattern mainly involves deficiency.

Formulas to treat postpartum depression are listed below, and the syndrome is further discussed in the following Anxiety section. The syndrome is mentioned in this text since many women experience emotional trauma during childbirth. Treatments with Chinese medicine significantly improve the condition, though in some cases there might be a need for Western medical attention. These must be identified and referred out as needed.

## Liver Qi Stagnation with or without Heat

### Pathophysiology

Emotional trauma and reliving its memory creates blockages and impedes the liver's ability to keep the channels open. The Hun's ability to courageously make decisions and act at the proper time is hindered. A patient feels depressed because of an inability to move forward. The qi stagnation can generate heat, and this sign will be detected.

The diagnostic signs/symptoms and treatment protocols are the same as in the Liver Qi Stagnation pattern or the Liver Heat/Fire pattern listed above in the Anger section.

## *Phlegm and Damp Accumulation with or without Heat*

### *Pathophysiology*

The liver qi stagnation causes an excess wood condition that overacts on the earth element; the spleen's function to transform fluids is weakened. Fluids accumulate and hinder qi flow, resulting in depression. This causes the Yi to become clouded, unable to take action and move forward; it "spins its wheels in the mud." The trauma memory becomes stuck in the phlegm (a stubborn pathogen). Once the phlegm is transformed, the trauma memory is released, the Yi is freed, and the depression lifts.

### *Diagnostic Signs*

| Face | Channel Palpation |
|---|---|
| • Flaccid, puffy muscle tone | • Slippery, hard, or tight sensation in the lung, spleen, and stomach channels (this can be shallow or hard depending on the chronicity of the issue) |
| • Greasy sheen to the face | |
| • Puffy upper eyelids | |
| • Yellowing of the face (especially on the upper eyelids, nose bridge, or around the mouth) | • Roughness or bumpiness in the fascia and/or slippery nodules in the lung, spleen, and stomach channels |
| • Tight, tense, contracted Shen | • Nodules with slippery sensations at SP-9 |
| *With heat:* | • Nodules, veins, tenderness at ST-40 |
| • Red, flushed face | • Tenderness and tightness at R-9 |
| • Redness around the mouth | • Pulsing at R-12 |
| • Redness under the nostrils | • Pulsing around the umbilicus (especially at R-6 and R-9) |
| | *With heat:* |
| | • Tenderness in the lung and large intestine channels |
| | • Nodules and tenderness at SP-2, PC-7, and ST-44 |

| Pulse | Tongue |
|---|---|
| • Slippery | • Puffy and swollen |
| • Tense and tight | • Scallops |
| • Engorged in the right middle position | • Thick, white coat |
| • Slow | *With heat:* |
| *With heat:* | • Red body |
| • Tense, tight, and rapid | • Thick, yellow, greasy coat |
| • Slippery and tense in the right middle position | |

| Physical Symptoms | Emotional Symptoms |
|---|---|
| • Fatigue | • Depression; lack of motivation |
| • Heaviness in the body | • Gloom |
| • Phlegm production | • Confusion |
| • Cough with phlegm; wheezing; asthma | • Worry |
| • Sinus congestion (with excess phlegm production) | • Obsession |
| • Tightness and fullness in the chest | • Mood swings |
| • Sluggish digestion, nausea, and poor appetite | • Constant examination of past events |
| • Bloating and fullness; weight gain (especially in upper arms and calves) | • Holding onto past events |
| | • Slow decision making |
| • Sugar and carbohydrate cravings | • Grief and sadness |
| • Puffy, round body | • Feeling as if a past grief experience just occurred |
| • Dizziness; vertigo | |
| • Poor concentration, slow decision making | • Withdrawal; isolation |
| • Chemical sensitivity | • Lack of confidence |
| *With heat:* | • Over-nurturing |
| • Insomnia; nightmares; waking early in morning | • Indecisiveness |
| | • Sensitivity to stimuli and emotionally reactive to chemicals |
| • Yellow/green phlegm | *With heat:* |
| • Nausea/vomiting; acid reflux; belching; bitter taste | • Irritability |
| | • Anxiety |
| • Excess appetite | • Anger |
| • Heat sensations | • Agitation |
| | • Manic behavior |
| | • Mood swings |

## Treatment Principle

Transform Phlegm and Dampness, Regulate the Qi, Benefit the Lung and Spleen, and Liberate the Yi and Po; Clear Heat if present.

## Acupuncture

| | |
|---|---|
| LU-5 and SP-9 and R-12 | Auricular: Upper and/or Lower Lung, Spleen, |
| LU-8 and LI-5 | Stomach, Liver, Shen Men, Brain |
| PC-5 and ST-40 | Infrared heat on the abdomen for patients without |
| LI-10 and R-11 | excess heat |
| LU-5 and R-17 | *With heat:* |
| SP-5 and ST-41 | SP-2 and ST-44 |
| SP-3 and SP-9 | LV-2 and ST-44 |
| SP-4 and ST-43 | PC-7 and LU-5 |
| R-9 and R-12 | LI-11 and LU-10 |
| DU-12 and UB-13 | Auricular: Point Zero |
| Ding Chuan (M-BW-1) | Bleed ear apex |
| DU-20 and DU-24 | |
| UB-13 or UB-18 and UB-20 | |
| UB-20 and UB-21 | |

## Herbal Formulas

| | |
|---|---|
| General Phlegm/Damp Accumulation | Di Tan Tang Modified (Scour Phlegm Decoction Modified) (Maclean and Lyttleton 2000, p.134) |
| Phlegm Heat | Huang Lian Wen Dan Tang (Warm Gallbladder Decoction with Coptis) (Maclean and Lyttleton 2000, p.134) – or – Shi Yi Wei Wen Dan Tang (Eleven Ingredient Decoction to Warm the Gallbladder) (Maclean and Lyttleton 2000, p.911) |
| Phlegm/Damp Accumulation in the Lungs | Er Chen Tang (Two-Cured Decoction) (*see modifications below*) |
| After Phlegm is Cleared | Liu Jun Zi Tang (Six-Gentlemen Decoction) to help support digestion |

### MODIFICATIONS TO ER CHEN TANG

| | |
|---|---|
| Qi Stagnation | Hou Po (Cortex Magnoliae Officinalis) Zhi Shi (Fructus Aurantii Immaturus) |
| Minor Phlegm Heat | Huang Qin (Radix Scutellariae) Gua Lou (Fructus Trichosanthis) Huang Lian (Rhizoma Coptidis) Zhu Ru (Caulis Bambusae in Taenia) Dan Nan Xing (Arisaema cum Bile) (Chen and Chen 2009, pp.1209–1210) |

## Affirmations

"My body is light and my mind is clear. My energy flows freely and my digestion is happy and strong in a harmonious rhythm."

"My body is light and my lungs are clear, feeling spacious. I am feeling confident and strong."

## Blood Stagnation

### Pathophysiology

Unresolved emotional trauma can eventually cause blood stagnation and results in severe depression inhibiting the minds of the organs—primarily the Hun, Shen, and Po. Also, a trauma memory relived with great intensity can impede blood flow and ultimately compromise the animation of the body. The expression of the Hun and Shen is blocked and patients experience extreme symptoms such as suicidal thoughts, intense mood swings, and even rage. The Hun's ability to make clear decisions and act appropriately is compromised, and the Shen's function to clearly perceive reality is clouded. The lung's function of moving the qi is reduced when the blood stagnates. The constraint of lung qi weakens the Po. The Po's ability to set boundaries and engage with the world shrinks and patients feel lost and disconnected. Long-term use of psychotropic medication can cause blood stagnation. Due to the severity of symptoms experienced by patients with this condition, they should also be referred to a counselor/psychologist and receive information on psychiatric crisis hotlines.

### Diagnostic Signs

**Face**

- Dusky, dark Shen
- A "checked out" look
- Absence of light in the eyes
- Dark temples
- Darkness down the side of the face to the jaw
- Dusky skin

**Channel Palpation**

- Bumpy, rough, dry channels (especially the liver, pericardium, and heart channels)
- Nodules are deeper, harder, and generally fixed
- Nodules at PC-4, LV-3, LV-5, LU-6, SP-8, SP-10, and HT-5
- Veins or dark areas present on the channels (especially around PC-4/LU-6, ST-36 to ST-38, SP-8, and SP-10)

**Pulse**

(Hammer 2001, p.628)

- Choppy
- Blood unclear; blood heat; blood thick
- Muffled
- Engorgement in the liver position
- Rough vibration at the blood depth
- Tense and ropy

**Tongue**

- Dusky
- Dark spots
- Engorged veins

| Physical Symptoms | Emotional Symptoms |
|---|---|
| • Insomnia | • Depression |
| • Body pains | • Suicidal thoughts |
| • Fatigue | • Severe mood swings |
| • Dry skin | • Rigidity |
| • Dry mouth | • Unclear perception |
| | • Easily cries |
| | • Angry outbursts; rage |

## Treatment Principle

Activate Qi and Blood Circulation, Relieve the Depression, Liberate the Hun, Stabilize the Shen, and Benefit the Po.

## Acupuncture

| | |
|---|---|
| PC-4 and LV-6 | SJ-6 and GB-34 |
| LI-4 and LV-3 | DU-20 |
| PC-6 and SP-4 | Auricular: Liver, Spleen, Heart, Shen Men, Lower |
| LU-6 and SP-8 or SP-10 | Lung |
| HT-5 and KD-6 | |

Cupping the upper back or shoulders.

## Herbal Formula

Xue Fu Zhu Yu Tang Modified (Drive out the Stasis in the Mansion of Blood Decoction, Modified) (Maclean and Lyttleton 2010, p.130)

| Postpartum Cases of Blood Stagnation | |
|---|---|
| With Cold | Sheng Hua Tang (Generation and Transformation Decoction) (Micleu 2002) |
| Without Cold | Ge Xia Zhu Yu Tang (Drive out Blood Stasis Below the Diaphragm Decoction) (Micleu 2002) |

*These postpartum cases can be serious, and women can present with suicidal thoughts, aggressive behavior, rage, and—in the most serious cases—infanticidal intent. Sometimes this can be a "psychiatric emergency" and requires Western medical attention.*

## Affirmation

"My blood is circulating freely in a harmonious rhythm; my spirit is free and I make decisions with ease. I am actively engaged in life."

## Qi and Blood Deficiency

### Pathophysiology

Emotional trauma initially scatters the qi and compromises the earth element. The spleen's function of transforming and transporting nutrients diminishes. This can be exacerbated if qi blockages arise, producing liver qi stagnation; the wood overacts on the earth. The resultant lack of nourishment leads to qi and blood deficiency and depression. Each time the trauma memory is relived, the condition worsens, causing a lack of blood and destabilizing the spirit. The Shen leaves the body. The primary treatment is tonification of qi and blood. In addition, the qi must be circulated and any phlegm and damp accumulation transformed. This diagnosis includes postpartum depression cases and others wherein patients have lost a significant amount of blood. However, most treatments for postpartum depression will be listed in the Anxiety section since the heart organ system is primarily affected.

### Diagnostic Signs

**Face**

- Hollow, sagging cheeks
- Pale, lined nose bridge
- Worry lines (vertical lines below the third-eye area)
- Pale nose tip (can be pinched)
- Pale upper lip line
- Slack, dry lip line
- Hollow upper lip area
- Lines around lips
- Puffiness and darkness in the inner canthus upper eyelid area
- Tight, tense, contracted Shen
- Lost look; unfocused; glazed, dazed eyes
- Eyeballs move slightly back and forth or in a circular fashion (frantic thought under a seemingly calm surface)
- Light in the eyes vibrates

**Channel Palpation**

- Weak, slippery, soft sensations in the heart, spleen, lung, and stomach channels
- Dryness in the spleen, heart, and liver channels (especially in the wrist and ankle/lower leg area) due to blood deficiency
- Soft and weak at SP-3, SP-6, ST-36, and R-6
- Nodules at SP-3, HT-7 to HT-5 area, and PC-6

**Pulse**

- Thin; thin yielding; thin feeble
- Smooth vibration
- Hollow
- Deep
- Reduced substance, especially in the middle position
- Thin; muffled at left distal position

**Tongue**

- Pale
- Puffy and enlarged
- Scallops
- Pale tip
- Crack to the tip

| Physical Symptoms | Emotional Symptoms |
|---|---|
| • Fatigue | • Depression |
| • Insomnia/difficulty falling asleep | • Lethargy |
| • Disturbing dreams | • Nervousness |
| • Blurred vision | • Anxiety |
| • Palpitations | • Over-seriousness |
| • Stammering; stuttering; muteness | • Worry |
| • Panic attacks | • Overthinking |
| • Dizziness | • Indecision |
| • Poor appetite; bloating and fullness | • Slow decision making |
| • Sugar and carbohydrate cravings | • Constant examination of past events |
| • Loose stools | • Confusion |
| • Tiredness after eating | • Inability to express emotions |
| • Incomplete digestion | • Mood swings |
| • Hemorrhoids | • Irritability |
| • Dry hair/skin/eyes/nails | • Sadness |
| • Bruising easily | • Smothering |
| • Prolonged menstrual cycles | • Over-nurturing |
| • Pale menstrual blood | • Under-nurturing |
| • Fatigue with exertion (and symptoms worsen) | • Hypersensitivity to stimuli |
| • Poor concentration | |
| • Compression issues: fallen arches; compressed vertebrae | |
| • Slow-healing wounds | |
| • Pitting edema | |

## Treatment Principle

Tonify Qi and Blood, Benefit the Digestion, Nourish the Heart, Calm and Anchor the Shen, Ground the Hun, and Liberate the Yi.

## Acupuncture

| | |
|---|---|
| ST-36 and R-6 | PC-6 and SP-4 |
| HT-7 and SP-3.5 or SP-6 | UB-13, UB-15, or UB-18 and UB-20 |
| SP-3 and SP-6 | 33.12 Ximen (Heart Gate) and LV-2 |
| SI-4 and R-4 | DU-20 and DU-24 |
| LI-10 and R-11 | Yin Tang (M-HN-3) and DU-20 |
| LU-9 and SP-6 | 1010.22 Bi Yi (Nasal Wing), right side for female |
| 44.10 Tianzong and ST-36 | and left side for male |
| SI-4 and GB-40 | Auricular: Heart, Spleen, Stomach, Upper |
| SI-4 and SP-3 | and Lower Lung, Brain, Anxiety, Shen Men, |
| PC-6 and GB-39 | Sympathetic |
| LV-3 and LV-8 | Infrared heat on the abdomen |

## Herbal Formulas

| Diagnosis | Formula |
| --- | --- |
| Qi and Blood Deficiency | Gui Pi Tang Modified (Restore the Spleen Decoction Modified) *Add:* Ye Jiao Teng (Polygomi Multiflora Caulis) 15–30g He Huan Pi (Albizziae Cortex) 12–15g (Maclean and Lyttleton 2000, pp.137–138) |
| Qi Deficiency (Blood is Stable) | Si Jun Zi Tang (Four-Gentlemen Decoction) (Chen and Chen 2009, p.522) – or – Bu Zhong Yi Qi Tang (Tonify the Middle and Augment the Qi Decoction) (Chen and Chen 2009, p.542) |
| Qi Deficiency with Mild Phlegm/ Damp Accumulation | Liu Jun Zi Tang (Six-Gentlemen Decoction) (Chen and Chen 2009, p.527) |
| **Postpartum Depression** | |
| Spleen Deficiency | Dang Gui Bu Xue Tang (Dang Gui Decoction to Supplement the Blood) (Maclean and Lyttleton 2010, p.139) or Gui Pi Tang |
| Heart Qi and Blood Deficiency (palpitations present) | Zhi Gan Cao Tang (Honey-Fried Licorice Decoction) (Micleu 2002) |

## Affirmations

"I am healthy and strong, calm and peaceful, thinking clearly, full of energy. My life-force is connected to the earth."

"My thoughts are clear and I am flowing harmoniously in the rhythm of life."

## Kidney Yang Deficiency

### Pathophysiology

Continued reliving of the trauma memory and chronic fear deplete the qi and lead to a waning of yang; both the kidney and spleen yang decline. The kidney yang fails to warm the spleen, resulting in fatigue and poor digestion. The Yi does not properly process thought, causing confusion. The weakened Zhi fails to manifest motivation and the patient is lethargic. Extreme exhaustion with signs of cold is the key indicator of yang-deficient depression. It is commonly found in middle-aged and older patients due to their lack of yang to propel the body and spirit forward. Warming and increasing the yang of the kidneys shift the apathy and feelings of lethargy and lift the depression. There are aspects of spleen yang deficiency in this pattern. However, the focus is on tonifying kidney yang to resolve the spleen signs. This diagnosis is typical of a trauma that has been passed down from a previous generation.

Refer to the Kidney Yang Deficiency pattern outlined in the Fear section above.

# Anxiety

Emotional trauma shocks the system, depletes the yin and blood, and leaves the spirit ungrounded. The unstable Shen is restless, creating anxiety. In time, the naturally buoyant and joyful Shen is exhausted and joy turns to sadness. Anxiety and sadness are the typical emotions experienced when the heart and Shen are affected, in addition to feeling nervous and melancholy, and having a sense of scattered energy. Frequently patients react by being overly serious or insatiable.

*Observing Natural Rhythms*

The heart circulates the blood in rhythm and houses the spirit. Emotional trauma disturbs this rhythm, which is intensified by continually reliving the trauma memory. Overstimulation disturbs the heart and the stillness of the heart mirror. To re-establish the clarity of the heart mirror, adopting a lifestyle of routine removes excess stress and allows the Shen to root in the body. Regular, scheduled mealtimes and bedtimes, daily meditation, and qigong help the heart to beat in a gentle rhythm. Many artists or "free spirits" find these recommendations unacceptable and rebel against such structure. However, by adapting this scheduled lifestyle, creative people will experience an increase in insight and inspiration. Unnecessary chaos is removed, leaving space for the spark of creativity to shine through.

Trauma and reliving the memory block the qi flow, congest the fluids, and constrain the Yi and Hun. This pattern generates phlegm-heat misting the heart and obstructs the Shen, resulting in anxiety. It is the only excess pattern mentioned below and commonly affects those with chemical sensitivities.

*Common Pathophysiology of Postpartum Depression*

Women suffering from postpartum depression are often diagnosed with heart deficiency. The uterus has a connection with the heart; blood loss during labor creates heart blood deficiency and/or blood stagnation. Women with this condition generally report feeling depressed and are commonly misdiagnosed with qi stagnation. The underlying issue of emotional instability relates to the heart pathology of yin, blood, and qi deficiency. The depression they feel is accompanied by anxiety. Treatment of the syndrome is described below, and many of the point combinations and Chinese herbal formulas used will be the same, unless otherwise noted.

## Heart Qi and Yin Deficiency

*Pathophysiology*

The heart holds the Shen, and when the body experiences a shock the qi is scattered and the Shen becomes ungrounded. Each time the trauma memory is relived, the stability of the heart is compromised; the qi and yin of the heart are depleted, resulting in intense anxiety and sensations of sadness. Without the qi and yin to stabilize the Shen, the person can feel scattered and nervous to the point of feeling overwhelmed by life. This ultimately distorts their perception of reality. Benefiting the qi and nourishing the yin stabilizes the heart and calms the spirit.

In this diagnostic pattern, the heart is the main organ system affected by the emotional trauma. The kidney system can become involved in chronic conditions when the kidney yin is deficient, giving rise to heat—the communication between the fire and water elements becomes compromised. The main differentiating aspect of a strictly heart qi and yin deficiency diagnosis is the lack of kidney pathological signs.

## Diagnostic Signs

| Face | Channel Palpation |
|---|---|
| • Dry skin | • Dryness on the heart, pericardium, and small intestine channels |
| • Dry, slightly red nose tip | • Nodules at HT-7, HT-6, PC-7, and KD-7 |
| • Pinched nose tip | |
| • Vertical or horizontal line on nose tip | |

| Pulse | Tongue |
|---|---|
| • Tight in left distal position | • Dry tip |
| • Muffled in the left distal position | • Crack to tip |

| Physical Symptoms | Emotional Symptoms |
|---|---|
| • Stammering; stuttering; muteness | • Nervousness |
| • Palpitations | • Anxiety |
| • Insomnia | • Over-seriousness |
| • Panic attacks | • Inability to express emotions |
| • Irritability | • Isolation |
| • Dry skin and mouth | |

## Treatment Principle

Nourish Heart Yin and Astringe Fluids, Tonify Heart Qi, Benefit Fluids, Calm the Shen, and Still the Heart Mirror.

## Acupuncture

| | |
|---|---|
| HT-6 and KD-7 | UB-15 and UB-23 |
| PC-7 and LV-3 | 33.12 Ximen (Heart Gate) and LV-2 |
| HT-7 and SP-6 | DU-20 and DU-24 |
| PC-6 and GB-39 | Yin Tang (M-HN-3) |
| SI-4 and GB-40 | Auricular: Heart, Anxiety, Shen Men, Sympathetic |

## Herbal Formula

Sheng Mai San (Generate the Pulse Powder)

**MODIFICATIONS TO SHENG MAI SAN**

| | |
|---|---|
| Irritability and insomnia | Suan Zao Ren (Semen Ziziphi Spinosae) and Bai Zi Ren (Semen Platycladi) |
| Yin deficiency | Substitute Xi Yang Shen (Radix Panacis Quinquefolii) for Ren Shen (Radix et Rhizoma Ginseng) |
| Patients with a faint pulse and risk of shock | Increase Ren Shen (Radix et Rhizoma Ginseng) to a large dose |
| *Postpartum Cases of Heart Yin Deficiency* | Gan Mai Da Zao Tang (Licorice, Wheat, and Jujube Decoction) |

*Source:* Adapted from Chen and Chen 2009, pp.554–555

## Affirmation

"I am at peace, gently moving through life, feeling loved and safe."

## Heart and Kidney Yin Deficiency with Heat

### Pathophysiology

Emotional trauma shocks the heart. As the trauma is relived, the yin is depleted, creating heat. The kidneys (water element) typically control the fire, but as the yin decreases, the fire goes unchecked, resulting in high anxiety levels, panic attacks, insomnia, and restlessness. The fluctuation between anxiety (caused by heat) and depression (due to deficiency) occurs due to the miscommunication between the heart and kidney. Patients feel different levels of cycling between the highs and lows.

Kidney signs and symptoms are seen in this pattern, such as low back and knee pain, proximal pulse changes, palpation changes on the kidney channel, and facial diagnostic signs in the kidney areas. Heat signs are also detected. As the yin declines, this pattern is frequently experienced by menopausal women due to the shift in the yin and yang balance.

## Diagnostic Signs

**Face**

- Flushed face
- Red, dry nose tip
- Pinched nose tip
- Redness in upper lip line
- Excessive joy lines; lines going into hairline
- Chin: wobbly, wrinkled, and dimpled; skin resembling an orange peel with redness and dryness
- Under the eyes: redness; redness on lower eyelids; dryness
- Face is red, especially in the cheeks
- Three-sided eyes
- Red and dry philtrum
- Thin ear cartilage
- Glazed look; sideways glance(s)

**Channel Palpation**

- Dryness with/without roughness on the heart, pericardium, small intestine, and kidney channels
- Nodules at HT-7, HT-6, and KD-7
- Grainy sensation and/or tenderness at PC-7
- Tenderness at PC-8, UB-14, UB-15, UB-23, KD-2, and HT-8
- Thickening at KD-7
- Dip at KD-7

**Pulse**

(Hammer 2001, p.405)

- Tight in left distal position
- Thin, deep, empty in left proximal position
- Rapid
- Both left distal and proximal positions are feeble-absent or tight

**Tongue**

- Red, dry tip and body
- Less coat
- Crack to tip
- Red; cracked; dry; less coat; mirror coat; saliva lines on sides
- Dip in the rear of the tongue body

**Physical Symptoms**

- Stammering; stuttering; muteness
- Shoulder or hip weakness
- Palpitations
- Insomnia with night sweats
- Panic attacks
- Fatigue
- Low back and knee pain
- Elbow pains
- Forgetfulness
- Tinnitus
- Five-center heat
- Dry skin and mouth

**Emotional Symptoms**

- Nervousness
- Anxiety
- Over-seriousness
- Inability to express emotions
- Mania
- Irritability
- Fright
- Easily startled
- Depression
- Sadness
- Isolation

## Treatment Principle

Nourish the Yin and Tonify the Blood, Benefit the Heart and Kidney, Calm and Root the Shen, and Benefit the Zhi.

*Acupuncture*

| | |
|---|---|
| HT-6 and KD-7 | UB-15 and UB-23 |
| PC-7 and LV-2 | 33.12 Ximen (Heart Gate) and KD-6 |
| HT-7 and SP-6 | DU-20 and DU-24 |
| R-4 and SP-6 | Yin Tang (M-HN-3) |
| PC-6 and GB-39 | Auricular: Heart, Anxiety, Shen Men, Kidney, |
| SI-4 and GB-40 | Sympathetic |

*Herbal Formula*

Tian Wang Bu Xin Dan (Emperor of Heaven's Special Pill to Tonify the Heart) (Chen and Chen 2009, p.725)

*Affirmation*

"I am at peace, gently moving through life, feeling loved and safe, rooted and balanced."

## Heart and Spleen *Qi* and Blood Deficiency

*Pathophysiology*

Emotional trauma and reliving its memory stir the spirit, depleting the heart qi and blood, causing anxiety, sadness, and depression, in addition to other physical symptoms related to the heart. Moreover, the earth element is weakened, affecting the spleen's ability to transform nutrients into blood. This reduces the heart blood. Worry and overthinking about the trauma further complicate the condition, hindering the Yi from processing clearly. Since the Yi governs the rhythm of the body to process nutrients, a vicious cycle occurs with the emotions disturbing the Yi and the dwindling blood supply stirring the emotions. The Shen is ungrounded, and dream-disturbed sleep is common, along with the emotional symptoms. The lack of sleep and limited replenishment of the blood compounds the issue.

A healthy heart emanates joy. When the heart is not full, sadness is felt. This emotion is a main component of heart pathology and is commonly confused with grief belonging to the lungs. The presence of heart signs and symptoms determines the origin of the sadness. Patients' emotions will wax and wane between sadness and anxiety—a yin and yang rhythm. As the qi and blood are tonified, the highs and lows will soften.

Many cases of emotional trauma have an aspect of heart blood and spleen deficiency. An ungrounded Shen and disturbed Yi commonly occur with the reliving of a trauma, and modern lifestyle choices exacerbate this condition. Poor dietary habits reduce the spleen's ability to transform nutrients into blood, and lack of sleep hinders the cleansing and generation of blood, resulting in a destabilized spirit. Blood loss in pregnancy makes this diagnosis common in postpartum depression.

Refer to the Qi and Blood Deficiency pattern outlined in the Depression section above.

## Heart and Gallbladder Qi Deficiency

### Pathophysiology

Most texts do not offer much explanation or description of likely patho-mechanisms of heart and gallbladder qi deficiency patterns. In the *Clinical Handbook of Internal Medicine, Vol. 3*, the authors assert that this condition is likely an acquired personality trait which might be brought on by trauma in the womb or in childhood (Maclean and Lyttleton 2010, p.909). Hammer, in *Chinese Pulse Diagnosis, Revised Edition*, describes the pattern based on the midday/midnight channel clock connection (Hammer 2001, p.562), which provides a partial explanation. However, clinicians are often looking for more.

### DIFFERENTIATING FEAR

> *The timid person is frightened before a danger, a coward*
> *during the time, and a courageous person afterward.*
>
> Johann Paul Friedrich Richter

Fright has many shades, from a person reacting to a horror movie, to being scared to speak in front of a group, to jumping at the sight of their shadow. Some people are haunted with a feeling of timidity and are generally skittish; these patients lack the courage to simply participate in life. As illustrated by the quotation above, a timid person does not need a dangerous situation to be afraid. In the Chinese physiological model, this absence of courage stems from a qi deficiency in the heart and gallbladder. The lack of heart qi fails to secure the Shen, and the weakness of the gallbladder exacerbates the situation by not keeping the Shen upright. The heart, housing the Shen, requires the yang qi from the gallbladder to maintain a calm Shen. Specifically, the gallbladder instills upright yang in the body, including the heart, to embolden movement through life.

If the gallbladder is compromised (or inherently deficient), then the patient will lack this boldness and will also startle easily. A kind of vicious cycle can follow in which the Shen becomes frightened regularly, thus further weakening the heart. Additional insight might be gleaned by considering the nature and relationships of the channels associated with the two organs.

## SAME MOVING CHANNEL PAIRING

The arm shao yin channel is coupled with the leg shao yang channel via the same moving pivot channel pairing. It is through this connection that the gallbladder supports the heart directly. Strong yang qi from the gallbladder supplies the heart with the fortitude to interact with the world with composure and clarity. If the gallbladder is weak, its decision-making abilities regarding fluid metabolism are compromised and phlegm is created that mists the heart. This phlegm distorts the heart mirror, causing the heart to over-react. Any damage to either organ will affect the other, resulting in timidity. Because of this relationship, shock can reverberate from one organ to the other. The initial weakness can begin *in utero* from a trauma experienced by the mother.

## ORIGIN OF FRIGHT BASED ON TRANSFERENCE VIA SHOCK TO THE CHANNEL

*In utero*, the organs are still developing, and disturbance to the heart could transfer to the gallbladder or vice versa. Other organs can be disturbed, but in this pattern it is the heart/gallbladder connection that is affected. Childhood trauma, or trauma experienced as an adult, agitates the heart and reverberates in the gallbladder. The pathogenic action can also stem from the gallbladder. Someone born with a weak gallbladder organ is susceptible to shock that would transmit to the heart. These traumas weaken both organs and result in qi deficiency.

## SHAO YANG PROVIDING QI TO PROTECT THE HEART

Strong qi in the gallbladder provides courage for making decisions, especially those based on digestion, that is, what nutrients to digest and how much (Wang and Robertson 2008, p.234). Processing trauma is part of this "digestive" function, as the gallbladder must be upright to foster fearlessness and decide what to take in and how to react. The heart benefits from this qi to maintain a calm Shen and to remain settled during a traumatic event. A weak gallbladder fails to properly aid digestion, resulting in phlegm and the inability to process traumas. Thus, phlegm mists the heart and traumas are trapped in the body, disrupting the Shen, causing timidity.

An additional level of complexity in this pattern arises from the shao yang–jue yin relationship. Upward movement of yang from shao yang supports the heart-protective function of the pericardium. In particular, the situation might be further aggravated by a concurrent abdication of the role determining what both enters and exits the heart. If the regulatory function of the pericardium is jeopardized, then the heart is susceptible to injury. Ample qi from the shao yang channel is essential to maintain this stability. The paired jue yin and shao yang also supplies the liver with courage. In the case of a traumatic event, the liver responds by maintaining open pathways to the heart. If the liver lacks the proper yang in these situations, the lack of clarity described above is further exacerbated. In both cases there is a unique kind of yang deficiency which compromises both heart shao yin and jue yin pivoting and closing movements.

The shao yang channel is comprised of the san jiao and gallbladder channels. The gallbladder is the yang organ involved in this pattern, not the san jiao. It is the qi from the gallbladder that is crucial in this pattern because of its connection with the heart via the same movement channel pairing. Another yang organ to discuss in this differentiation is the small intestine.

### Yin and Yang Channel Pairing

The small intestine, the yang paired organ of the heart, supplies the heart with abundant blood to stabilize the Shen and clear heat. In anxiety, due to blood deficiency and heat, the small intestine fails to build blood to cool and stabilize the Shen. Heat and blood deficient signs would comprise this pattern. The Heart and Gallbladder Qi Deficiency pattern is different in that it involves cold and phlegm. The gallbladder fails to provide the movement, warmth, and clear fluids required to steady the Shen. To identify this pattern, there are several unique diagnostic signs to note.

### Recognizing Essential Diagnostics

Observing puffiness at GB-40, thinning or missing outer eyebrows, and paleness on the left side of the tongue with a thick tongue coating (especially on the left side) are some key diagnostic signs that indicate gallbladder deficiency. Signs of heart deficiency include soft sensations palpating the heart channel, a pale and/or pinched nose tip, a deep, slippery, and thin quality of the pulse in the left distal position (Hammer 2001, p.404), and a slightly pale tongue tip with white coating. Another important determining factor in this diagnosis is how a patient's sleep is affected. Specifically, they wake due to fright and startle easily when sleeping. This is due to the unsteadiness of the Shen. Typically, the patient would report experiencing a shock. The pattern is commonly treated with the Chinese herbal formula Wen Dan Tang (Warm the Gallbladder Decoction).

### Understanding the Pattern through Treatment

Dr. Wang believed it was important to follow the original version of Wen Dan Tang (Warm the Gallbladder Decoction) encouraged by Sun Si Miao in his book *Important Formulas Worth a Thousand Gold Pieces*. This approach calls for the increase of Sheng Jiang (Rhizoma Zingiberis Officinalis) to 12 grams to open and warm the gallbladder (Wang and Robertson 2008, p.234). Sheng Jiang improves circulation and warms the yang. This allows the gallbladder to provide yang qi and clear fluids to the heart to endure a shock.

Acupuncture point prescriptions follow a similar approach. Tonifying GB-40, the source point, increases yuan qi to bolster courage and decision making. The fortified qi travels to the heart (via their channel connection) to secure the Shen.

## Resolving Heart and Gallbladder Qi Deficiency

Benefiting both the heart and gallbladder reduces fright and anxiety and ultimately equips the patient with a solid foundation with which to process future trauma. The pathological signs and symptoms disappear as treatment progresses and the patient will then have the steadfastness to react in and navigate through subsequent stressful events. As Ralph Waldo Emerson encourages, "Don't be too timid or squeamish about your actions. All life is an experiment. The more experiments you make, the better."

### Diagnostic Signs

| Face | Channel Palpation |
|---|---|
| • Thinning or missing outer eyebrows<br>• Pale nose tip<br>• Pinched nose tip | • Puffiness at GB-40<br>• Weak; slippery; soft sensations in the heart and gallbladder channels<br>• Roughness or bumpiness in the gallbladder and heart channels due to qi deficiency<br>• Nodules at HT-7 and GB-40 |

| Pulse<br>(Hammer 2001, p.563) | Tongue |
|---|---|
| • Deep and thin in the left distal position<br>• Tense and slippery in the gallbladder position<br>• Feeble in the right middle position | • Normal color, possibly a pale tip or paleness on the left side<br>• Thick coating on the left side<br>• Lacerations on the side |

| Physical Symptoms | Emotional Symptoms |
|---|---|
| • Insomnia; nightmares; awakening startled and frightened<br>• Restlessness<br>• Palpitations<br>• Sighing<br>• Blurred vision and dizziness<br>• Panic attacks | • Easily startled<br>• Fearfulness<br>• Anxiety<br>• Worry<br>• Phobias<br>• Timidity<br>• Quick temper |

### Treatment Principle

Calm the Shen, Benefit and Warm the Gallbladder, Benefit the Hun, and Restore the Upright Position of the Gallbladder.

*Acupuncture*

| HT-7 and GB-40 | Auricular: Shen Men, Heart, Gallbladder, |
| PC-6 and GB-39 | Sympathetic |
| UB-15 and UB-19 | Infrared heat on the abdomen |

*Herbal Formula*

Wen Dan Tang (Warm the Gallbladder Decoction) (Chen and Chen 2009, pp.1213–1214)

*Note:* Use the classical dose of 12g for Sheng Jiang (Rhizoma Zingiberis Officinalis).

*Affirmation*

"I am calm and courageous. I make wonderful decisions and am at peace. I am safe and protected."

## Heart Fire

*Pathophysiology*

Reliving emotional trauma excites the body, creates fire, and stirs the heart. The fire agitates the Shen, giving rise to anxiety. The heart fire blazes uncontrolled by the kidney water and patients experience nervousness, anxiety, and a sense of being scattered. The heart mirror is disturbed and a patient's perceptions become distorted, causing hallucinations. The heart no longer circulates blood smoothly, and sleep disturbances are common. Until the heat is cleared, the Shen will be restless. Conditions such as mania and psychosis are seen in this pathology.

Patients exhibiting heart fire can be suffering from serious mental imbalances. These cases are less common in typical outpatient Chinese medicine clinics, and the author has minimal experience in treating cases of severe heart fire. Many of the signs and symptoms below are therefore included from other sources. Patients with strong heart fire are usually already hospitalized. However, there are less extreme cases of heart fire, and for those practitioners who treat in-patient cases, the information below is applicable.

## Diagnostic Signs

### Face

- Red nose tip
- Flushed face
- Joy lines into the hairline
- Red eyes
- Darting eyes
- Four-sided eyes
- Red lower eyelids
- Intense Shen
- Sideways glance(s)

### Channel Palpation

- Tenderness and/or roughness in the heart, pericardium, small intestine, san jiao, and gallbladder channels
- Hardness and/or nodules and/or tenderness at HT-8, PC-8, HT-7, PC-7, SJ-5, and GB-41

### Pulse
(Hammer 2001, pp.589–590)

- Rapid, tense pulse
- Heart Full quality
- Reduced substance in the left proximal position if the kidney yin is deficient

### Tongue
(Kirschbaum 2000, p.117)

- Red points on the tip of the tongue (*Note:* Not to be confused with wind-heat invasion where the points are fresher, coarser, bigger, and generally extend into the upper third of the tongue)

### Physical Symptoms
(Maclean and Lyttleton 2000, p.838)

- Decreased mental acuity
- Insomnia; frequently awakening with nightmares/fright
- Agitation; restlessness; uptight
- Obsessive thinking
- Excessive talking
- Bitter taste in the mouth
- Mouth and tongue ulcers
- Palpitations
- Thirst and desiring cold fluids
- Concentrated or painful urination

### Emotional Symptoms

- Anxiety
- Nervousness
- Scattered
- Worry
- Mania

## Treatment Principle

Clear Heart Fire, and Calm and Settle the Shen.

*Acupuncture*

| | |
|---|---|
| HT-8 and KD-2 | Yin Tang (M-HN-3) |
| PC-8 and GB-41 | An Mian (N-HN-54) |
| HT-9 and SP-2 | UB-15 and UB-23 |
| HT-7 and KD-7 | DU-20 and DU-24 |
| PC-7 and SP-6 | Auricular: Shen Men, Sympathetic, Heart, Point |
| SJ-5 and GB-41 | Zero, Anxiety, Neurasthenia Point and Area |
| LI-11 and ST-44 | Bleed ear apex |
| HT-7 and KD-6 | |

*Herbal Formula*

Huang Lian Jie Du Tang (Coptis and Scute Combination) Modified (Maclean and Lyttleton 2000, p.838)

*Affirmation*

"My body is still and I am feeling peaceful."

## Phlegm Heat

*Pathophysiology*

Blocked channels from trauma limit the circulation of fluids and qi, which generate phlegm and heat. The reliving of the trauma memory constrains the Hun. Instead of living in the present and making decisions, the Hun/liver are congested and overact on the digestion and the Yi. This reduces the spleen's ability to transform fluids and contributes to the phlegm accumulation. The weakened Yi fails to process clearly, creating stagnation and generating heat. Each time the patient relives the trauma memory, the Yi's function is reduced and the accumulation of unclear fluid worsens.

This unclear fluid mists the heart, which disturbs the heart mirror, causing anxiety; the Shen is unable to clearly perceive its surroundings. The heat heightens anxiety by stirring the Shen and increases nervousness and panic attacks. Patients suffering from chemical sensitivity commonly experience this pathology because chemicals engender phlegm.

## Diagnostic Signs

### Face

- Flaccid muscle tone
- Puffy areas
- Greasy sheen
- Puffy yellow upper eyelids
- Tight, tense, contracted Shen
- Red, flushed face
- Yellowing and horizontal lines in the nose bridge area
- Redness around the mouth and under the nostrils

### Channel Palpation

- Slippery, hard, or tight sensation in the spleen and stomach channels. This can be shallow or deep depending on the chronicity of the issue
- Roughness or bumpiness in the fascia of the spleen and stomach channels
- Slippery nodules in the spleen and stomach channels
- Nodules and tenderness at SP-2, SP-9, ST-44, and PC-7
- Nodules; engorged veins; tenderness at ST-40
- Tenderness and tightness at R-9
- Pulsing around the umbilicus, especially at R-6 and R-9

### Pulse

- Slippery and rapid
- Tense, tight
- Engorged in the right middle position
- Slippery and tense in the left proximal position

### Tongue

- Red, puffy, and swollen
- Scallops
- Thick, yellow, greasy coat

### Physical Symptoms

- Fatigue
- Heaviness in the body
- Dizziness/vertigo
- Palpitations
- Insomnia; waking early in morning
- Phlegm that is yellow/green
- Sluggish digestion and hunger
- Sugar and carbohydrate cravings
- Nausea/vomiting
- Acid reflux; belching; bitter taste
- Bloating and fullness; weight gain
- Puffy, round body
- Poor concentration

### Emotional Symptoms

- Anxiety
- Nervousness
- Depression

## Treatment Principle

Clear Heat, Transform Phlegm and Dampness, Benefit the Digestion, Calm and Clarify the Shen, and Liberate the Yi and Hun.

## *Acupuncture*

| | |
|---|---|
| SP-9 and ST-40 and R-12 | LU-5 and LV-2 |
| SP-2 and ST-44 | DU-20 and DU-24 |
| HT-8 and SP-5 | Auricular: Shen Men, Sympathetic, Heart, |
| PC-8 and GB-41 | Stomach, Spleen, Liver |
| HT-5 and ST-41 | Bleed ear apex |
| PC-5 and GB-34 | |

## *Herbal Formula*

Shi Yi Wei Wen Dan Tang (Eleven Ingredient Decoction to Warm the Gallbladder) (Maclean and Lyttleton 2000, p.911)

## *Affirmation*

"My body is light and my mind is clear. My energy flows freely and my digestion is happy and strong in a harmonious rhythm."

# Worry

The Yi, the mind of the spleen, is responsible for processing thought. Thinking constantly about a trauma memory hinders the function of the spleen and its ability to transform and transport nutrients within the body. The production and movement of qi and blood result in constraint and/or deficiency. Worry and unclear thinking are the byproducts of a trauma memory and resolve when the Yi's ability to process clearly is re-established. Poor dietary choices and sedentary lifestyles exacerbate the condition; nutrition along with exercise and action-based living play key roles in treatment. Regulating and benefiting the earth element restores the Yi and clarity. For many patients, free the constraint before implementing tonification.

## *Spleen and Stomach Qi Stagnation*

### *Pathophysiology*

Worry and excessive thought, stemming from a trauma memory, inhibit the spleen and stomach's qi dynamic of processing nutrients and thoughts. This constrains the Yi, resulting in mood swings. Signs of deficiency may be present, but the stagnation must first be cleared so as not to cause further constraint. For elderly or immune-compromised patients, include some tonification treatment to support the earth element when moving qi.

## Diagnostic Signs

| Face | Channel Palpation |
|---|---|
| • Full, dark, overly moist lips | • Shallow hardness or tightness in the spleen and stomach channels |
| • Darkening and yellowing above the upper lip | |
| • Yellowing or darkening in the nose bridge area | • Roughness or bumpiness in the spleen and stomach channels |
| • Lines in the nose bridge area | • Nodules at ST-40, SP-9, and LU-5 |
| *With heat:* | *With heat:* |
| • Red lips | • Nodules at ST-44 |
| • Lost look; unfocused; glazed eyes | |
| • Puffy face, eyelids, lips, and lower cheeks | |

| Pulse | Tongue |
|---|---|
| • Tense, tight, and slippery quality | • Thick tongue coating |
| • Engorgement in the right middle position | *With heat:* |
| *With heat:* | • Red edges |
| • Rapid | |

| Physical Symptoms | Emotional Symptoms |
|---|---|
| • Bloating; fullness; nausea | • Worry; obsession |
| • Incomplete digestion | • Mood swings |
| • Weight gain—especially in the mid-body, upper arms, and calves | • Constant examination of past events |
| • Fatigue | • Slow decision making |
| • Problems concentrating | • Holding on to past events |
| *With heat:* | • Over-nurturing |
| • Mouth sores; bad breath; excessive thirst and hunger | • Indecisiveness |
| • Eating to fill void; stress eating | *With heat:* |
| | • Irritability |

## Treatment Principle

Regulate the Qi Dynamic of the Spleen and Stomach, Benefit the Digestion, and Free the Yi; Clear Heat if needed.

## Acupuncture

| | |
|---|---|
| LU-5 and SP-9 | Cupping on R-8 |
| ST-40 and R-12 | *With heat:* |
| ST-25 and SP-15 | PC-7 and ST-44 |
| PC-6 and SP-4 | Bleed ST-36 to ST-38 area |
| DU-20 and ST-36 | Bleed ear apex |
| UB-20 and UB-21 | |
| Auricular: Spleen, Stomach, Shen Men, Brain | |

## Herbal Formulas

| Diagnosis | Formula |
| --- | --- |
| Spleen and Stomach Qi Stagnation | Zhi Zhu Wan (Immature Bitter Orange and Atractylodes Macrocephala Pill) (Chen and Chen 2009, p.1274) |
| With Heat | Xie Huang San (Drain the Yellow Powder)<br>*With irritability add:*<br>Deng Xin Cao (Medulla Junci)<br>Chi Fu Ling (Poria Rubra) (Chen and Chen 2009, p.396) |

## Affirmation

"I freely move through life with clarity and action. I am in the present moment, safe and nurtured."

## Spleen and Heart Qi and Blood Deficiency

*Pathophysiology*

Constant thoughts of the trauma memory weaken the spleen and its ability to provide nourishment to the body. This results in weight regulation and nutrient absorption issues. If the condition is caught quickly, simply tonifying the spleen qi is all that is needed; however, blood deficiency is commonly concurrent. The lack of blood affects the Shen and the heart mirror, unsettling the spirit and making the heart mirror susceptible to the winds of emotion. Women suffering from postpartum depression frequently experience worry and obsessive thoughts, due to the strain on digestion during pregnancy and the loss of blood during childbirth.

Refer to the Qi and Blood Deficiency pattern outlined in the Depression section above.

## Spleen Yang Deficiency

*Pathophysiology*

Ruminating on the trauma memory exhausts the qi and the yang wanes. The symptoms and signs of this pattern are similar to the Spleen Qi Deficiency diagnosis and include cold signs. The Yi is frozen and the thoughts are stuck. Warming the yang and dispelling cold are needed to resolve the worry and confusion. Since the yang from the kidneys provides warmth for the spleen to function, Kidney Yang Deficiency is frequently part of this pattern. Thus, kidney signs and symptoms are commonly concurrent.

## Diagnostic Signs

| | |
|---|---|
| **Face** *Similar to Spleen Qi Deficiency and include:* | **Channel Palpation** *Similar to Spleen Qi Deficiency and include:* |
| • Paler skin | • Cold sensations when palpating the abdomen |
| • A deeper look of tiredness | • Nodules at SP-3 and SP-9 will be more fixed and deep |
| • Blue tint to the nose bridge | |
| • Increased hanging/sagging skin on the cheeks | • Soft/weak areas at ST-36, SP-3, SP-7 to SP-8, SP-6, and R-6 are deep and feel cold |
| • Eyes look frozen and the Shen has a frigid appearance | • Potential tenderness at KD-3 |

| | |
|---|---|
| **Pulse** (Hammer 2001, p.628) | **Tongue** |
| • Slow; deep; feeble-absent | • Pale |
| • Empty in proximal positions | • Swollen |
| • Changes in qualities | • Scalloped |
| • Scattered | |

| | |
|---|---|
| **Physical Symptoms** *Similar to Spleen Qi Deficiency with:* | **Emotional Symptoms** *Similar to Spleen Qi Deficiency with:* |
| • Cold hands and feet; body feels cold | • Extreme mental fatigue |
| • Sensitivity to cold foods and drinks | • Withdrawn |
| • Watery diarrhea | • Apathy |
| • Stomach pain relieved by warmth | • Strong feelings of hopelessness |

## Treatment Principle

Warm the Spleen Yang, Dispel Cold, Benefit the Spleen, Strengthen the Yi, and Tonify the Yang.

## Acupuncture

Similar acupuncture protocols to Spleen Qi Deficiency, incorporating infrared heat on the abdomen or using moxa on SP-3, SP-15, and R-6, and using moxa with salt on R-8.

## Herbal Formula

Fu Zi Li Zhong Wan (Prepared Aconite Pill to Regulate the Middle) (Chen and Chen 2009, p.463)

## Affirmation

"I am powerful and strong. My body and mind are in a harmonious rhythm and my thoughts are clear. A red/golden ball is warm and glowing in my lower belly."

### *Phlegm and Damp Accumulation with or without Heat*

*Pathophysiology*

Obsessive thinking caused by reliving trauma memory bogs down the spleen's ability to process fluids clearly and generates phlegm and damp accumulation; the Yi is constrained. This condition includes both spleen deficient and phlegm accumulation signs. The accumulation can collect in the lungs and/or in the spleen and stomach. The fluid accumulation can also percolate and produce heat, which further complicates the situation. If heat is present, it must be cleared gently to preserve the fluid balance. For those cases where the phlegm accumulation is coupled with heat, the additional signs and symptoms are listed.

The treatment generally focuses on regulating the fluid metabolism before tonifying the spleen. Utilizing points that calm spirit and soothe the trauma memory helps to set the Yi in its appropriate cadence.

Refer to the Phlegm and Damp Accumulation with or without Heat pattern in the Depression section above.

# Grief

> *A gem cannot be polished without friction*
> *nor a man perfected without trials.*
>
> *Chinese proverb*

Initially, emotional trauma blocks qi flow and hinders the lung's ability to regulate qi. Qi and blood stagnate in the lungs and bring about a heavy feeling of grief and/or a sense of lack. Over time, this weakens the lungs and creates deficiency. If the trauma is recent, regulating qi and blood is sufficient. However, most patients seek care long after a trauma has occurred and have some form of lung deficiency. Patients are not encouraged to dredge up the emotion of grief, but if it surfaces, releasing the pent-up energy through tears offers a healthy way to disengage the emotion.

### *Stabilizing the Po*

The lungs are the most external of the five zang organs and are highly susceptible to stressful events. Experiencing trauma and reliving its memory scatter the qi, causing a feeling of emptiness. This leaves a patient feeling less present in their body; their sense of having a secure place in the world is diminished. The Po is weakened, along with a person's ability to maintain boundaries with their environment. They tend to withdraw, lack self-esteem, have extreme sensitivity, feel deep grief, cry frequently, strive for perfection, and may feel completely disconnected. Coughing, asthma, frequent colds, sinus infections, and similar frequently occur.

## Lung Qi Stagnation

### Pathophysiology

The gasp, when a shock is experienced, stops the smooth rhythmic flow of the breathing and hinders the lungs' ability to regulate the qi. This qi stagnation affects the heart (since it relies on smooth qi flow to circulate the blood) and the liver. The heart counts on the lungs to maintain smooth qi flow to uphold "buoyancy." When there is a shock and tightening of the chest, the "lighthearted" feeling is compromised, causing sadness.

The blocked qi can also result in anger due to the natural flow between the lungs and liver. The lungs descend qi and the liver ascends qi—creating a tai ji-like movement. When deep grief is experienced, this flow is reduced and lung/liver signs and symptoms occur. Grief is a normal emotion and doesn't always require treatment, but if it is not processed and lingers, it will eventually weaken the lungs. To address the stagnation, both the lungs and liver require attention to restore the qi flow.

### Diagnostic Signs

| Face | Channel Palpation |
|---|---|
| • Dull Shen (lack of sparkle) | • Weak and slippery, soft sensations, or tightness and roughness in the lung channel |
| • Tired Shen | |
| • Hollow cheeks | • Nodules throughout the lung and large intestine channels |
| • Gray skin color | |
| • Lines in the wei qi area | • Nodules and tenderness at LU-6, LU-5, LI-6 through LI-11, and LV-3 |
| • Darkening and a pale hue in the wei qi area | |
| • Pale, gray, or darker look to the entire nose | |
| • Dark purpose lines | |
| • Darkening in the third-eye area | |
| • Swelling and darkening of the lower lip | |
| • Swelling under the eyes ("unshed tears") | |

| Pulse | Tongue |
|---|---|
| (Hammer 2001, p.550) | • Swelling in the anterior third of the tongue |
| • Flat and feeble in left and right distal positions | |

| Physical Symptoms | Emotional Symptoms |
|---|---|
| • Cough; chest tightness; wheezing | • Grief and sadness |
| • Small amount of phlegm production; difficulty in expectorating | • Feeling as if the past grief experience just occurred |
| • "Plum pit qi" | • Irritability |
| • Shallow breathing/shortness of breath | • Isolation |
| • Overall joint pain | • Lack of confidence |
| • Frequent crying | |
| • Constantly plugged nose | |
| • Sensitivity to environmental toxins | |
| • Asthma | |
| • Constipation | |

## Treatment Principle

Regulate the Lung and Liver Qi, Direct Qi Downwards, Stabilize and Benefit the Po, Liberate the Hun, and Ventilate the Lung.

## Acupuncture

| | |
|---|---|
| LU-5 and SP-9 | PC-5 and UB-65 |
| LU-6 and LV-5 | R-17 and R-22 |
| LU-5 and LV-3 | LU-3 and SP-4 |
| LI-4 and LV-3 | 1010.20 Shuijin |
| LI-6 and GB-34 | Auricular: Upper and Lower Lung, Shen Men, |
| LI-5 and GB-38 | Liver, Sympathetic |

## Herbal Formulas

| Possible Formulas |
|---|
| Zhi Sou San (Stop Coughing Powder) (Maclean and Lyttleton 2000, p.78) |
| Shen Mi Tang (Mysterious Decoction) |
| Si Mo Tang (Four Milled-Herbs Decoction) (Chen and Chen 2009, pp.848–849) |

*Note:* Zhi Sou San is clinically effective for treating grief that causes lung qi stagnation. This formula re-establishes proper qi flow and opens the lungs. The herbs regulate the qi, directing it downwards and upwards. Moreover, deep-seated grief can be interpreted as wind continually affecting the lungs. Jing Jie (Herba seu Flos Schizonepetae Tenuifolia), a herb in the formula, resolves internal wind. The dosing of the formula can be modified, based on the amount of fluid accumulation in the lung. The formula is contraindicated for lung yin deficiency or lung heat.

## Affirmation

"I am grateful for my life and am breathing deeply, feeling relaxed and confident."

# Lung Qi and / or Yin Deficiency

## Pathophysiology

The lungs are delicate and susceptible to dryness and exhaustion. Grief that is not processed and released slowly depletes the metal element. Reliving the trauma memory can trigger grief, exhausting the qi and fluids, causing chronic coughing, asthma, skin issues, and a weak immune system, among other ailments. Emotionally, patients feel isolated from the world and withdraw; their self-confidence wanes, and feelings of vulnerability and hypersensitivity increase. Patients have either qi or yin deficiency; the main differentiating factor is a presence of dryness with yin deficiency.

## Diagnostic Signs

**Face**

*Lung Deficiency:*

- Hollow, lined cheeks in the wei qi area
- Darkening and/or pale in the wei qi area
- Dull, deadened Shen, lacking sparkle
- Tired Shen
- Pale, ashen gray skin color
- Slack lower lip

*Qi Deficient signs:*

- Pale face

*Yin Deficient signs:*

- Dryness in the wei qi area
- Dryness and lines on the nose
- Dry lips
- Dryness and lack of life to the skin
- Flushed face

**Channel Palpation**

*Lung Qi Deficiency:*

- Weak and slippery/soft sensations in the lung and large intestine channels
- A rough or bumpy quality in the lung and large intestine channels
- Dip and weak sensation at LI-10; frequently tender
- Soft, weak areas on the lung channel

*Lung Yin Deficiency:*

- Dry sensations in the lung and large intestine channels

## Pulse

*Lung Qi Deficiency:*

- "Right distal position is Feeble, Slippery, Rough Vibration, and a Slow rate, with Change in Qualities and Intensity" (Hammer 2001, p.424)
- "The Special Lung position is Tight, Wiry, and Slippery, Rough Vibration, and Change in Intensity" (Hammer 2001, p.424)

*Lung Yin Deficiency:*

- "Tight-Wiry, Slippery, Rough Vibration, Change in Intensity, and a slightly Rapid rate" (Hammer 2001, p.424)
- "The Special Lung position is Wiry, Slippery, Rough Vibration, and Change in Intensity" (Hammer 2001, p.424)

## Tongue

*Lung Qi Deficiency:*

- Depression and/or slightly pale in the anterior third of the tongue body

*Lung Yin Deficiency:*

- Cracks and dryness in the anterior third of the tongue body

## Physical Symptoms

- Loss of smell
- Cough; chest tightness; wheezing
- Weak, small voice
- Shallow breathing; shortness of breath
- Hunched shoulders and slumped-over posture
- Overall joint pain
- Frequent crying
- Constantly plugged nose
- Sensitivity to environmental toxins
- Asthma
- Constipation
- Skin infections; slow healing skin

*Qi Deficiency:*

- Frequent colds
- Tire easily with exertion
- Weak cough; clear mucus
- Spontaneous sweating

*Yin Deficiency:*

- Dry cough with little mucus (if mucus is present, yellow and sticky)
- Dry skin/mouth/throat/stools
- Night sweats, five-center heat
- Excessive thirst

## Emotional Symptoms

- Grief
- Sadness
- Feeling as if the past grief experience just occurred
- Irritation
- Withdrawn
- Feeling of isolation
- Lack of confidence

## Treatment Principle

Benefit the Lung, Strengthen the Po, Tonify the Lung Qi, and/or Nourish the Lung Yin.

## Acupuncture

| | |
|---|---|
| LU-9 and UB-64 | *Qi Deficiency:* |
| LU-7 and KD-6 | LU-9 and KD-3 |
| LI-10 and R-11 | UB-43 and UB-13 |
| ST-36 and R-6 | 1010.22 Bi Yi (Nasal Wing), right side for female |
| LU-1 and SP-6 | and left side for male |
| LU-3 and SP-3 | Infrared heat on the lower abdomen for patients |
| UB-13 and DU-12 | without excess heat |
| 1010.20 Shuijin | *Yin Deficiency:* |
| DU-20, DU-24, and Ah Shi 2 cun lateral to DU-24 | LU-9 and KD-7 |
| Auricular: Upper and Lower Lung, Shen Men | |

## Herbal Formulas

| Diagnosis | Formula (with or without modifications) |
|---|---|
| Lung Qi Deficiency | Bu Fei Tang (Tonify the Lung Decoction) (Chen and Chen 2009, p.560) |
| Lung Yin Deficiency | Bai He Gu Jin Tang (Lily Bulb Decoction to Preserve the Metal)<br>*With heat add:*<br>Zhi Mu (Rhizoma Anemarrhenae)<br>Yu Xing Cao (Herba Houttuyniae) (Chen and Chen 2009, pp.1036–1037) |
| Chronic Grief Exhausting the Yin | Bu Fei E Jiao Tang (Tonify the Lung Decoction with Ass-Hide Gelatin) (Chen and Chen 2009, p.1039) |
| Lung Qi and Yin Deficiency | Sheng Mai San (Generate the Pulse Powder)<br>*With irritability and insomnia add:*<br>Suan Zao Ren (Semen Ziziphi Spinosae)<br>Bai Zi Ren (Semen Platycladi)<br>*More yin deficiency than qi deficiency:*<br>Substitute Xi Yang Shen (Radix Panacis Quinquefolii) for Ren Shen (Radix et Rhizoma Ginseng)<br>*Faint pulse and risk of shock:*<br>Increase Ren Shen (Radix et Rhizoma Ginseng) to a large dose (Chen and Chen 2009, pp.554–555) |

## Affirmation

"I am at peace gently moving through life, feeling strong, confident, and connected to my environment."

### *Phlegm and Damp Accumulation*

*Pathophysiology*

Long-term grief inhibits the circulation of fluids in the lungs, causing phlegm and dampness accumulation. This commonly results in a stubborn chronic cough or sinus congestion. In some patients, the phlegm will generate heat. Treating the tai yin channel resolves the phlegm/dampness and allows the body to process the trauma. Dietary choices play a major role in the resolution of this pattern, and nutritional counseling is important.

Refer to the Phlegm and Damp Accumulation pattern presented in the Worry section above.

## Mood Swings

Reliving a trauma memory causes a host of emotions, and some patients can suffer extreme mood swings. The emotions surge between yin feelings (depression, sadness, worry, and fear) and yang feelings (anxiety, mania, anger, and rage). The yin feelings suppress and block qi, and the yang feelings arouse qi. The energy in the organ systems fluctuates greatly and needs to be regulated. For these patients, there is a combination of heat with deficiency or accumulation. The possible diagnoses are:

- Liver Qi Stagnation with Heat

- Blood Stagnation with Heat

- Phlegm and Damp Accumulation with Heat

- Heart and Kidney Yin Deficiency with Heat.

### *Liver Qi Stagnation with Heat*

*Pathophysiology*

The liver organ system maintains the channel flow, keeping the pathways open. When the liver qi stagnates, movement is depressed, tension and heat build, and yang rises, resulting in anger. The flow can become so blocked and the Hun so constrained that rage flares up and explosive reactions ensue. Cycling between depression and anger/rage characterizes the condition. By freeing the qi stagnation and clearing the heat/fire, the Hun is liberated.

Refer to the Liver Qi Stagnation with Heat pattern in the Depression section above.

### Blood Stagnation with Heat

*Pathophysiology*

Patients suffer chronic stagnation when a trauma goes unresolved for several years. Blood stagnation develops, which is exacerbated in those patients taking pharmaceutical medication. The stagnation generates heat, giving rise to fluctuations in moods; patients cycle between depression and anxiety/manic behavior. Each time the trauma memory is triggered, heat and pressure increase in the channels, creating vocal or violent outbursts. Signs of blood stagnation and a history of chronically reliving an emotional trauma confirm the diagnosis.

Refer to the Blood Stagnation pattern in the Depression section above.

### Phlegm and Damp Heat Accumulation with Heat

*Pathophysiology*

Congested fluids bog down the body and generate feelings of depression, sadness, worry, and lethargy. When the fluid accumulation stews long enough, heat produces the yang feelings of anxiety, irritation, and anger—the emotions cycle between the suppressed and expressed. Diagnosing this pattern can be easy when the phlegm signs are obvious, but sometimes the phlegm is subtle and hidden. Channel palpation and pulse diagnosis are some of the best techniques used to uncover this pattern.

Refer to the Phlegm and Damp Accumulation with Heat pattern in the Depression section above.

### Heart and Kidney Yin Deficiency with Heat

*Pathophysiology*

The communication between the heart and kidney balances the fire and water of the body. When the yin becomes deficient, the fire is no longer managed by the water, giving rise to heat and anxiety. The deficiency causes the body to feel tired at the core, but the uncontrolled heat produces restlessness. Patients fluctuate between these extremes. Women going through menopause frequently experience this oscillation due to the sea of yin waning in older age. Heat flares up unrestrained by the fluid deficiency. Any patient with yin deficiency is susceptible to a resurgence of a trauma that was suppressed. The rising fire due to yin deficiency releases the trauma memory.

Refer to the Heart and Kidney Yin Deficiency with Heat pattern in the Anxiety section above.

## Summary of the Emotional Symptoms

Emotional trauma uniquely affects the qi dynamic of each organ system and involves multiple emotions, organ systems, and pathogens. The layers of trauma are uncovered as treatment progresses, shedding light on hidden emotions and pathogens. As the qi dynamic is restored for one organ system, another might show a need for balancing when the emotional symptoms change. Generally, starting with the primary organ system involved will bring the most balance and—at times—secondary and tertiary patterns resolve.

## BEHAVIORAL SYMPTOMS

Disharmony of the five spirits creates unhealthy reactions to emotional trauma and its memory. Patients can shut down, get trapped in negative thought patterns, and/or harm themselves. Behaviors are reflections of the unprocessed trauma disturbing the spirits of the organ systems. All warriors have scars, and Chinese medicine balances the disharmony to allow the scar of trauma to heal, no longer causing behavioral patterns.

## Avoidance/Disassociation

The emotional trauma and its memory can overwhelm a patient's ability to face the world or people, places, and activities that remind them of their trauma. They feel like crawling into a hole and shutting out life—a yin activity—caused by either qi/yang deficiency or qi and blood stagnation. Each mind/spirit plays a role in a person's ability to engage life. The table below summarizes the spirit pathophysiology, some general symptoms, and possible diagnoses.

**AVOIDANCE/DISASSOCIATION AND THE FIVE MINDS**

| Mind | Avoidance/Disassociation | Common Signs/ Symptoms | Common Diagnoses |
|------|--------------------------|------------------------|------------------|
| Zhi | Fear from the trauma weakens the Zhi and therefore the drive and stability to engage. | Low back and knee pain; urinary issues; deep proximal pulses; markings on the chin and under the eyes; dip in the back of the tongue. | 1. Qi Stagnation<br>2. Kidney Qi Deficiency<br>3. Kidney Yin Deficiency<br>4. Kidney Yang Deficiency<br>5. Heart and Kidney Yin Deficiency with Heat |
| Hun | The Hun is constrained or destabilized, hindering the courage to engage. | Darkness and green in the temples; curled tongue sides; tenderness at LV-2 and LV-3; hypochondriac pain. | 1. Qi Stagnation<br>2. Blood Stagnation<br>3. Liver Yin/Blood Deficiency |

| Mind | Avoidance/Disassociation | Common Signs/ Symptoms | Common Diagnoses | | |
|------|--------------------------|------------------------|------------------|---|---|
| Shen | The heart mirror is distorted, causing the Shen to misperceive the environment and be overwhelmed and retreat. | Heightened anxiety and panic attacks; nodules between HT-7 and HT-4. | 1. | Heart Qi and Yin Deficiency | |
| | | | 2. | Heart Qi and Blood Deficiency | |
| | | | 3. | Heart and Gallbladder Qi Deficiency | |
| | | | 4. | Phlegm Heat | |
| | | | 5. | Blood Stagnation | |
| Yi | Constantly thinking about the trauma weakens the Yi, causing inaction. | Digestive disorders; rumination; nodules between SP-3 and SP-4. | 1. | Spleen and Stomach Qi Stagnation | |
| | | | 2. | Spleen Qi and Blood Deficiency | |
| | | | 3. | Phlegm Damp Accumulation | |
| Po | The Po and a person's self-esteem are destabilized, resulting in a desire to withdraw. | Hypersensitivity; hollowness and lines in the cheeks; cough; wheeze; nodules in the lung channel. | 1. | Lung Qi Deficiency | |
| | | | 2. | Lung Yin Deficiency | |
| | | | 3. | Phlegm Damp Accumulation | |

# Negative Thinking

The five spirits work in harmony to support positive thoughts. An imbalance in any of the five elements can lead to a patient feeling hopelessness, lack of joy, and unable to see the positive. Negative thoughts take hold of the patient and their overall approach to life. The table below differentiates the effect of trauma on the five elements. The diagnostic patterns are similar to those of avoidance.

**THE IMBALANCES OF THE FIVE ELEMENTS CAUSING NEGATIVE THINKING**

| Water | Wood | Fire | Earth | Metal |
|-------|------|------|-------|-------|
| Fear weakens the will power, leading to an inability to resist negative thinking. | The wood element is either blocked or depleted and a person feels overwhelmed, trapped, and unable to decide—causing a negative view of the world. | The joy of life is dampened by the trauma and its memory, leading a patient down a pathway of negative thinking. The heart mirror is distorted. | Ruminating on the trauma can cause a tendency toward victimization and being bogged down by life. | The hopeful quality of the metal element is depleted and negative thoughts take hold. |

Lifestyle recommendations play a significant role in transforming negative thinking. The Shaking Qigong Form "trashes out" the negative thoughts. Positive affirmations take the place of negative thoughts, and gratitude journaling increases positivity.


## Self-Destructive Actions

The triggering of a trauma memory can bring about self-destructive behavior. Reliving the memory creates heat and fire, which rise and stir the spirit, causing self-destructive acts. Accumulated phlegm exacerbates the situation by muddling the spirit. Evaluate the signs and symptoms to determine the nature of the heat and fire (excess and/or deficiency) and the organ systems affected. The primary diagnoses are:

- Liver Heat/Fire

- Heart Heat/Fire

- Yin Deficiency with Heat

- Phlegm Damp Accumulation with Heat

- Blood Stagnation.

**THE VARIOUS EFFECTS OF HEAT AND PHLEGM ON THE ZANG ORGANS**

| Kidney | Liver | Heart | Spleen | Lungs |
| --- | --- | --- | --- | --- |
| Heat depletes the kidney yin and the will to care for the self. | Heat destabilizes the Hun, resulting in reckless decision making and self-harm. | Heat/phlegm disrupts the heart mirror. The perception of self-worth is distorted. | Heat/phlegm disturbs the processing ability of the Yi. Thoughts are muddled and the capacity to nourish the self is weakened. | Heat constrains the lungs and depletes the fluids, which can lead to heat in the upper jiao and disturb the heart. |

*Treatment Tips*

- Integrate the "Soothing the Trauma Memory" protocol into specific organ/channel treatments.

- Calm the spirit by incorporating the auricular acupuncture points Shen Men and Point Zero.

- Bleed the ear apex to clear heat and vent pressure in the channels.

- Teach the patient Metta meditation to shift their behavior from self-harm to positive thoughts and self-love.

- Encourage the patient to focus on hobbies and/or their natural talents to transform their negative reactions into constructive behavior.

Cutting oneself is one manifestation of a self-destructive act. The patient cuts themselves, generally subconsciously, to release the heat and pressure building inside their body. This is an extreme form of self-destructive behavior (which is becoming increasingly prevalent in teenagers), and any patient exhibiting this behavior requires treatment with compassion to prevent any further self-harm. Counseling is essential, and the patient should also see a Western medical doctor to evaluate (and treat if necessary) the wounds for infection. Chinese medicine is an effective part of an integrated team to address this issue. Employing suitable treatment methods to vent the heat relieves the heat/fire pattern and rectifies the imbalance.

## Summary of the Behavioral Symptoms

Treatments are not meant to cause a release of strong emotions. However, as the channels and organ systems rebalance, old trapped trauma is freed and an emotional reaction can occur. Some patients require a staged approach involving the use of the "Gathering the Qi" and "Soothing the Trauma Memory" protocols between individualized organ system treatments. The finesse of the practitioner to understand each patient's constitution and to harmonize the macrocosm with the microcosm yields a smooth transformation.

## PHYSICAL SYMPTOMS

### Insomnia

The yang energy wanes as night falls. Adequate yin secures the spirit; the body rests and regenerates. Emotional trauma and its memory frequently disturb this delicate balance, resulting in waking and restlessness at night. Identifying key diagnostic indicators verifies the type of imbalance causing insomnia.

*Key Diagnostic Indicators*

1. Difficulty falling asleep signifies qi and blood deficiency.

2. Wakefulness between 1 and 3 am is caused by liver stagnation.

3. Sleeping for approximately five hours and then waking reflects a heart organ system disharmony.

4. Waking with heat and night sweats involves a diagnosis of heat, due either to excess or deficiency.

5. Waking at night needing to have a bowel movement is a sign of internal heat. *Note: This is not to be confused with early morning diarrhea belonging to kidney yang deficiency.*

6. Bloating and digestive distress at night indicates the Spleen and Stomach Qi Stagnation pattern.

7. Nightmares and disturbing dreams are caused by heat and qi/blood stagnation.

8. Being startled easily and waking with fright belongs to the Heart and Gallbladder Qi Deficiency pattern.

9. Dreaming of routine and mundane events denotes spleen deficiency.

10. Dreams of one or multiple elements (water, wood, fire, etc.) indicate which organ system is involved.

## Causes of Insomnia

- Liver Qi Stagnation with or without Heat/Fire

- Heart Fire

- Spleen and Stomach Qi Stagnation

- Phlegm Accumulation with Heat

- Blood Stagnation

- Heart and Spleen Qi and Blood Deficiency

- Heart and Kidney Yin Deficiency with Heat

- Heart and Gallbladder Qi Deficiency

- Yin and Blood Deficiency.

(Maclean and Lyttleton 2000, p.860)

## Acupuncture Treatment Tips

The "Soothing the Trauma Memory" protocol and the auricular acupuncture points (Shen Men, Neurological Area, Neurological Point, and Sympathetic) can be incorporated into specific treatments for the various causes of insomnia.

## Deep Sleep Helpful Hints

1. Maintain regular bedtime (making sure to sleep between 11 pm and 3 am).

2. Avoid caffeine in the afternoon/evening.

3. Avoid eating large meals one to two hours before bed.

4. Discontinue screen use (cell phones, TV, computers, etc.) one hour before bed.

5. Drink a small cup of herbal tea, such as chamomile, to settle the body and mind.

6. Gently stretch or read to relax the body and allow the yin energy to build.

7. Dim the lights one hour before bed and sleep in a darkened, cool room.

8. Take flower essences and diffuse essential oils with calming properties.

9. Keep a notepad near the bed to write down and release thoughts arising during the night.

10. Meditate before bedtime.

## Panic Attacks

The Mayo Clinic defines a panic attack as "a sudden episode of intense fear that triggers severe physical reactions when there is no real danger or apparent cause. Panic attacks can be frightening. When panic attacks occur, one might think they are losing control, having a heart attack or even dying" (Mayo Clinic 2017b).

*Symptom Groups and Elements Affected*

- Fear, chest pain, and palpitations = water and fire elements

- Shortness of breath and tightness in the chest = fire and metal elements

- Trembling or shaking and numbness = wood element

- Digestive upset (abdominal pain and nausea) = wood and earth elements

- Feeling detached from reality = metal and fire elements.

Fear and anxiety are common emotions felt, both during the attack and when anticipating another. The "Soothing the Trauma Memory" protocol addresses these emotions and reduces the intensity of the trauma memory, thus diminishing the intensity of future attacks. Auricular acupuncture points—Anxiety, Shen Men, Point Zero, and Sympathetic—are effective points to add to a treatment. Identify the main symptoms of the attack to accurately determine the cause of the pattern. (For a treatment plan refer to the Anxiety section above.)

*Chinese Herbal Formula*

Gan Mai Da Zao Tang Modified (Licorice, Wheat, and Jujube Decoction Modified) settles the restless qi and can be further modified based on the underlying pattern of the panic attacks. Patients can take this during an attack to calm themselves.

*Tips for Soothing the Attack*

- Practice deep breathing techniques focusing on the lower Dantian.

- Utilize EFT.

- Take flower essences and diffuse essential oils with calming properties.

These self-care tips provide the patient with something they can do for themselves, empowering them in the process. These are not to take the place of Western medicine treatment. Patients with severe attacks need to consult a Western medical physician to possibly integrate a biomedical approach to this pattern. Seeing a counselor or psychotherapist is important for expressing the underlying trauma triggered during the attack.

## Emotional Reactivity

The winds of emotion stir with the trauma memory and excite the various organ systems, causing emotional reactivity. Each emotional reaction generally correlates to a certain organ system. Acupuncture points addressing the organ system are coupled with the "Soothing the Trauma Memory" treatment to reduce the severity of emotional reactivity. If the patient reacts strongly to a trauma memory causing their qi to scatter, use the "Gathering the Qi" treatment to stabilize their qi.

CORRELATION OF EMOTIONAL REACTIVITY SYMPTOMS TO
THE ORGAN SYSTEMS IN CHINESE MEDICINE

| Symptoms listed by the Mayo Clinic (2017a) | Organ System Primarily Involved in Chinese Medicine |
|---|---|
| Always being on guard for danger. | Kidney/Urinary Bladder |
| Irritability, angry outbursts, or aggressive/self-destructive behavior, such as drinking too much or driving too fast. | Liver/Gallbladder |
| Being easily startled or frightened. | Heart/Pericardium/Gallbladder |
| Trouble concentrating. | Spleen/Stomach |
| Overwhelming guilt or shame. | Lung/Large Intestine |

A study, published in the journal *Biological Psychiatry*, determined that patients with PTSD were more likely to perceive a world full of threat. Researchers examined 44 soldiers from the Canadian Armed Forces, 22 with PTSD and 22 without. The soldiers were given neuropsychology and clinical exams using certain words. Words related to combat were mixed in with neutral words. All soldiers reacted to the combat words, but the response was heightened for those with PTSD. The visual cortex area of the brain had greater activation for the soldiers with a PTSD diagnosis, showing that patients suffering with PTSD "may literally see a world more populated by traumatic cues, contributing to a positive feedback loop that perpetuates the effects of trauma" (Todd *et al.* 2015).

The trauma memory in patients can change their perception of the world, and these negative thoughts perpetuate the reliving of the trauma. Softening the trauma memory and clearing the heart mirror shifts negative perceptions and stops the feedback loop. Working with the shao yin channel system is essential to returning the patient to a positive view of the world. Helping the patient discover which activities and interests resonate for them brings joy into their life, generating positivity.

Restoring blood and fluids plays a crucial role in resolving emotional reactivity. The vessels must be full of blood and fluids to hold the Shen and maintain an environment not easily stirred by the winds of emotion. Reliving the trauma exhausts the blood and fluids, creating space in the vessels. For each pattern, include some acupuncture points and Chinese herbs that nourish blood and fluids to stabilize the spirit. The primary emotion the patient is feeling guides the differential, along with the symptoms and signs.

*General Diagnoses*

- Heat/Fire

- Qi Stagnation

- Phlegm Accumulation

- Blood Stagnation

- Yin/Blood Deficiency.

*Soothing Emotional Reactivity Self-Care Treatment Tips*

- Practice deep breathing techniques and focus on the lower Dantian.

- Utilize the "Transforming the Emotional Surge" visualization.

- Use EFT.

- Take flower essences and diffuse essential oils with properties associated with the patient's specific emotions to reduce the reactivity.

- For patients lacking a rooted Shen due to blood and/or fluid deficiency, increase protein and fish oil intake.

- Increase the amount of rest and downtime.

## Fatigue

Reliving a trauma memory both exhausts and blocks the body's energy. Differentiating between stagnation and true deficiency is essential. Simply noting the qualities of the pulse and state of the tongue reveals the cause of fatigue in most patients.

*Pathology (can be due to an excess and/or deficient condition)*

- Qi and/or Blood Stagnation

- Phlegm/Damp Accumulation

- Qi, Blood, Yin, and/or Yang Deficiency.

A balanced diet, exercise, meditation, and other lifestyle factors are crucial to build and maintain energy. In addition, help a patient find their passion and life purpose. Facial diagnosis plays a large role in this discovery. By applying facial diagnosis, the practitioner can point out the patient's specific features relating to their inherent talents and abilities. With each successful treatment to build energy, the patient's clarity in realizing their purpose increases. As they begin to manifest their purpose, they start to fully access their Jing and their core energy.

Many patients function on nervous energy and complain of increased tiredness after Chinese medicine treatment. The nervous energy (false fire) gives the patient an artificial sense of strength, yet when this false fire is cleared they feel tired. They experience their true energy level and must understand that time is needed to restore their depleted reserves. Educate the patient about this process so that they comprehend the necessity of, as Brian LaForgia describes, "refilling the aquifers."[2] As treatments progress and their energy is built up, the patient feels a solid source of strength. This base provides a foundation on which to endure future reliving of memories and prevents the leakage of energy.

---

2   Personal communication with Brian LaForgia, L.Ac.

## Poor Concentration

The Yi is frequently derailed by the trauma memory, causing confusion and poor concentration.

*Pathology*

- Spleen Deficiency

- Wood overacting on Earth, that is, Liver Stagnation and Spleen Deficiency

- Phlegm/Damp Accumulation.

The Yi requires a routine lifestyle to establish a steady rhythm. Observing routine mealtimes, a bed time, and other daily schedules encourages a harmonious flow. Follow a diet benefiting the earth element. Enjoying daily exercise to activate the muscles enlivens the Yi and improves concentration. Taking action in life clears the mind and stops the patient's thoughts from "spinning in the mud." Once a decision is made, the Yi is free to process another thought. Akin to throwing sand on railroad tracks, action provides traction to propel the train of thought, keeping the Yi moving on down the tracks.

## Body Pains

Body sensitivity and chronic pain are commonly experienced in those patients suffering from emotional trauma and PTSD (Mostoufi *et al.* 2014). The initial trauma disrupts qi flow in the channels and causes pain and sensitivity. The blockage worsens with reliving the trauma memory and depletes the body's energy. Several patterns of disharmony are involved in body pains.

Blockage in the channel and organ flow can be due to excess and/or deficiency. Channel palpation is a key diagnostic tool used to identify the primary channels causing the pains, that is, nodules at yuan-source points as opposed to shu-stream points. The different emotions triggered by the pain(s) also offer clues to the diagnosis. Emotional trauma can reside deep in the channels buried under several layers of blockage. Encouraging the patient to continue with treatment and educating them about the depth of the trauma helps them to remain hopeful. The blockages eventually resolve with consistent treatment and lifestyle modifications.

*Resolving Body Pain Self-Care Tips*

- Apply acupressure on the shu-stream points.

- Protect the body from external pathogens such as wind/damp/cold.

- Avoid sleeping with an open window or fan blowing air on the neck.

- Practice the Shaking Qigong Form to "trash out" blockages and pathogens.

- Pat down the limbs and torso to move the qi and clear stagnation.

- Practice loving-kindness meditations to stop the loop of negative thoughts about the body; that is, clear negative self-talk like "bad knee" or "stubborn elbow."

- Utilize EFT (especially when pains arise).

- Apply topical liniments/salves (Zheng Gu Shui and Tiger Balm).

- Soak in warm Epsom salt baths.

Pharmaceutical pain medications are helpful in certain situations and can be taken during Chinese medicine treatment. When initiating treatment, have the patient maintain their current regimen of medication to gauge treatment effectiveness. Patients are frequently tempted to abruptly stop using their medication once they feel relief from the pain(s). This practice leads to a rebound of pain, complicating the situation. As the pains subside, the patient can consult with their prescribing physician about tapering off the medication(s). If possible, establish communication between Chinese medicine and Western medicine practitioners. This is optimal for fostering better patient care.

## Sensory Organ Impairment

The trauma memory can be triggered by a sensory stimulation and affect the functioning of a sensory organ. Chinese medicine categorizes each sensory organ by a corresponding internal organ system. The kidneys open to the ears, the liver to the eyes, the heart to the tongue, the spleen to the mouth, and the lungs to the nose. The sensory organ affected provides a clue as to the root of the trauma memory. A patient experiencing visual changes when reliving a trauma memory might have a disturbance in the liver organ system. In contrast, a patient whose smell is weakened may have an issue with the lung organ system. However, this is not a steadfast rule; flexibility is needed when diagnosing the effects on the sensory organs.

### *Identifying the Channel Pathway Affected*

Sensory sensations are not just related to organ systems, but also to channel pathways. Several channels innervate each sensory organ. For example, if auditory cues trigger a trauma memory, the large intestine, san jiao, gallbladder, and small intestine channels need to be evaluated to identify which are affected.

*Using Multiple Treatment Modalities*

Acupuncture, dietary/lifestyle modifications, and Chinese herbal formulas effectively treat the sensory organs. The author rarely uses Chinese herbal formulas to treat sensory conditions, finding acupuncture and dietary/lifestyle modifications sufficient.

*Acupuncture to Treat Sensory Triggers*

Instead of simply selecting a few points for "excess," accurately determine the channel(s) involved. After diagnosing the affected channel(s), utilize both distal and local points synergistically to restore harmony in the sensory organs. Generally, a point combination includes an arm point, a leg point, and a local point. If the sensory organ condition is unilateral, the distal point is chosen on the opposite side and the guiding/directing points are on the same side. For example, for a person with a visual disturbance in the right eye, needle LV-2 on the left, and needle LI-4 and GB-14 on the right. Consider the heavenly stems and earthly branches when crafting a point prescription.

## Auditory Sensations

- A combat veteran hears the whoosh of incoming mortars and takes cover, then realizes he is not in Afghanistan, but in a grocery store parking lot hearing a small jet flying low overhead.

- A recently divorced woman experiences tinnitus every time she is reminded of her ex-husband.

Auditory sensations commonly trigger the trauma memory, *and* the memory itself can obstruct hearing. Both conditions respond well to Chinese medicine treatment. Sounds can elicit emotions (especially fear), and the underlying emotions triggered by the trauma can cause hearing problems such as tinnitus or deafness.

*Tinnitus and Trauma*

Directing treatment to the ears softens the intensity of the auditory trigger. One study, published in the *Journal of Holistic Health* in 2016, proved the effectiveness of treating PTSD-related tinnitus in war veterans with acupuncture (Arhin *et al.* 2016). Differentiation is essential to resolve the tinnitus or auditory triggers.

## TINNITUS PATHOLOGY AND ETIOLOGY

| Common Diagnoses | Etiology |
|---|---|
| Kidney Deficiency | Fear from the trauma depletes the kidneys. |
| Liver Yang Rising | Liver qi stagnation creates heat, leading to yang rising. |
| Blood Stagnation | The trauma creates severe blockage in the channels, causing blood stagnation. |
| Phlegm/Damp Accumulation | The Yi, damaged from rumination on the trauma, produces phlegm and dampness in the ears. |
| Qi and Blood Deficiency | Reliving the trauma exhausts the qi and blood. |
| Channel Involvement due to Stagnation and/or Deficiency | The trauma and its memory affect certain channels innervating the ears. |

## Channel Pathways to the Ears

- San Jiao

- Gallbladder

- Urinary Bladder (Deadman and Al-Khafaji 2007, p.251)

- Heart

- Kidney

- Pericardium

- Large Intestine

- Stomach (Deadman and Al-Khafaji 2007, p.126)

- Small Intestine.

(Wang and Robertson 2008, pp.591–604)

## TINNITUS DIFFERENTIATION

| High-pitched | Excess |
|---|---|
| Low-pitched | Deficiency |
| Water or ocean-like sound | Phlegm/Damp Accumulation |

## Acupuncture

| Qi Stagnation: | With heat: | Phlegm/Damp: | Deficiency: |
|---|---|---|---|
| SJ-3 and KD-1 | SJ-5 and GB-41 | ST-40 and SP-9 and | SJ-4 and KD-3 |
| SJ-6 and GB-34 | SI-2 and LI-11 | R-12 | SI-4 and KD-6 |
| PC-6 and KD-9 | PC-7 and ST-44 | PC-5 and GB-34 | PC-6 and KD-7 |
| SJ-10 and KD-10 | HT-8 and KD-2 | | UB-15 and UB-23 |
| PC-6 and GB-38 | | Blood Stagnation: | LI-10 and GB-39 |
| LI-4 and LI-6 | | GB-20 and SP-10 | ST-36 and SP-6 |
| SI-3 and SI-8 | | GB-39 and SP-6 | HT-7 and KD-3 |
| HT-5 and KD-6 | | | |

| Guide points | Local points |
|---|---|
| SJ-3, SI-3, LI-4, KD-3, or ST-36 | SJ-21, SI-19, GB-2, SJ-17, or GB-8 |
| Auricular points: Ear, Kidney | |

## Self-Care Tips for Resolving Tinnitus

- Practice the *hai hei* kidney massage in the Shaking Qigong Form.

- If the condition is due to heat rising, avoid alcohol, spicy foods, rich meats, and sugar.

- For conditions due to spleen deficiency or phlegm/damp accumulation, avoid cold and raw foods.

- For kidney deficiency, eat seaweed, green leafy vegetables, animal kidney, pig ears, and soups.

- Protect the body from external pathogens such as wind/damp/cold.

## Case Study: Stress Causing Tinnitus

A 54-year-old patient, "Glenice," reported high-pitched tinnitus after starting a new job. Adjusting to her new work environment was incredibly stressful, especially interacting with her overbearing boss. Her constant tinnitus—in the right ear only—worsened when she was at work. She had darkness under her eyes, a scared, vacant Shen, tinnitus markings on her ear (diagonal lines on the ear lobe—not to be confused with the vertical lines associated with blood pressure), nodules at SJ-5, PC-6, and GB-41, a deep, thin, slightly choppy pulse with engorgement at the liver pulse position, and a red, dusky tongue color with a yellow coat. Potential environmental triggers were ruled out, and the diagnosis was yang rising due to kidney yin deficiency.

The patient reported feeling grounded and not intensely triggered by trauma; therefore treatment addressing specific channels started immediately. Prior to needling, acupressure diagnosis (checking which points reduced the tinnitus with pressure) was used to determine the points to select. GB-41 and KD-1 were the most helpful. Pressure on SJ-5 had no effect. KD-1, the jing-well point, was needled bi-laterally to open the ear and clear the channel. GB-41 on the left side was paired with SJ-3 and SJ-21 on the right side. Needling GB-41 cleared heat, while SJ-3 and SJ-21 directed the treatment to her right ear.

After the first treatment, KD-1 was replaced with KD-4 (the luo-connecting point) because the tinnitus reduced when the point was pressed (luo-connecting points open the channels and remove stagnation). By the fourth treatment, Glenice only experienced tinnitus in the evenings and her yellow tongue coating disappeared. The treatment focus shifted to nourishing yin and KD-4 was replaced with KD-7 (the mother point on the water channel). As she improved, her Shen began to glow, the tinnitus markings on her ear became less apparent (Figure 4.1), the nodules on the channels reduced, and her pulse was fuller. By her seventh treatment, Glenice barely noticed the tinnitus and the treatments were tapered off until her condition resolved.

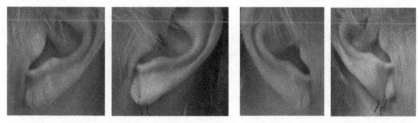

*Figure 4.1 Tinnitus Markings: left ear before, left ear after, right ear before, and right ear after*

### Summary of Auditory Sensations

Tinnitus and hearing loss are some of the most difficult conditions to treat. If there is physical damage or hearing loss due to aging, the treatment effectiveness is minimal to none. Educate patients about the challenges of treating hearing issues. Significant results are rarely seen in one or two treatments. Reducing the intensity of the memory restores accurate auditory perception. The quieter the spirit, the more a person can hear.

## Visual Disturbances

- A woman sees a red truck headed straight for her. After a few deep breaths, she realizes it is only changing lanes and is not the same truck that collided with her last year.

- An elderly man suffers from blurry vision every time he remembers the flood that destroyed his home several years earlier.

*Perception is a clash of mind and eye, the eye believing
what it sees, the mind seeing what it believes.*

Robert Brault

Patients with PTSD and emotional trauma often have visual disturbances and hallucinations when the trauma memory is provoked. Visual disturbances can range from mild, blurry vision to full hallucinations. Patients require a full work-up with an ophthalmologist to rule out any organic issues before receiving Chinese medicine treatment. They must also undergo a psychological evaluation and be encouraged to see a psychiatrist or psychologist for routine treatment and counseling.

*Persons appear to us according to the light we
throw upon them from our own minds.*

Laura Ingalls Wilder

The liver organ system opens and directs blood to the eyes; imbalances in this system commonly cause visual disturbances. This is not the only channel to consider, but is one to begin with and rule out. Liver blood stagnation, heat, and/or deficiency hinder the nourishment of the eyes. The triggering of the trauma memory usually affects the blood and can easily disturb the vision. However, the liver blood is only one factor. Additionally, the heart mirror, stirred by the memory, reflects unclearly and distorts vision. Blockages in any of the channels to the eyes can impair the vision. Therefore, employ meticulous diagnostic skill to tease out the root.

Once a clear diagnosis is formulated, use a point prescription combining distal and local acupuncture points. A short list is offered in the table below to provide ideas for clearing heat, opening channel flow, and generating blood. The "Soothing the Trauma Memory" protocol restores proper visual perceptions and is commonly added to the differentiated point combinations. Choosing two distal points and two local points is sufficient. LI-4 is a wonderful distal guiding point and can be shown to patients for self-acupressure care between treatments.

**VISUAL DISTURBANCE PATHOLOGY AND ETIOLOGY**

| Common Diagnoses | Etiology |
| --- | --- |
| Blood Heat | Reliving the trauma generates heat that disturbs the heart mirror and distorts vision. |
| Qi/Blood Stagnation | Blockage in the channels resulting from trauma impedes circulation to the eyes and causes visual changes. |
| Yin/Blood Deficiency with Internal Wind | The triggering of the trauma memory depletes yin and blood and generates wind that distorts vision. |

*Channel Pathways to the Eyes*

- Liver

- Heart

- Stomach

- Small Intestine

- Urinary Bladder

- San Jiao

- Gallbladder

- Ren

- Du

- Yin Qiao

- Yang Qiao.

(Wang and Robertson 2008, pp.591–606)

*Acupuncture*

| Blood Heat: | Qi/Blood Stagnation: | Yin/Blood Deficiency: |
|---|---|---|
| LI-11 and LV-2 | LI-4 and LV-3 | SI-4 and ST-36 |
| HT-8 and GB-41 | LI-6 and LV-5 | SI-4 and R-4 |
| PC-7 and ST-44 | SI-3 and ST-43 | LV-8 and GB-40 |
| SJ-5 and LV-2 | UB-7 and UB-62 | LV-3 and GB-39 |
| Bleed LV-1, GB-44, or the ear apex | SJ-6 and GB-34 | SI-6 and KD-6 |

| Guide points | Local points |
|---|---|
| LI-4, SI-3, or SJ-3 | GB-14, UB-1, UB-2, Tai Yang (M-HN-9), Yin |
| Auricular points: Eye, Liver | Tang (M-HN-3), or ST-2 |

Stimulating the point 55.02 Huaguyi (Flower Bone One), of the Master Tung family acupuncture system, successfully treats various eye conditions. This includes visual disturbances due to emotional trauma. The four-point unit is on the bottom of the foot between the first two metatarsals, opposite the liver channel. Adjacent to the kidney channel, the point set is akin to directing water to the wood element to support the eyes. When needled mindfully, the patient experiences minimal discomfort.

*Self-Care Tips for Benefiting the Eyes*

- Increase consumption of protein, beets, spinach, carrots, animal liver, animal heart, nuts, seeds, and bone broth.

- Drink either the "Root of Inspiration" or "Super Blood and Qi" soup to benefit yin and blood.

- Increase fish oil intake (for those adventurous patients, eating fish eyes is a classic prescription).

- Reduce activities that strain the eyes, for example screen time.

- Emphasize "shaking the eyes" in the Shaking Qigong Form to improve the vision.

- Benefit the wood element by exercising and spending time in nature to activate the blood.

- Gently tap on the acupuncture points around the eyes.

*The Trauma Memory Causing Patients to "See Things"*

Many patients involved in car accidents experience mild hallucinations following the accident. They imagine cars coming toward them or pulling out in front of them. They feel anxious while driving and feel angry and stifled by their lack of courage to get behind the wheel. Usually there is a combination of jue yin and shao yin channel involvement. Several patients regain their driving confidence and their clear perception after Chinese medicine treatment. Acupuncture prescriptions begin with the "Gathering the Qi" to settle the qi after the accident, and then shift to the "Soothing the Trauma Memory" protocol to calm their Shen. And, finally, the point combinations listed above resolve the issue completely.

> *When you change the way you look at*
> *things, the things you look at change.*
>
> Wayne Dyer

## Case Study: Imaginary Cars

A 35-year-old patient, "Lucile," continued to "see" cars pulling out in front of her after suffering a major car accident. She sought Chinese medicine treatment and was diagnosed with Scattered Qi, Liver Qi Stagnation, and Blood Deficiency. First the "Gathering the Qi" protocol was used, followed by incorporating the "Soothing the Trauma Memory" protocol. Her treatment occurred in February (the heavenly stem is Jia), relating to the gallbladder. GB-14 and GB-39—coupled with the "Soothing the Trauma Memory" protocol—resolved her paranoid visions and she could drive confidently after three treatments. The use of local and distal points worked synergistically to quickly restore accurate perception.

## Case Study: Quickly Restoring Proper Vision

A 53-year-old man, "Joey," came in with a recent case of strabismus. He had experienced a stressful event and woke with his eyes crossed. His condition started five days before seeking help. The use of UB-2 and ST-36 resolved the condition in one treatment. Joey was treated in October (the heavenly stem is Wu and the earthly branch is Xu—both relating to the stomach organ). The stomach channel travels to the eyes, and ST-36 is frequently used to support healthy qi and blood flow to the eyes. ST-36 was activated to stabilize his qi, blood, and eyesight. The stimulation of UB-2 guided the treatment and benefited his eyes.

### *Speech Disorders*

- A mother becomes "tongue tied" every time she recounts the traumatic delivery of her son.

The shock of an emotional trauma upsets the Shen and can create speech disorders. The heart opens to the tongue and governs speech and expression. When reminded of past trauma, patients frequently feel powerless and are rendered speechless or incoherent. Chinese medicine effectively stabilizes and calms the Shen, which re-establishes clear speech. Disturbance of speech indicates a significant shock, and patients require evaluation by a Western physician.

**SPEECH DISORDER PATHOLOGY AND ETIOLOGY**

| Common Diagnoses | Etiology |
|---|---|
| Heart and Kidney Yin Deficiency | The shock of the trauma disturbs the heart and affects expression. This can be compounded by fear exhausting the kidneys, which affects heart and kidney communication. |
| Heart and Spleen Qi and Blood Deficiency | The trauma unsettles the Shen and disrupts speech. Reliving the trauma weakens the spleen and the musculature of the tongue. The spleen is associated with speech issues involving the movement of the tongue to form words (Wang and Robertson 2008, p.616). |
| Blood Stagnation | Blockages created by the trauma affect the microcirculation and the ability to speak clearly. |

## Channel Pathways to the Tongue

- Spleen

- Heart

- Kidney

- Ren

- Du

- Yin Wei

- Yin Qiao

(Wang and Robertson 2008, pp.594–598, 613)

## Acupuncture

| Heart and Kidney Involvement: | Spleen Involvement: | Blood Stagnation: |
|---|---|---|
| HT-5 and KD-6 | SI-8 and SP-9 | HT-5 and KD-6 |
| HT-4 or HT-6 and KD-7 | SI-4 and SP-6 | SP-9 and KD-9 |
| HT-6 and GB-39 | SI-6 and SP-5 | SP-10 and KD-8 |
| HT-7 and SP-6 | SP-3 and ST-36 | |
| HT-7 and KD-3 | SP-1 and ST-41 | |
| HT-3 and GB-34 | | |
| HT-4 and GB-38 | | |
| HT-7 and GB-40 | | |
| HT-8 and KD-2 | | |

| Guide points | Local points |
|---|---|
| HT-7, KD-7, and SP-5<br>Auricular point: Stomach | R-23, R-24, R-22, or 1010.20 Shuijin |

## Self-Care Tips for Resolving Speech Disorders

- Increase expressive activities, for example journaling and singing.

- Emphasize "shaking of the tongue" during the Shaking Qigong Form.

- Utilize flower essences and essential oils that aid in expression.

- Increase consumption of protein, beets, spinach, carrots, animal liver, animal heart, nuts, seeds, and bone broth.

**NUTRITIONAL SUGGESTIONS**

| | |
|---|---|
| Heart and Kidney Deficiency | • Increase consumption of green vegetables, seaweed, high quality meat, deer, buffalo, salmon, and bitter foods. |
| | • Drink "Great Communicator" clear broth soup. |
| | • Avoid hot spicy foods and fluids, including alcohol, coffee, sugar, rich meats, and shellfish. |
| Spleen Deficiency | • Eat a bland diet consisting of warm, whole-cooked foods, smaller meals, and clear broth soups; cook food slowly. |
| | • Observe regular mealtimes; chew food thoroughly; eat when relaxed; no working while eating; and avoid stressful conversations at mealtime. |
| | • Avoid smoothies, juices, dairy products, wheat, refined sugars, greasy foods, tofu, and cold-natured foods. |

Speech disorders due to trauma respond well to frequent treatments. Integrating care is an important part of the treatment process. Once the heart, kidney, and spleen are functioning harmoniously, the patient can clearly express their inner beauty.

> *Self-expression must pass into*
> *communication for its fulfillment.*
>
> *Pearl S. Buck*

## Changes in Taste and Food Sensitivities

- A woman bites a nectarine and the taste of the fruit triggers the memory of the day her son was hospitalized with leukemia.

Taste can link a patient with the trauma memory and cause them to relive it.

### The Earth and the Mouth

The spleen—the earth element—opens to the mouth and governs taste. Emotional trauma disrupts the rhythm of the earth element and causes changes in taste and, in some cases, food sensitivities. Patients can report tasting certain flavors after a trauma and experience digestion problems, poor appetite, and/or food cravings. Specific foods can trigger and intensify the trauma memory. The tastes a patient describes relate to the five elements and aid in determining the organ system affected. For example, if a memory is triggered by bitter foods, the heart is likely affected, rather than a memory triggered by sour foods resulting in a liver system imbalance. Eating disorders can be triggered by a trauma memory and would fall into this category. (Patients who are experiencing eating disorders must seek counseling. The combination of Chinese medicine and psychological care is essential to bring resolution to this difficult issue.)

Typically, begin treatment with the earth element; focus acupuncture points on the leg tai yin and yang ming channels. For cases involving other channels traveling to the mouth, consider the luo-connecting points or the shu-stream points. As with other conditions relating to the senses, a distal pair added to a guide and local point is recommended. The point prescriptions vary based on the root cause of excess or deficiency.

**TASTE AND FOOD SENSITIVITY PATHOLOGY AND ETIOLOGY**

| Common Diagnoses | Etiology |
|---|---|
| Spleen and Stomach Qi Stagnation | The rumination on the trauma memory stagnates qi in the digestive system, affecting the ability to taste. |
| Spleen Deficiency | Reliving the trauma memory depletes the spleen, leading to food cravings (especially sugar) and taste sensitivity. |
| Phlegm/Damp Accumulation with/without Heat | A weakened spleen due to trauma generates phlegm and damp that obstructs taste. |

## Channel Pathways to the Tongue, Mouth, and Lips

- Spleen

- Stomach

- Kidney

- Liver

- Large Intestine

- Ren

- Chong

- Du

- Yin Qiao

- Yin Wei.

(Wang and Robertson 2008, pp.598, 602–604, and 617)

## *Acupuncture*

*Distal points relating to the spleen:*
ST-36 and SP-9
SI-4 and SP-3
SP-3 and SP-9
SP-4 and ST-43
SP-3 and R-12
SP-5 and ST-44
R-12 and SP-9 and ST-40
Auricular points: Shen Men and Stomach
Cupping *Shen Que* R-8

*Note:* The auricular points Shen Men and Stomach effectively treat food cravings.

| Guide points | Local points |
|---|---|
| SP-3, SP-4, and ST-36 | R-24 |
| Auricular points: Spleen and Stomach | |

## *Self-Care Tips for Restoring Taste*

- Eat warm, simple, whole-cooked meals; use sauces and spices minimally; eat high quality meats; chew food thoroughly.

- Drink one cup of "Super Qi and Blood" clear broth soup daily.

- Enjoy small meals; follow a regular mealtime schedule; eat when relaxed; no working while eating; and avoid stressful conversations when eating.

- Avoid raw foods, smoothies, juices, dairy products, wheat, refined sugars, greasy foods, tofu, and cold-natured foods.

## **Olfactory Impairment**

- A man smells jasmine perfume and is reminded of his ex-wife and their traumatic divorce.

- A woman experiences a total loss of smell after being given a terminal diagnosis.

The sense of smell is governed by the lungs, the most external of the zang organs. After an emotional trauma, patients may experience a reduction in the sensitivity of smell or they might develop hypersensitivity. In some cases, the patient completely loses their sense of smell. The metal element is sensitive, and specific smells triggering the trauma memory hinder the Po by constraining or weakening its function. Stabilizing the Po and benefiting the lungs restores the sense of smell and a person's ability to establish clear boundaries with their environment.

### Reducing Chemical Sensitivity

Patients can become sensitive to chemicals following trauma and experience physical and emotional reactions. Laundry detergents, pesticides, perfumes, body lotions, deodorizers, and many more can trigger the trauma memory, causing emotional surges and physical ailments (including skin rashes and neurological conditions). Scientists link emotional changes to chemical sensitivity and believe chemical sensitivity "is not a functional or psychologic illness or a belief system of the patient" (Ross 1992). With the increased use of chemicals in our environment, this condition is prevalent. Clinically, many patients who suffer from chemical sensitivity report experiencing emotional trauma.

Dietrich Klinghardt (an expert in the field of treating Lyme disease) correlates toxin accumulation with emotional trauma. He finds that, once the trauma is resolved, toxins clear at a faster rate. Klinghardt compares certain emotions to the functions of organs (e.g., anger affects liver function, and fear distresses the kidneys). He describes a vicious cycle wherein emotions decrease blood flow to the organs, which in turn leads to a build-up of toxins. The increased toxins further damage the organs (Klinghardt 2009). Chinese medicine can both transform the emotional trauma and improve circulation of qi and blood.

---

## Case Study: Trauma Causing the Loss of the Sense of Smell

There are documented cases where people have experienced an emotional trauma and were left with only the ability to smell pesticides, cleaning products, perfumes, and similar. A 38-year-old man, "Hector," was under tremendous stress, going through a divorce, while caring for his physically and mentally challenged daughter. During this time, his sense of smell changed and left him only able to smell pesticides and laundry products. He was treated using LI-20 and Yin Tang, coupled with ST-36 and SP-9. After six sessions, Hector's ability to properly smell returned and his sensitivity to chemicals reduced.

---

### Inheriting Trauma via Smell

Western medical research links the triggering of traumatic memories and smell. Researchers have also proved that traumatic memories can be passed down generationally. One study using mice (humans and mice share a similar genetic blueprint, having 99% of genes in common) showed that the mice trained to fear a specific scent passed this fear down two generations. The mice were exposed to a cherry blossom scent and given an electric shock and developed a fear of the smell. Mice of the next two generations exhibited the same reaction to the smell. The mice had a startle reaction to the smell, and receptors associated with the specific scent in their brain became enlarged (Wolynn 2016, pp.35–37).

> *For the sense of smell, almost more than any other, has the*
> *power to recall memories and it's a pity we use it so little.*
>
> Rachel Carson

An evaluation by an otolaryngologist (Ear, Nose, and Throat Physician) is needed to determine any physical damage to the sinuses or nasal obstruction. This information assists with the diagnosis in Chinese medicine. Not all cases of olfactory impairment are due solely to a lung imbalance—they can stem from other organ systems or from blocked channels that have pathways to the nose. Acupuncture treatment for cases involving a lung imbalance focuses on the tai yin and yang ming channels. Select a distal point pair along with a guide point and one or two local points. If only one nostril is affected, follow the protocol of the distal points on the opposite side and the guide and local points on the same side.

**OLFACTORY IMPAIRMENT PATHOLOGY AND ETIOLOGY**

| Common Diagnoses | Etiology |
|---|---|
| Lung Qi Stagnation | The emotional trauma impedes lung qi flow, causing olfactory impairment. |
| Lung Qi and Yin Deficiency | Reliving the trauma memory exhausts the lung qi and yin, creating olfactory impairment. |
| Phlegm/Damp Accumulation | Toxins generate phlegm and damp, block the lungs, and affect the sense of smell. |
| Heat Toxin Accumulation | Environmental toxins and blockages created by the trauma lead to accumulated heat in the lungs that damage the sense of smell. |

## Channel Pathways to the Nose

- Stomach

- Large Intestine

- Urinary Bladder

- Small Intestine

- Yin Qiao

- Heart divergent channel

- Kidney divergent channel

- Du

(Wang and Robertson 2008, pp.592–593, 595, 619)

## Acupuncture

| Lung Qi Stagnation: | Lung Qi and Yin Deficiency: | Phlegm/Damp Accumulation: |
|---|---|---|
| LU-8 and LI-5 | LU-9 and UB-64 | LI-6 and ST-40 |
| LU-7 and LI-6 | LU-7 and KD-6 | LU-8 and ST-40 |
| LU-5 and LI-11 | LI-4 and ST-36 | *Heat Accumulation:* |
| LU-3 and LI-18 | LI-10 and ST-36 | LU-11 and LI-1 |
| LU-10 and LI-3 | HT-7 and ST-36 | LU-6 and LI-11 |
| LU-6 and UB-63 | | Bleed ear apex or DU-10 (with cup) |

| Guide points | Local points |
|---|---|
| LI-4 or 11.17 Mu (Wood point) | LI-20, DU-26, Yin Tang (M-HN-3), 1010.20 |
| Auricular points: Upper or Lower Lung and Nose | Shui Jin, 1010.21 Yuhuo (Jade Fire), or 1010.22 Biyi (Nasal Wing) |

*Note:* 11.17 Mu (Wood point) is a two-point unit and only the proximal point is needed for cases involving the sinuses. This point is used in the Master Tung Family Lineage system for a runny nose due to a common cold (Young 2005, p.20). Clinically, it is effective for treating olfactory triggers of the trauma memory.

### Activating the Master Tung Point 1010.20 Shui Jin to Restore Proper Smell

1010.20 is indicated for kidney disease and breathing issues (Young 2005, pp.148–149). Because of its connection to the kidney, it can address the fear involving certain smells and help the lungs to grasp the qi in breathing disorders. Thus, patients suffering from chemical sensitivity and smells that trigger a trauma memory benefit from the stimulation of this point. Proper needling technique is crucial to obtain the maximum effect. A 36-gauge, 1½ cun needle is inserted at 1010.20 and angled subcutaneously toward the zygoma (approximately toward ST-7) (Young 2008, p.229).

### Bleeding Ling Tai DU-10

Heat and toxins frequently accumulate in the blood and impair the lungs' function. When the patient is exposed to a triggering smell, this can act like a toxin and cause lung dysfunction. Bleeding DU-10 clears heat and toxin (Deadman and Al-Khafaji 1998, pp.541–542).

## Case Study: Toxins Triggering Trauma

A 60-year-old woman, "Francine," was exposed to mold and household chemicals that triggered memories of childhood abuse. Abuse, especially experienced during childhood, damages the Po and the ability to maintain healthy boundaries with the environment. Francine's exposure to toxins further destabilized her Po and caused physical and emotional symptoms. The detrimental physiological effects of the chemicals created tangible issues and activated the emotions she experienced as a child. She moved out of the house that was contaminated with the mold and chemicals, but still developed an intense chemical sensitivity to laundry detergents, perfumes, pesticides, cleaning agents, and deodorants. Interestingly, perfume and cologne caused emotional symptoms (anxiety, anger, reactivity, and crying easily), while cleaning agents and pesticides caused physical symptoms (coughing, extreme fatigue, dizziness, muscle twitching, and confusion). She experienced these symptoms daily; they would be activated when someone wearing perfume simply walked by her or if she drove by a field recently sprayed with pesticide.

Treatment began with the "Gathering the Qi" protocol, followed by the "Soothing the Trauma Memory" protocol. Once Francine's qi was centered and the intensity of the trauma memory reduced, she was given the diagnosis of Lung Qi Deficiency with Heat Phlegm Toxin Accumulation. She had a red-colored tongue (red prickles on the front third) with a yellow, greasy coat, and a slippery pulse. Nodules were detected between the lung and pericardium channels at the level of LU-6.

Primarily, points on the tai yin and yang ming channels were used over several months. LU-5, ST-40, and 1010.20 (Shui Jin) were some of the main points incorporated into consecutive treatments. The physical and emotional symptoms lessened but Francine still experienced some intense flare-ups around chemicals; her tongue remained red with a greasy, yellow coat. Treatment was modified to include bleeding DU-10 to clear the phlegm heat toxin accumulation. Francine reported significant relief with the treatment and, after three sessions, the frequency of her reactions to chemicals was reduced from several times a week to a few times per month.

### Utilizing Essential Oils to Stabilize the Spirit

Scents can transport a person into the past and trigger memories. Each smell can create different emotional responses: positive, neutral, or negative. Scientists published a study in *Psychological Science* in 2015, explaining how smells can elicit both positive and negative responses. For many years, science has proved that odors caused negative emotions, but this study suggested odors could cause a happy state of mind as well (de Groot *et al.* 2015). The use of essential oils is an example of how scents stabilize and elevate mood. In addition to using oils to improve the emotional state, strengthening the function of the nose by using acupuncture points frees the patient from reliving the trauma memory and allows them to be in the present moment.

### Summary of Sensory Impairment

The heart mirror, when clear, accurately perceives the world. As Morihei Ueshiba explains, "Polish the heart, free the six senses and let them function without obstruction, and your entire body will glow" (Ueshiba 2007, p.60). The Shen is easily disturbed by emotional trauma, and the senses can become muddled. These sensory symptoms provide clues as to the main causes of the difficulties affecting the organ systems. Bringing harmony to the senses allows the body, mind, and spirit to flourish.

### Summary of the Physical Symptoms

Many patients feel more comfortable discussing physical ailments than delving into their emotional state. As their physical symptoms reduce, generally any emotional imbalance corrects and the impact of the emotional trauma on the body (both physically and emotionally) resolves. Patients experience significant treatment on multi-dimensional levels and gain trust in Chinese medicine and in their practitioner, which frequently leads to open discussions about emotions and feelings. This transformation comprises part of the overall evolution of their self-awareness and expansion of their energy field.

Moreover, Chinese medicine's ability to treat the physical symptoms of emotional trauma wins the trust of professionals in other medical fields. Western medicine practitioners who specialize in emotional trauma become receptive to Chinese medicine when they observe positive physical symptom results of this complex syndrome. This can encourage collaboration. As Chinese medicine treatment grows in prevalence, may the teamwork between the various types of medicine thrive.

## SUMMARY OF DIFFERENTIATING THE EMOTIONAL, BEHAVIORAL, AND PHYSICAL SYMPTOMS OF TRAUMA

> *When the sun is shining I can do anything; no mountain*
> *is too high, no trouble too difficult to overcome.*
>
> *Wilma Rudolph*

Wilma Rudolph was the first American woman to win three gold medals in a single Olympics. Winning three gold medals is remarkable, and in Rudolph's case her background made her accomplishment phenomenal. Rudolph was a sickly child who had to wear a brace on her left leg. She overcame her disability and went on to win medals in track and field. This degree of determination is required of both the patient and practitioner in the process of resolving emotional trauma.

Patients usually have a combination of emotional, behavioral, and physical issues. The proficiency to determine the main organ system involved correlates with the speed of recovery. In some cases, after the trauma is resolved, the patient experiences a similar stressful event. The patient will seem to be a magnet for a certain type of trauma. There are techniques to help the patient shift their energy/consciousness so that they face future traumatic events with a strong constitution and unwavering spirit. They transform old patterns of reactivity and fully process future traumas, unencumbered on their life's journey. The next step in the treatment of emotional trauma is to ameliorate the degree of impact on the body from future traumatic events.

## References

Arhin, A.O., Gallop, K., Mann, J., Cannon, S., Tran, K., and Wang, M.C. (2016) "Acupuncture as a treatment option in treating posttraumatic stress disorder-related tinnitus in war veterans: a case presentation." *J. Holist. Nurs. 34*, 1, 56–63.

Chen, J., and Chen, T. (2009) *Chinese Herbal Formulas and Applications*. City of Industry, CA: Art of Medicine Press.

de Groot, J.H., Smeets, M.A., Rowson, M.J., Bulsing, P.J., *et al.* (2015) "A sniff of happiness." *Psychol. Sci. 26*, 6, 684–700.

Deadman, P., and Al-Khafaji, M. (1998) *A Manual of Acupuncture*. Hove: Journal of Chinese Medicine Publications.

Deadman, P., and Al-Khafaji, M. (2007) *A Manual of Acupuncture* (Second Edition). Hove: Journal of Chinese Medicine Publications.

Hammer, L. (2001) *Chinese Pulse Diagnosis, Revised Edition*. Seattle: Eastland Press.

Kirschbaum, B. (2000) *Atlas of Chinese Tongue Diagnosis*. Seattle: Eastland Press.

Klinghardt, D. (2009) *Microbes, Toxins, Unresolved Emotional Conflicts: A Unifying Theory*. Available at www.publichealthalert.org/dietrich-klinghardt---microbes-toxins-unresolved-emotional-conflicts-a-unifying-theory.html, accessed on 30 May 2017.

Maclean, W., and Lyttleton, J. (2000) *Clinical Handbook of Internal Medicine, Vol. 1*. Sydney: University of Western Sydney.

Maclean, W., and Lyttleton, J. (2010) *Clinical Handbook of Internal Medicine, Vol. 3*. Sydney: University of Western Sydney.

Mayo Clinic (2017a) *Post-Traumatic Stress Disorder*. Available at www.mayoclinic.org/diseases-conditions/post-traumatic-stress-disorder/basics/risk-factors/con-20022540, accessed on 19 May 2017.

Mayo Clinic (2017b) *Panic Attacks and Panic Disorder*. Available at www.mayoclinic.org/diseases-conditions/panic-attacks/basics/symptoms/con-20020825, accessed on 30 May 2017.

Micleu, C. (2002) *Birth and Beyond*. Lecture at OCOM, February 2002.

Mostoufi, S., Godfrey, K.M., Ahumada, S.M., Hossain, N., *et al.* (2014) "Pain sensitivity in posttraumatic stress disorder and other anxiety disorders: a preliminary case control study." *Ann. Gen. Psychiatry 13*, 1, 31.

National Institute of Mental Health (2016) *Post-Traumatic Stress Disorder*. Available at www.nimh.nih.gov/health/topics/post-traumatic-stress-disorder-ptsd/index.shtml, accessed on 19 May 2017.

Ross, G.H. (1992) "Treatment options in multiple chemical sensitivity." *Toxicol. Ind. Health 8*, 4, 87–94.

Todd, R.M., MacDonald, M.J., Sedge, P., Robertson, A., *et al.* (2015) "Soldiers with posttraumatic stress disorder see a world full of threat: magnetoencephalography reveals enhanced tuning to combat-related cues." *Biol. Psychiatry 78*, 12, 821–829.

Ueshiba, M. (2007) *The Art of Peace* (trans. J. Stevens). Boulder, CO: Shambhala.

Wang, J.-Y., and Robertson, J. (2008) *Applied Channel Theory in Chinese Medicine.* Seattle: Eastland Press.

Wolynn, M. (2016) *It Didn't Start with You.* New York: Viking.

Yanping, S. (2004) "The application of modified xiao yao san in the treatment of gynaecological diseases." *J. of Chin. Med. 74*, 19–23.

Young, W.-C. (2005) *Tung's Acupuncture.* Taipei: Chih-Yuan Book Store.

Young, W.-C. (2008) *Lectures on Tung's Acupuncture Points Study.* Rowland Heights, CA: American Chinese Medicine Cultural Center.

# CHAPTER 5

# Prevention of Emotional Trauma

Emotional trauma is part of the human experience. For many people the trauma is processed and becomes a thing of the past—just a distant memory carrying no emotional weight. However, for others the trauma becomes trapped in the body and the person is unable to move on. Processing emotional trauma is akin to traversing a forest or clearing a hurdle. People become stuck, unable to advance along their path or overcome obstacles. Chinese medicine provides a light with which to navigate the dark woods, and good track shoes for jumping the hurdle. Thus, the person moves into the future without carrying the burden of the emotional trauma. If the trauma is not overcome, it becomes PTSD, and continues to disturb the body physiology and deplete its energy. The person is hindered from realizing their full potential.

## Trauma as a Vehicle for Transformation

The process of resolving emotional trauma serves as a catalyst to open the heart, reduce the ego, and shed the armor. After the transformation, the person's ability to connect with the universe is enhanced. They can discover their personal balance of heavenly pursuits and earthly pleasures to completely embody and express the spirit of the universe. Each emotional trauma has a theme relating to an individual's faulty belief system: for example, "I am not safe around dogs," "All male authority figures will try to take advantage of me," and "All women will leave me." This theme will cycle throughout their life and present similar traumas until the "lesson" is learned. Chinese medicine prevents the trauma from cycling again and again by assisting the patient to completely resolve the trauma.

## Preventive Measures to Surmount Future Trauma

In the future, other traumas might occur and bring up other faulty beliefs. A patient might have processed and dealt with their "mother" issues, yet still have issues regarding money. Chinese medicine stabilizes the patient so that they can process each trauma smoothly. Emotional trauma scatters the qi, creates blockages in the channels, and generates heat. This is ultimately an alchemical-type process wherein one produces gold from raw material. Processing and releasing each traumatic event refines the gold in each person, until they eventually become pure. Then the gold continues to be polished. Preventive treatments and lifestyle modifications halt the tarnishing of this beautiful metal caused by future emotional trauma. As each trauma is processed, the gold shines brighter. There are several examples throughout history of people going through the heroine's or hero's journey to be transformed into an enlightened way of being. Siddhartha is such a story. Chinese medicine stands by and supports the person as they sit under the Bodhi tree.

## Intervention is Needed to Resolve Trauma

The old adages "this too shall pass" and "time heals all wounds" speak to the resolution of emotional trauma. Over time, emotional trauma might not reduce on its own, but may hole up deep in the organs and channels to rise again later in a patient's life. A study in the *Journal of the Association of Psychological Science* proved that major life stressors do not commonly resolve on their own and treatment is needed (Infurna and Luthar 2016).

Full resolution of emotional trauma *is* possible, in addition to finding ways of identifying potential upcoming trauma. Typically, trauma is experienced in cycles, and Chinese medicine can determine the trauma patterns. Treatment plans are established to prevent trauma in the patient's life and in future generations. These include building the Zheng qi (the body's ability to resist disease), helping patients identify their path, and uncovering their talents. Dr. Bessel Van der Kolk, a leading psychiatrist in the field of emotional trauma, emphasizes the idea of restoring a patient's inner compass and helping them to imagine a way to make a situation better (Van der Kolk 2014, p.98). When a person can see a positive way out of their trauma, they are able to move forward. As they advance in life, they experience successes, and with each success become freer from the pull of the trauma.

## The Dark Night of the Soul

Emotional trauma is inevitable as life brings trials and tribulations. However, not everyone develops PTSD after experiencing trauma. Essentially, energy leaks out and creates a space where emotional trauma can reside. When a person's energy is clear and strong, there is no container to hold the trauma. Not everyone who witnesses or hears about a traumatic event will be wounded or affected long term. Those who have cleared old belief systems and have shifted their perspective will flow through traumatic events with grace and not continue to be charged by the trauma.

Joseph Campbell describes a ritual in Australia:

> "Now, when a boy gets to be, you know, a little bit ungovernable, one fine day the men come in, and they're naked except for stripes of white down that has been stuck on their bodies, and stripes with their men's blood. They used their own blood for gluing this on. And they're swinging the bull-roarers, which are the voice of the spirits, and they come as spirits. The boy will try to take refuge with his mother; she'll pretend to try to protect him. The men just take him away, a mother's no good from then on, you see, he's no longer a little boy." (Moyers 1988)

Boys' rites of passage to adulthood simulate the dark night. Emotional trauma facilitates the transformation of consciousness to fully open the patient's true self. Trauma does not only occur during adolescence. This example illustrates how the perception of an emotional trauma can shift one from a sense of being a victim to one on a path toward empowerment.

## *Removing Blockages of Potential*

Resolving emotional trauma clears blockages and brings a person closer to realizing their potential. If the trauma is not fully dealt with, the universe has an uncanny way of manifesting another trauma later in life to accentuate those aspects needing to be addressed and cleared. The trauma pokes at areas of sensitivity until the charge is released. Many patients work at length to avoid situations and personalities highlighting their specific sensitivities.

Michael Singer, in his book *The Untethered Soul* (Singer 2007), relates this idea to a thorn in the skin that continues to be poked and irritated by certain triggers. He provides the metaphor of people dealing with such a thorn by devising ways to prevent it from being disturbed, like building some apparatus to enclose it. Then the apparatus becomes irritated and the person builds another protective device until they are ultimately in a bubble. Eventually the bubble gets bothered, and so on. Simply removing the thorn sidesteps all this isolating effort. Chinese medicine works at the body level to reduce the charge of the "thorn" and lessen the reaction to future stressful events.

## *Identification with Emotional Trauma*

Patients can identify with old trauma and the reactions the emotions evoke. Transforming the energy is resisted since they believe their identity will become lost. They can become addicted to the trauma memory and have difficulty letting go. Helping them to see how the transformation will ultimately improve their life is essential. Once they begin to feel the benefits of the metamorphosis, this can encourage them to continue. Getting stuck in the trauma and attempting to fight the flow of life is common in humans. Joseph Campbell reflects, "We must be willing to get rid of the life we've planned, so as to have the life that is waiting for us" (Moyers 1988). When patients embrace this idea, and allow for the divine guidance of life, they can easily move forward.

Completing the lesson to be learned by the trauma assures clearing of the sensitivity and allows the individual to be fully present on their path. Chinese medicine facial diagnosis is used to determine the different ages at which a trauma occurred and will reoccur. This will help one figure out the timeline of the trauma and fully incorporate the lesson.

## Determining the Trauma Cycle and Faulty Belief Systems

### Detecting Cycles with Facial Diagnosis

Chinese Facial Diagnosis provides detailed information regarding significant impacts in a person's life, whether past or future. The Facial Age Map shows where each age is represented on the face and, if a marking is present, the Jing has somehow been affected. Scanning a person's ears and face reveals the ages where they did not fully have use of their Jing. A trauma or event of some magnitude is the cause of a marking on the Facial Age Map. The map will determine at which specific ages the Jing was affected. The practitioner, using compassionate questioning, is responsible for investigating which type of trauma/event occurred, for example a loss, a sense of repression, the feeling of being a victim, and a strong feeling of guilt.

Accounting for each marking on the Facial Age Map in a patient's past aids in identifying their pattern. Once each of these has been discussed, the pattern (generally involving a faulty belief system) is determined and can be extrapolated to understand which type of trauma might be experienced again. Many patients have markings on the Facial Age Map representing future ages. For example, a 35-year-old man might have a horizontal line at age 60. This line indicates an upcoming stressful event. The event can be prevented, or at least minimized, once the current pattern is resolved. After treatment, these future age markings should soften, thus confirming the practitioner's diagnosis. The fading of the markers represents the weakening of the power of the faulty belief system tied to the cycle.

### Observing the Five Minds to Identify Faulty Belief Systems

Traumas affect belief systems. Each person operates within their own, which influences their choices, actions, and inactions. Research has shown that belief systems are established by age six (Take Charge Counseling n.d.). Each belief becomes ingrained in the subconscious through the teen years. The famous Adverse Childhood Experiences (ACEs) Study conducted by the Centers for Disease Control and Kaiser-Permanente found direct correlations between stressors experienced in childhood and chronic disease, health risk behaviors, and mental illness. Liver disease, alcoholism, heart disease, poor academic achievement, depression, and suicide attempts are some of the many issues adults experience because of stress suffered in childhood (Centers for Disease Control and Prevention 1997). Traumas reside in the organs/channels, and the events occurring in the past set the stage for upcoming traumas. Observing the balance of the five elements reveals the nature of the limiting beliefs.

### The Kidneys and the Zhi

Belief systems linked to the emotion of fear negatively affect the Zhi and cause a freezing or sinking effect. When a person recoils from life or is unclear as to their life path due to a belief system, the Zhi is weak. Strengthening the Zhi shifts the tendency to shrink from life. Thus, when faced with a similar trauma, the patient sees it as manageable and they perceive future traumas as a way to forge their path, providing clarity in their life's destiny. Each trauma tests the will and gives rise to an inner strength when they successfully meet a challenge.

Conversely, some people hold belief systems that cause them to react with stubbornness and they refuse to flow with a situation. Their Zhi is stagnant and needs to move with life's changes. Working with channels to support the Zhi will bring about this transformation.

### The Liver and the Hun

Beliefs of timidity and indecisiveness mark a discordant Hun (Wang and Robertson 2008, p.163) and commonly cause a patient to have excessive anger or hate. Left untreated, this will lead to depression and inaction or cause a person to become overly responsible (Bridges 2012, p.293). Once harmonized, the patient perceives trauma as an opportunity to act and display courage. The patient begins to feel empowered by such an event, happy at the chance to make decisions, and they refrain from acting overly responsible. The faulty belief system is resolved and it no longer holds them prisoner, as the tissue memory has shifted.

## The Heart and the Shen

Any held beliefs causing anxiety, nervousness, or seriousness suggest a disharmonious Shen (Bridges 2012, p.293). The belief system clouds perception and impairs insight. The patient sees the trauma in a negative light and feels "victimized" by life. Stabilizing the Shen revitalizes their perception of trauma—they perceive challenging events as a means toward insight and creativity.

Trauma often causes patients to believe they are not creative—supporting their Shen allows them to tap into their inventiveness and gain insights from future stressful events. In other cases, patients hold a faulty belief that life must always be thrilling. The Shen becomes agitated by a trauma and excites the body. Patients can mistake this excitement for a positive feeling of "being alive" and seek drama and exhilaration. "Adrenaline junkies," patients always looking for the next big thing, fall into this category. Calming the Shen allows them to extend the happy feeling received from an enjoyable event (transforming the belief) rather than chasing another quick high. Fostering enjoyment benefits the Shen, so when faced with a stressful event, the Shen remains stable and prevents being unsettled by any future trauma.

## The Spleen and the Yi

Processing intent and digesting ideas belongs to the Yi, the mind of the spleen (Wang and Robertson 2008, pp.74–75). Belief systems eliciting feelings of worry, confusion, and sympathy are indicators of a disturbed Yi. Patients with a Yi disharmony react with indecision, confusion, over- or under-nurturing, or by smothering others (Bridges 2012, p.293). Once balanced, patients trust their instincts, choose the right action, and no longer spin their wheels. Their perception of a stressful event shifts from confusion to a call to act and get into rhythm.

## The Lungs and the Po

The Po establishes healthy boundaries with the environment and the people in it (Maclean and Lyttleton 2010, p.98). The lungs have the ability to let go and regulate the qi within the body. Responding to a trauma with feelings of grief or lack shows the involvement of the Po. Belief systems involve perfectionism, lack of self-esteem, grandiosity, and claustrophobia (Bridges 2012, p.293). Patients who tend to glorify events or feel smothered by an event display this disharmony. Their beliefs cause boundary issues and an inability to move on from a traumatic event. When these old beliefs are transformed and the patient has redefined boundaries, the energy is fully shored up in the lung system. The secure Po interprets trauma as an instrument to shed old energy and let go of the drama.

## Case Study: Recalling Janis from Chapter 2

From an early age, Janis developed the faulty belief that she did not have clear boundaries with her environment (deficient Po). Her near-fatal bout with measles, being forbidden to interact with her father in public, turmoil with her mother's alcohol abuse, her brother leaving home, and her being raped all fed into her thinking that she could not establish a clear barrier between herself and her surroundings. Janis's metal element was compromised. During her twenties, she exerted herself and created parameters with others and with life. She stopped using drugs, went to college, and eventually became a teacher. However, she still did not see herself as one who could write and publish a book. Instead of following her dream of writing, she took a job as an accountant.

The choice was not her fault and she was not to blame. This could have been a learned pattern of overcompensating to be responsible and was identified by interpreting markings observed on the Facial Age Map. These markings correlated with the ages of Janis's different traumas. These traumas had influenced her belief systems and, thus, she felt a lack of empowerment to stand on her own as a writer. Janis had created some boundaries, but to put herself "out there" as a published author was inconceivable to her. The Po establishes boundaries and provides a sense of individuation. For Janis, she felt vulnerable and unable to take the step to this next level of Po strength.

Once an individual's trauma pattern is identified, a specific treatment plan can be created. The plan includes changing belief systems affecting the minds of the organs so that there is not a continual triggering of the traumas.

Janis's lungs and large intestine reflected weakness by her respiratory distress and colon issues. Treatments to benefit her earth and water elements built up her metal element/Po, giving her the ability to realize her dream—she published her first book. By stepping out as a writer and sharing her story with the world, her Po increased and her lungs strengthened. The age marker at age 61 softened and she avoided a major traumatic event. Yet, there was still a marker at age 73.

When reviewing the markers with Janis and asking what happened at each age, the marker at 73 was pointed out. Her Shen instantly changed. Her skin turned pale and a frozen look came into her eyes. Janis felt fear. She disclosed that both her parents died at age 73 and she had been worried about that age. Janis had become a writer and had another book in production, but was still having strong psychic experiences wherein she would lose herself. She described the experiences as periods of possession or channeling, where other spirits would talk through her. This could last for minutes or hours. Janis would lose consciousness and have no recollection about the events— another form of surrendering boundaries.

Her Po was still showing signs of weakness and allowing other energies to invade her body. Additional treatments were needed to build up her Po and transform her perception of being vulnerable to other energies. Janis was still playing out the old belief of not having clear boundaries with her environment. Even though there had been many successful transformations, she had yet to process an additional layer of this pattern. Work to shift her thoughts, claim her power, and stop the faulty belief loop was the next essential step to prevent a future trauma at age 73.

Over the course of several months, the "Gathering the Qi" and "Soothing the Trauma Memory" protocols were applied, followed later by treatments using yuan-source and jing-river points on the metal and earth channels. In addition to acupuncture and shamanic drumming treatments, Janis was encouraged to complete her next book. She had started a series on women with strong voices. These women had presences in history and Janis was working on the first of the series: Mary Magdalene. This was a shift for Janis from sharing her personal life-stories with the public to sharing information about a powerful historic figure. Janis was removing herself from baring personal information. This change established yet another boundary with the world. By writing about such a strong woman, Janis could embody Magdalene's compelling energy.

During treatments, the age marker at 73 was observed and faded over time. Age markers are dynamic and can change in microseconds. When Janis spoke about Magdalene, the marker notably softened. This indicated that the potential trauma, coming up at 73 should be just a "small bump in the road." Janis could see how the adverse experiences in her life had been gifts; she could fully transform and become a writer. Through treatment and lifestyle modifications, Janis reconstructed her interpretation of past traumas and strengthened her energy to confront future traumas.

## Clearing Faulty Beliefs and Stopping the Trauma Cycle

Emotional traumas will continue to impact the patient until imbalances in each of the mind/spirit energies are resolved and the patient "wakes up," realizing their potential. A fully realized patient recognizes that traumas are helpful in breaking the walls around their energy field and letting light in. With each transformation of a trauma, the power of faulty beliefs wanes. Eventually the patient stands in complete harmony with life and the universal energy field. This is not to say the patient will never again experience trauma. However, when faced with trauma, their new skill and perspective allow them to move through it with grace.

Future traumas affect them less deeply and become further removed from their experience. For example, a trauma pattern centered around abandonment issues will reduce in intensity. Situations of abandonment become more detached as the patient lets go of the belief. At first, they might experience abandonment from a parent, followed by a spouse. As the belief lessens, the next trauma might involve a friendship and then an acquaintance until the intensity of each event is deflated to less and less intimate relationships. The organ energy harmonizes, the faulty beliefsno longer carry a charge, and the trauma cycle is broken, which results in the patient no longer attracting that type of trauma.

## Transforming the Perception of an Emotional Trauma

### *Thoughts Attracting Energy*

Our thoughts act like magnets. Focusing on a fear or worry of what will happen manifests that very thing. If one believes they will be abandoned, they will attract a person who will do so—a self-fulfilling prophecy. The patient is not to blame and should not feel guilty about a pattern replaying itself. The belief is generally subconscious and ingrained in tissue memory. The minds of the organs are in a loop and will perceive or react to events based on the belief systems.

An event experienced by one person can be interpreted completely differently by another. For example, the loss of a job can be viewed as a chance to start a brand-new path full of adventure, but to another person it can be experienced as a confirmation of unworthiness—they will never find a better job. Each time a trauma is experienced, the belief system comes to the surface and plays out again. Once this belief system is cleared and the subconscious program is no longer running, the energetic attraction disappears. The body operates efficiently and the trauma memory will not be triggered. The patient perceives the world accurately, not based on the emotional tendencies created by past trauma.

### *Reclaiming Power*

Shifting the internal mindscape allows the patient to feel empowered by the inevitable change in life. Nelson Mandela observes, "May your choices reflect your hopes, not your fears." Encourage the patient to switch their view of trauma, from an event taking their power to seeing it as a natural change in life leading to increased enlightenment. Experiencing emotion from a trauma is expected, but not to the extent where it rocks the person's core. Life will bring what it may, but when the patient has clear channels and the minds of the organs are in harmony, a traumatic event will make a smaller impact.

## Addiction to Trauma

Changing a pattern can be likened to changing the walking route a person has been taking to work for several years. At first, they will be aware of getting up in the morning and heading out, walking on a different set of streets. But after a few days, they arise not fully present, and find themselves on the old streets they took for years.

## Reducing the Attraction and Ingrained Nature of Trauma

The trauma memory can be resolved and the number of triggers lessened. However, the feelings and charges provoked in the body by the memory are addictive. The identification with being a trauma victim, the excitement felt from reliving it, the habit of experiencing it, and the sense of routine it gives—all play into drawing the patient back into trauma addiction. Dr. Van der Kolk describes many patients seeking reactions or charges to light up the trauma in order to feel alive (Van der Kolk 2014, p.85). The "fight-or-flight" response triggered when reliving a trauma memory provides a false sense of aliveness or excitement. Living in peace without the trauma memory can feel boring at times, or even like being numb. Shifting away from a state of heightened awareness is challenging.

Any pattern, whether it is a trauma memory, asthma, or Crohn's disease, is similar to driving a tractor in a groove or rut. Chinese medicine seeks to steer a patient away from the groove. Each treatment guides their path further away from the old groove. However, they are used to driving in that groove and will veer back toward it, especially early on in treatment. Helping the patient become comfortable with moving in a different direction is the key to stopping the addiction. If they can find positive ways to feel alive and secure, they will drop the old pattern much more easily.

## Addressing the Habit Loop

Unfortunately, this is much more difficult than simply turning a wheel on a tractor and heading off into the sunset. In Chinese medicine, the channels and organs are accustomed to certain routine and continue to follow a certain cycle until they are harmonized. In Western medicine, advancements in brain research have shown how addiction is wired in the brain. The striatum plays a significant role in habits and behavior. The nucleus accumbens is connected to the limbic system and influences impulsive behavior (Korb 2015, pp.24–25). These aspects of the brain are regulated by neurochemicals that cause addictive behavior. The neurochemicals are released with stress, anxiety, and excitement. Before the patient is even aware of it, they are back in the trauma memory loop.

Alex Korb suggests ways to change habit loops through behavior-altering techniques such as: identifying triggers, developing a routine, getting plenty of rest, deep breathing, and other stress-reducing activities (Korb 2015, pp.63–73). These are similar to the suggestions in Chinese medicine. In addition to these, reducing the heat in the body will also curb the addiction to trauma. The trauma memory is like gasoline, and any extra heat will ignite the thrill it brings. Lifestyle and dietary changes reduce heat and successfully decrease cravings. To treat addiction with acupuncture, utilize the emotional trauma treatment protocols ("Gathering the Qi" and "Soothing the Trauma Memory") with the addition of the auricular acupuncture points that reduce cravings.

### Building a Sense of Self-Love

The trauma memory can provide a sense of security to a person: an identity. Once the memory is transformed and it is no longer a major part of their life, the patient can feel lost—they have lived with it for so long. Even though it hindered them from having access to all their energy, they can feel a deep sense of insecurity by its absence. If the patient can gain a new perspective on their situation, the longing to go back down the path of the trauma memory can be switched off.

## Opening the Third Eye

In the book *Opening the Dragon Gate*, Ancestor Lu said, "The opening to the eye to heaven is the mystery of mysteries, the opening of openings, the way to join inside and outside… Those who open it live long… Maintaining sincerity is subtle activity; there is an even subtler marvel of marvels, which is when all ruminations are set aside" (Chen and Zheng 1996, p.167). Once the trauma is transformed, it is essential for patients to continue to keep their third eye open. (For methods to maintain an open third eye, refer to the Wood Element subsection below.) Finding their purpose, they can move forward and not become mired in the trauma memory. Connecting to the human family, and being of service in whatever capacity they have been destined, allows them to be a part of the community—open to feeling love.

After they have navigated the dark night and walked into the light of love, they need to continue without turning back. Using the wisdom learned in the process (transforming fear), feeling compassion for others in a negative situation (transforming anger), enjoying life (transforming anxiety), connecting with others (transforming over-thinking), and being thankful (transforming grief) for making it through the dark night allow the patient to reflect and refract like a diamond.

### Love Heals All Wounds

Love is healing. Chinese medicine treatments transform trauma, center the patient, establish clear communication between the organs and channels, and remove pathogens. The patient's body, mind, and spirit function at a higher level and merge with the universal energy. Therefore, a patient has a greater capacity to emanate love and be a rainbow of inspiration.

In the film *Red Beard*, the chief doctor assigned a 12-year-old patient to his intern. The child had been severely emotionally traumatized and had fallen sick, suffering from a high fever. The intern treated the girl for the fever, but in the process of treating her, he became overcome with exhaustion. The girl nurses *him* back to health and, by doing so, learns to trust and love again. By caring for someone and helping, she shifted her story from a traumatized girl mad at the world to a girl useful to others. She had lived in a state of anger and distrust but, through finding a way to step into a new way of being, was transformed into an empowered, caring, and helpful girl. She found her purpose and embraced a role of kindness.

"The world can be heaven or it can be hell." This is a statement from a monk living in the Zhong Nan Mountains in the documentary movie *Amongst White Clouds*. He explains that, even though there are clouds in the sky, the sun is always shining on the other side. How the patient perceives their history and story can either lift or deflate their energy.

## Case Study: Living to Full Potential

A 65-year-old woman, "Bethanie," sought treatment for a partial shoulder tendon tear. She shuffled into the clinic disheveled and with an aura of defeat. Bethanie said she had "given up" and was not interested in really doing anything. She used to weave rugs but was no longer able due to the pain. Her interest in weaving waned and she felt despondent. Bethanie was encouraged to design and choose colors for a new rug. A few weeks after starting treatment, she was coming into the clinic dressed well and with a sparkle in her eyes. Her shoulder pain was significantly reduced and she had cleaned and re-organized her weaving room. Bethanie started weaving and brought in some of her previously made rugs to display in the clinic. One of her rugs was purchased, which lifted her spirits and inspired more creations. Bethanie got back onto her path, acknowledging her gift of weaving and sharing her beauty with the world.

## Unresolved Emotional Trauma Affects Future Generations

Trauma victims can pass on their trauma genetically (Yehuda *et al.* 2015). By clearing trauma and the charge of a particular belief system, it is possible to prevent passing the trauma on to future generations. Western medical research in epigenetics has shown that memories and traumatic experiences can be transferred up to five generations (Houri-Ze'evi and Rechavi 2016). In Chinese medicine, the Jing contains the genetic information, and this can be passed on to each generation via the Chong mai (Farrell 2016, p.67).

## Discoveries through Epigenetics

Attitudes, personality, emotional make-up, and belief systems are all part of the Jing that is inherited. Strengths and imbalances are passed on. The imbalances can be corrected to prevent them from continuing in a patient's offspring. Cellular biologist Bruce Lipton demonstrated in his research that emotions experienced by a mother can be transferred to her children through non-coding DNA (Lipton n.d.; Wolynn 2016, p.29). The field of epigenetics has significantly increased our understanding of how traumas are passed on to subsequent generations.

Inherited traumas can cause future generations to repeat behavioral cycles and emotions experienced by their parents. For example, a mother feels anger and resentment due to marrying a controlling man. Her first daughter might follow her mother's pattern by marrying a controlling man, and her second daughter might have anger issues (Wolynn 2016, p.47). The mother's pattern was not brought to light and cleared; thus her behavior and emotions were passed on to her daughters.

## Western Psychology Interpretation of Intergenerational Trauma

A stressful experience is stored in the tissues until it is processed and transformed. Both Sigmund Freud and Carl Jung believed that traumas are stored in the unconscious until they are recognized and dealt with (Wolynn 2016, pp.15–16). These traumatic experiences do not just evaporate. Modern technology and genetic research is now proving these 100-year-old Western psychology theories to be true. Mark Wolynn (Director and Founder of the Family Constellation Institute) writes in his book *It Didn't Start with You* about trauma passed down through the generations. Wolynn explains, "Recent developments in the fields of cellular biology, neurobiology, epigenetics, and developmental psychology underscore the importance of exploring at least three generations of family history in order to understand the mechanism behind patterns of trauma and suffering that repeat" (Wolynn 2016, p.16).

## DNA and Jing-Holding Traumas

Lipton explains that traumas are inherited through the non-coding DNA, and a person responds to experiences based on how their parents reacted to similar types of events. A parent who suffered PTSD from witnessing an explosion could have a child who shudders every time they hear a loud noise (Wolynn 2016, pp.29–30). Scientists are gaining a deeper understanding of how the traumas manifest themselves. Research suggests that latent trauma passed to a future generation "turns on" under stress (Kellermann 2013).

Epigenetic modifications of DNA methylation tend to be what is studied most in cases of inheriting PTSD. Research suggests that psychosocial stress alters the patterns in DNA methylation (Almli *et al.* 2014; Yehuda *et al.* 2016). DNA is comparable to the Jing in Chinese medicine. Jing (essence) is stored in the kidneys, and pre-natal Jing holds the genetic information of the parents that is passed on to their children (Wiseman and Feng 1998, p.324). The Jing governs the growth, development, and the constitution of the offspring (Wiseman and Feng 1998, pp.178–179). An unresolved trauma experienced by a parent can be carried on to future generations in the Jing. Addressing the kidneys is one approach to resolving inherited trauma.

### Inheriting Trauma through Low Cortisol and the Concept of Kidney Deficiency

Rachel Yehuda, professor of psychiatry and neuroscience at Mount Sinai School of Medicine in New York and a leading expert in PTSD, has published several studies indicating how trauma is inherited. In addition to DNA, Yehuda's research indicates that low levels of cortisol are a factor that predisposes a person to PTSD symptoms. Studies of veterans, children of Holocaust survivors, and pregnant mothers suffering from PTSD after the World Trade Center attacks showed that all had a common denominator of low cortisol levels (Wolynn 2016, pp.19–20). Another study by Eric Nestler, published in the *Journal of American Medicine*, echoed similar findings regarding pregnant mothers and their children after the 9/11 attacks (Wolynn 2016, p.32). These low cortisol levels can be correlated to the concept of kidney deficiency in Chinese medicine. The research conducted by Yehuda supports the idea of fear affecting the water element in the next generation.

Yehuda proves how this hormonal similarity connects a child to their parents and grandparents. Her studies illustrate that PTSD symptoms are passed genetically, as opposed to the children being traumatized by witnessing their parents having symptoms or from hearing their parents' stories (Wolynn 2016, pp.19–20). Moreover, a parent suffering from PTSD is three times more likely to have a child who experiences PTSD symptoms (Wolynn 2016, p.19).

### Proving Ancient Beliefs of Stress during Pregnancy with Western Medicine

For millennia, Chinese medicine theories have discussed the importance of a mother's emotional state during pregnancy. They have held that anger, fear, grief, and so on experienced by the mother can be transferred to the fetus during gestation. The condition of "fetal fright" is an example of an emotional disturbance startling the fetus (Wiseman and Feng 1998, p.198). Lipton's and Yehuda's biological research has proven that a mother's emotions can be passed biochemically to the fetus (Wolynn 2016, p.27) and the child can react similarly to a comparable stressful experience after they were born (Wolynn 2016, pp.27 and 29). This correlates to the Chinese medicine theory of the Chong vessel being responsible for passing traumas to the next generation. The "sea of blood" holds the genetic information and, as Western medicine research has proven, the blood from the placenta connects with the mother's emotional state.

## Trauma of Three Generations in One Mother

Viewing transgenerational trauma from an embryological position, the passing on of emotions can happen before conception. An unfertilized egg shares a cellular environment with both a person's mother and grandmother (Wolynn 2016, p.25). A trauma experienced by a person's grandmother when pregnant with the person's mother affects the unfertilized egg (Wolynn 2016, p.25). In contrast, sperm develop during adolescence and throughout adulthood. A father encountering stress months before conception transmits this to his sperm. In both cases, the emotions felt before fertilization are transferred to the child (Wolynn 2016, p.26).

## Mirroring Similar Behaviors as Parents

Western medical studies of children born to combat veterans have shown that these children mirror their parents' behavioral and emotional issues (Wolynn 2016, p.32). Suicide rates were shown to be higher in children of Australian Vietnam War veterans (Wolynn 2016, p.32). Bert Hellinger, a German psychotherapist, states that each person bears a "family consciousness" and people carry feelings, symptoms, behaviors, and hardships unconsciously as if they were their own (Wolynn 2016, pp.44–46). However, inherited behavior can also be a gift. Animals have the instinct to run from fire. This is an example of passing on traits that can save a life. Trauma experienced and processed by a previous generation can result in them becoming resilient to certain stressors, and that quality can be passed on to later generations (Nauert 2016). Yet, many traumas are not fully processed and emotional responses are inherited.

Interestingly, the type of emotional responses can be different based on whether the PTSD is passed down from the mother or the father. In Yehuda's research, she and her team have shown that children inheriting PTSD from the mother will tend to be anxious and those inheriting from the father will tend to disassociate (Wolynn 2016, pp.33–34). These findings can be interpreted through the lens of Chinese medicine. The child inheriting trauma from the mother exhibits yin deficiency pattern behavior, tending to be anxious and restless. Those inheriting traumas from the father, by comparison, disassociate—a yang deficiency type response.

## Resolving Inherited Trauma with Chinese Medicine

For patients who are anxious and unsettled due to inherited trauma from their mother, emphasize the "Gathering the Qi" protocol to connect the patient to Mother Earth. Also, activate points on the Ren vessel (in addition to R-12) to build self-love. Traumas passed down by the father can be cleared using the Du vessel. This vessel instills courage in the patient to engage in activities in the world and exhibit more yang. Utilize the "Soothing the Trauma Memory" protocol to treat the father energy and connect them to Father Sky. Once these general imbalances are addressed, the Chong vessel and kidney organ can be treated.

The Chong vessel holds generational trauma; thus, the vessel can be used to transform the trauma (Farrell 2016, p.68). Stimulating SP-4 (the opening point) along with KD-16 (a point on the Chong vessel) unblocks the trauma and frequently causes the patient to feel emotions (some might display anxiety, while others become sad) which allow the practitioner to make an accurate, differentiated diagnosis. The practitioner can then focus on treating the specific channels affected for the individual. Activating the Chong vessel is a deep treatment and it is imperative the practitioner has gathered the qi of the patient before embarking on this unwinding of old trauma.

Patients processing inherited trauma—or any trauma—tend to have emotional sensations arise. This is normal and is where Chinese medicine can excel in helping patients to feel safe and calm during the dark night of the soul. Therapist Mark Wolynn explains the importance of patients feeling the sensations experienced by their ancestors in order to process the old trauma (Wolynn 2016, p.22). Because working through the trauma is an intense process, having patients see a therapist, along with receiving Chinese medicine treatment, is highly recommended.

## Practicing Qigong/Meditations to Resolve Intergenerational Trauma

Qigong and meditations focused on sending positive energy to future generations help to break the belief system cycle. Having the patient feel the energy in their heart and send love forward transfers clear, positive energy to future generations. Master Zhongxian Wu teaches the Three Treasures Qigong Form. As part of this form the participant sends grateful and positive qi to the seven generations of the past and to the future. (The reader is encouraged to study this form with Master Wu and experience its healing power.)

The connection to seven generations is also part of many Native American traditions. Made popular by the Iroquois, many Native nations believe that what occurs in the current generation affects up to seven succeeding generations. When a patient comprehends their lineage connection, the importance of life's challenges is realized. They understand how resolving trauma provides succeeding generations with a healthy set of tools to face future trauma. As Wolynn eloquently states, "traumas we inherit…forge a legacy of strength and resilience that can be felt for generations to come" (Wolynn 2016, p.24).

Situations will arise that will test the individual and any belief systems that have an emotional charge. This requires healthy, strong energy to stay clear when faced with these traumas. Maintaining proper Zheng qi ensures clear flowing channels, healthy qi and blood, and the ability to re-balance after a traumatic event.

## Zheng Qi and the Four Corrects

> *The glory is not in never falling, but*
> *rising every time you fall.*
>
> *Chinese proverb*

Maintaining upright qi is vital in life; inevitably there will be trials and tribulations along the way. Gathering and nourishing Zheng qi is an essential part of resolving old trauma and preventing the harmful effects of future occurrences. The Four Corrects ensure strong Zheng qi and maintain general health in the body, thus preventing trauma from taking hold, disrupting the system, and causing a relapse. As mentioned earlier, emotional trauma is experienced by many, but not everyone develops chronic symptoms.

A common phrase in Chinese medicine is "Zheng qi nei cun, Xie bu ke gan," which translates as "When Zheng qi gathers within, then the evil is harmless." Upholding the Four Corrects (breath, posture, presence, and intention) gathers the Zheng qi within and allows negative/undesirable energy to simply flow around and over a healthy energy field.

**Correct breath** is merely rooting the breath in the lower Dantian or in the middle Dantian. (Generally, it is recommended to focus the breath in the lower Dantian, but some texts encourage women to gather their breath in the middle Dantian; Cleary 1989, p.19.) The main action is following the breath and staying centered in the breath. Breathe in the universal light with all the pores of the skin and the lungs and then exhale the energy into the lower Dantian—a basic yet powerful way to maintain one's strength. The breath, ruled by the lungs, establishes clear boundaries and keeps the energy within.

**Correct posture** is another method for holding energy and maintaining confidence. Upright posture consists of the head held upright, shoulders relaxed, spine straight, and limbs full of energy. The body is neither stiff nor lifeless. Studies have shown that patients who maintain an upright posture have increased confidence and self-assurance. One study, published in the *Global Journal of Health Science*, measured low back pain and self-liberation of operating room nurses and found that both improved with proper posture (Moazzami *et al.* 2015). An article in the *Indian Journal of Occupational Environment Medicine* compiled the results of several studies verifying proper body posture as a significant factor in preventing chronic diseases (Sharma and Majumdar 2009). When the posture is correct, the patient's energy field is strong. Patients are encouraged to observe their body position by looking in the mirror to correct bad posture habits—what might feel correct to the patient is commonly *not* accurate.

**Correct presence** is about being in the present moment. Mindfulness is discussed in many traditions, and its practice offers great strength since tendencies to live in the past or future draw energy away from the body and compromise the potential. EFT and specific meditations are effective in bringing one's attention to the present. Meditations included in Thich Nhat Hanh's book *Peace is Every Step* exemplify the interdependence of correct breath, posture, and intention in nurturing mindfulness.

**Correct intention** involves following a virtuous path. An example of correct intention is a practitioner who is fully invested in healing rather than looking for fame, wealth, and attention. Any action in life requires an intention. Leading a positive lifestyle, following a path of bringing love, and embodying grace all nourish a correct intention. A person who has ill intentions attracts negativity and follows a path of destruction, thus leaking their energy.

Life will always bring a myriad of emotions and feelings—this is a natural occurrence. It is when the energy is compromised that the winds of emotion will stir and create chronic issues. Maintaining strong Zheng qi allows a person to process stressful events and not become muddled by the winds of change and emotion. Each emotion will be felt, processed, and released, enabling the patient to be enriched by each experience. Such a simple idea, but it can be a lifelong challenge to pursue.

## Lifestyle and Dietary Changes to Transcend Future Trauma

> *Harmony makes small things grow, lack*
> *of it makes great things decay.*
>
> Sallust

In a world obsessed with smart phones and bombarded by stimuli, it is crucial to create a stable environment externally and internally for the Shen to be settled. Over the last hundred years, humans have been exposed to an increasing amount of information and chaos. This alone scatters qi and makes it challenging to center after a stressful event. Utilizing the ancient lifestyle recommendations from Chinese medicine provides people with stability.

The five elements/spirits, when operating harmoniously, maintain a secure internal environment. They enable a patient to deal with trauma and change; the stronger the overall system, the quicker the recovery from future trauma. Each element can be strengthened with different types of activities, thoughts, and dietary changes (for the specific clear broth soups indicated below, refer to Appendix 2 for the recipes). Simple yet powerful techniques transform faulty beliefs, resolve the charge of a trauma, and clear the patient's energy field. As the elements are balanced, the patient gains clearer perspective and a greater understanding of ways to transcend the emotional triggering of future trauma.

## Water Element

### Accessing Internal Wisdom

Emotional trauma hinders a patient's natural progression in life. They can sink and shrink from their full potential. Tapping into their inherent wisdom and learning to flow with the changes in life transforms the fear and allows them to see from a new perspective (Bridges 2012, p.293). This wisdom is always available and effortlessly accessed with certain methods.

Suggest the patient engage in spiritual practice, whatever their spiritual or religious beliefs. A mystical experience, such as witnessing the beauty of nature in the northern lights, helps patients gain a broader perspective on life and encourages them to stand and face fears with confidence. Feeling part of a bigger energy helps to diffuse fears and takes them out of victim drama. Many patients feel beaten down by trauma and shrink away from their life's calling. Future trauma is inevitable, but with access to their wisdom it is powerless.

Meditation and other stillness exercises provide space for the inner intelligence to emerge. Having patients simply lie down in a quiet room provides them with a chance to tune in to their intuitiveness. Getting rest, avoiding overdoing, and simply "doing nothing" will protect the essence and allow for regeneration of energy.[1] As the patient becomes aware of their path and internal calling, they can maintain determination when faced with future emotional traumas.

Scientists proved the positive effects of silence by studying the hippocampus in mice. An article published in the journal *Brain Structural Function* found that mice exposed to periods of silence regenerated nerve cells in the hippocampus, whereas mice exposed to continuous sound did not (Kirste *et al.* 2015). The hippocampus (located in the limbic system) is associated with forming new memories and connecting emotions and senses. In Chinese medicine, the brain is the sea of marrow and is

---

1    Teaching to the author by Lillian Bridges.

nourished by the kidneys. Thus, Western medicine diagnostics verify the benefits of stillness in tonifying the kidneys. Meditation and other exercises that bring quiet are key components in strengthening the water element. Besides quiet, the water likes easy, flowing activities.

### Going with the Flow

Sometimes people can be overzealous about their path and become stubborn, preventing a natural flow. They burn out their kidney energy by pushing and refusing to let experiences guide them. The energy of the water element is exhausted and their life force is compromised.

Emotional traumas are intensified when a patient forces outcomes and fights against the flow. Changing the approach from exerting effort to acceptance will reduce the intensity of future traumas. A patient learns that when a trauma occurs they can flow through it and the emotion will pass (conserving the kidney energy), instead of resisting and exacerbating the reaction. The patient visualizes and senses the feeling(s) surfacing from a trauma to allow it to move and clear from the body (e.g., "Transforming the Emotional Surge" visualization). When a person simply experiences the emotion and does not give power to it, the charge will eventually dissipate.

**NUTRITIONAL RECOMMENDATIONS TO SUPPORT THE WATER ELEMENT**

| General Recommendations | Recommended Foods | Foods to Avoid |
|---|---|---|
| • Focus on adequate hydration.<br>• Consume one to two cups of clear broth soup per day.<br>• Increase fish oil. | • Clear broth soups, green leafy vegetables, seaweed, deer, buffalo, and salmon.<br>• *To nourish yin:* a cup of Xi Yang Shen (American Ginseng) once a day.<br>• *To tonify yang:* warm cooked foods, warm drinks, and lamb.<br>• "The Great Communicator," "Nourishing True Yin," "The Root of Inspiration," and "Fortify the Will" soups. | • Spicy foods and fluids, including alcohol, coffee, sugar, rich meats, and shellfish.<br>• Drying foods such as crackers, chips, and breads. |

## Wood Element

### Nurturing Compassion

Feelings of anger and hate are associated with the wood element and bring responses such as depression, overdoing, exaggerated responsibility, and rising energy. Fostering kindness and compassion reconstructs a patient's attitude; future trauma will not elicit such reactions (Bridges 2012, p.293). The Hun manages a person's courage to act and keeps the pathways open. Compassion, when fully felt and practiced, has such depth. Mark Twain explains, "Kindness is the language which the deaf can hear and the blind can see." This energy is felt and allows for an open flow of qi. When open, a patient can embody the magic of nature to change—they can be flexible when faced with a trauma. Instead of stopping action or doing too much, they can move in harmony with the inevitable changes in life.

Patients, ruled by rising qi, react in anger when they experience a trauma. Loving-kindness, known as Metta meditations, dispels this energy. Being compassionate with themselves and others softens the fight of the wood energy and transforms it into flexibility and healthy courage. Patients can spend time in nature feeling the power of the plants and trees. By observing the growth and magic of nature, they embody the adaptability of the wood element. When future trauma occurs, the person can emulate the flexibility of the wood element and be like a vine—growing around seeming blockages in their path and finding a new route.

## Standing Rooted in the Earth with a Smile

The Standing Qigong Form is an additional way to feel the upright energy of wood. This posture benefits wood, and upright posture in general builds confidence and sound decision making. As noted earlier, posture is one of the Four Corrects of healthy Zheng qi. In his book *The Upward Spiral*, Alex Korb describes several studies linking posture and decision making. Researchers in Germany, Spain, and Texas found that people in upright postures were decisive and confident. In tests, those that held confident postures—as opposed to those with doubtful postures—were decisive, believed in what they were writing about themselves, and were less likely to give up on difficult tests (Brinol, Petty, and Wagner 2009; Fischer *et al.* 2011; Riskind and Gotay 1982).

Practicing upright posture allows a patient to confront a future trauma confidently and clear the tendency to react negatively. The patient will feel encouraged to move through the trauma and reduce the charge of the anger. In addition to posture positively affecting emotions, facial expressions alter mood. Participants in one study, published in the medical journal *Frontiers of Psychology*, were shown pictures of people either furrowing their brow or smiling. They were then asked to measure their feelings toward the two types of expressions. The pictures of people furrowing their brow elicited anger (Hyniewska and Sato 2015).

## Seeing the Forest through the Trees

In Chinese facial diagnosis, the brow is interpreted as the liver (wood element), and vertical lines in the seat of the stamp indicate irritation or anger. Encourage patients to relax this area and expand their third eye. They can accomplish this by imagining clear open space, releasing tension in their body, setting an intention to remove themselves from the details of life, and feeling their connection to the human family and the universe. Refraining from prolonged screen time (smart phones, computer screens, TV, etc.) assists with softening this area. Widening the third eye helps the patient to remove themselves from drama and observe the situation from a higher perspective, therefore reducing the impact of the emotions felt. Opening oneself to a new outlook facilitates the movement of the wood energy and keeps the pathways clear. Another way to cultivate openness is through exercise.

### Enjoying the Benefits of Movement

The wood element requires action. The amount and type of exercise depends on the constitution of the patient. Those who have a strong wood element, that is, thick eyebrows and a strong jaw, benefit greatly from vigorous exercise. Patients with thinner eyebrows and a less-defined jaw respond better to gentle stretching, walking, and yoga. When the qi and blood are circulating, the Hun can respond to external stimuli—such as emotional trauma—in a positive way. The Hun can calmly assess the situation and act in harmony with the body and mind to prevent the trauma from lodging in the body. The trauma, like wind, will pass through rather than hide in the channels or organs. The liver regulates the blood and keeps the blood free of toxins (traumas can be viewed as toxins); thus a healthy liver will clear out these pathogens.

Multiple research studies have shown that exercise benefits the brain, stimulates the neuro-receptors, and produces many of the neurochemicals that support mood (Galdino *et al.* 2014; Nabkasorn *et al.* 2006). An article in *Psychiatry Research* concluded that physical exercise reduced the symptoms of PTSD—including depression—after researchers examined data from several studies (Rosenbaum *et al.* 2015).

### Replenishing the Blood

During the night, the liver processes the blood, cleansing it of toxins. Sleeping between 11 pm and 3 am (the "liver time") is essential to allow the liver to replenish the blood. One study published in *Behavioral Sleep Medicine* measured the moods in females who slept eight hours compared with those who had less than five hours. The group with less sleep had significantly higher levels of anger, depression, and confusion (Romney *et al.* 2016). The blood houses the spirit. When the blood is deficient, the vessels are not filled and there is space for wind (e.g., emotions from trauma) to enter, leading to the feelings mentioned above. Sufficient sleep enriches the blood, fills the vessels, and inhibits wind invasion.

**NUTRITIONAL RECOMMENDATIONS TO SUPPORT THE WOOD ELEMENT**

| General Recommendations | Recommended Foods | Foods to Avoid |
| --- | --- | --- |
| • Eat less and avoid heavy meals.<br>• Eat dinner earlier in the evening.<br>• Avoid stressful conversation or thoughts.<br>• Consume protein throughout the day (variety of meat, nuts, seeds, tofu, and beets) to build blood and root the spirit. | • Gou Qi Zi to supplement the liver blood; adding to soups, tea, or rice porridge.<br>• *If heat accumulates:* beets, celery, mung beans, peppermint, chrysanthemum, dandelion, and cucumber.<br>• *If blood stagnates:* the spices turmeric, garlic, cayenne, and rosemary; red wine in moderation (Maclean and Lyttleton 2002, p.886).<br>• "Determined Leader" soup. | • Heat-generating foods and fluids, including spicy foods, alcohol, coffee, sugar, rich meats, and shellfish.<br>• Astringent or cloying foods. |

## Fire Element

### Making the Fun Last

Joy is the healthy emotion of the fire element and is commonly confused with excitement. The heart likes to be lifted and buoyant, which enjoyment—in moderation—does. Many people crave or are addicted to excitement and look for the next "big" thing. This is a concern since it strains the fire element. Lillian Bridges speaks of stretching joy like taffy to draw out the lift of an enjoyable event, experience, food, conversation, and so on. Reducing overexciting activities such as television, screen time, video games, and stimulating images removes distraction from finding the pleasure in the simple joys of life.

A large spike in joy is inevitably followed by the downward dip of sadness; the higher the peak, the lower the valley. When feeling sadness and overexcitement, the fire element reacts with anxiety, nervousness, seriousness, and a sense of being scattered. Transforming these reactions with happiness and unconditional love stabilizes the Shen (Bridges 2012, p.293). Nurturing enjoyment bolsters the Shen and supports the spirit when faced with future emotional trauma.

### Serenading the Fire

Singing improves the fire element by opening the tongue (the sensory organ associated with the heart) and expressing oneself. This frees the heart and allows for a smooth flow of energy. Researchers conducted a study of amateur and professional singers and found that oxytocin levels and cardio function increased in both groups while performing/singing. Interestingly, the amateur group reported an increase in well-being whereas the professionals did not. However, the professionals could maintain stronger "heart–brain" connections than the amateurs (Grape *et al.* 2003).

### Lighting the Fire

The fire element likes new experiences and travel. Looking at the world through child-like wonder elevates the spirit and keeps the heart light.[2] Communication and expression support an open heart, which allows for the smooth movement of blood. Researchers in Malaysia studied patients with congenital heart defects (CHD) and found that "positive interaction and affectionate support, which include elements of fun, relaxation, love, and care, should be included in the care of adult patients with CHD" (Tye, Kandavello, and Gan 2017). Another study, mentioned in the book *The Upward Spiral*, revealed that anxiety and stress hormones reduced after talking with a friend (Hendrichs *et al.* 2003). Social interactions benefit the fire element and ultimately calm the Shen. When future emotional trauma occurs, the Shen remains grounded and the heart mirror accurately reflects reality—enabling the patient to view future trauma with a healthy perspective.

### Maintaining Rhythm

The heart pumps the blood throughout the body and holds the spirit. A steady rhythm keeps the spirit secure and enables the person to withstand trauma that would otherwise destabilize the energy for a prolonged period. Following schedules, limiting excitement, and fostering love establishes regular rhythm. Many traumas (no matter how strong a person's spirit) are still able to unsettle the Shen. However, when a person's spirit is rooted, the energy stabilizes quickly, leaving no residual effect.

### Keeping the Shen Happy

When a person engages in an activity in which they excel, their level of happiness increases. Joseph Campbell explains, "Find a place inside where there's joy, and the joy will burn out the pain" (Moyers 1988). Whichever activity brings comfort and smiles to a person (placing a person into "the zone") will lift their heart, build their spirit, and keep them moving in rhythm through life. Any level of trauma can be dealt with as the Shen spirals upward.

---

2    Teaching to the author by Lillian Bridges.

**NUTRITIONAL RECOMMENDATIONS TO SUPPORT THE FIRE ELEMENT**

| General Recommendations | Recommended Foods | Foods to Avoid |
|---|---|---|
| • Choose foods that build and support blood.<br>• Consume protein at each meal to steady the spirit. | • *If heat accumulates:* clear broth soups, broccoli, cucumber, zucchini, apple, pear, mung beans, alfalfa sprouts, kelp, and barley (Maclean and Lyttleton 2002, p.883).<br>• "The Great Communicator" and "The Root of Inspiration" soups. | • Heat-generating foods and fluids, including spicy foods, caffeine, refined sugar, chocolate, and alcohol. |

## Earth Element

### Taking Action

The earth element tends to the emotions of worry, bewilderment, and sympathy, and reacts with indecision, over- or under-nurturing, and smothering. Taking action, following instinct, and caring for oneself transforms these reactions (Bridges 2012, p.293). As Mark Twain pointed out, "The secret of getting ahead is getting started." Listening to "the gut" and acting on intuition sets a natural rhythm for the processing of ideas and emotions. Current scientific research supports this notion. Recent studies on the microbiome show how the bacteria in the gut interact with the environment and hint at the gut being part of decision making (Ursell *et al.* 2012). Bobby Robson stated, "Practice makes permanent," which is true regarding the Yi to act and follow instinct. When the Yi becomes accustomed to paying attention to instinct, the less likely it will be to "spin out" when confronted with a future emotional trauma. Moreover, research has shown that making a "good" decision over a "best" decision reduces depression and worry. The Yi requires a steady pace to process thoughts in a healthy manner. In his book *The Upward Spiral*, author Alex Korb describes the entanglement in debating every possible decision. If a person simply makes *a* decision, happiness increases, lifting depression (Korb 2015, p.94).

### Practicing Positive Outcome Imagery

Teaching patients to generate positive imagery and self-talk will help prevent trauma from making a lasting impact. Researchers worked with individuals suffering from generalized anxiety disorder (GAD) who experienced a high level of worry. They trained a group of the subjects to use images and verbal cues of positive outcomes related to their worries and the other cohort to simply generate positive images and expressions. The results, published in *Behavior Research and Therapy*, showed that both groups benefited. Visualizing and verbalizing positive ideation effectively counteracted worry (Eagleson *et al.* 2016).

## Taking Time for the Self

Nurturing is a trait of the earth element. When out of balance, patients will over-nurture (or smother) others and deplete their own body's energy by giving too much to others. This behavior is commonly seen in mothers who overindulge their children to the point that the mother becomes physically sick. On the face, lines above the upper lip (over-nurturing lines) are one indication of such behavior. Helping patients learn how to mother themselves (e.g., taking spa weekends or an afternoon off) transforms this syndrome. Other methods to benefit the earth element are: sitting and enjoying conversations, baking bread, following routines, and wearing loose, comfortable clothing.[3]

At the opposite end of the spectrum are people who react by under-nurturing others. These patients can transform this behavior by doing activities with the community and helping others.

## Hugging it Out

Hugging releases oxytocin, relieves stress, and benefits the earth element. A study published in *Biological Psychology* examined blood levels in 59 premenopausal women after exposure to warm contact with their spouses, ending with a hug. Their blood pressure reduced and oxytocin levels increased (Light, Grewen, and Amico 2005). Connecting with others enables a person to feel calm and centered in the face of an emotional trauma.

**NUTRITIONAL RECOMMENDATIONS TO SUPPORT THE EARTH ELEMENT**

| General Recommendations | Recommended Foods | Foods to Avoid |
|---|---|---|
| • Eat a bland diet, warm, simple whole foods, slow cooked, clear broth soups, and high quality meats.<br>• Chew food thoroughly, eat smaller meals, observe regular mealtimes, eat when relaxed, and avoid working and reading while eating or having stressful conversations.<br>• Take a leisurely stroll after mealtimes. | • *If phlegm/damp accumulates:* buckwheat, aduki beans, rye, barley, onion, turnip, radish, fresh ginger, and mustard.<br>• *If phlegm heat accumulates:* bamboo shoots, radish, kelp and seaweed, turnip, and shitake mushrooms (Maclean and Lyttleton 2002, pp.880–881, 883, and 885).<br>• "Super Qi and Blood" soup. | • Raw foods, smoothies, juices, dairy products, wheat, refined sugars, ice cream, carbohydrates, beer, rich meats, greasy foods, tofu, and cold-natured foods. |

---

3    Teaching to the author by Lillian Bridges.

## *Metal Element*

### *Utilizing the Power of Gratitude*

Emotional trauma can occur due to the lack of something, for example love, attention, and time. This loss affects the metal element and elicits grief and inadequacy. The person reacts by feeling a lack of self-esteem or responds with perfectionism, grandiosity, or claustrophobia. Gratitude is one method to transform these reactions (Bridges 2012, p.293).

A Western medical research study verified the power of gratitude by showing how the brain responded to this feeling in Holocaust survivors. Each survivor was asked to remember any gift they received during the war, for example food, shelter, protection, and clothing. They underwent brain imaging and, as they brought back these memories, there was enhanced brain activity in the anterior cingulate cortex (part of the emotional brain) and medial pre-frontal cortex (an aspect of the logical brain). Clear communication between these lobes is essential for emotional stability and supports feelings of gratitude to improve mental health (Fox *et al.* 2015).

Keeping a gratitude journal or writing letters of appreciation reduces depression and pain. In a six-month-long study, published in *Primary Health Care Research and Development*, participants wrote gratitude letters. At the end of the period, the subjects reported increased energy and a higher number of daily accomplishments, and there were measured improvements in mental and physical health (Lambert D'raven, Moliver, and Thompson 2015). Gratitude journaling (e.g., writing down three thankful things a day) trains the brain to see additional things one can be thankful for, which releases dopamine (Zahn *et al.* 2009). In addition to gratitude, mindfulness and deep breathing transform grief and loss (Bridges 2012, p.293).

### *Feeling Alive in the Moment*

When a person lives fully in the moment and finds beauty in the simple pleasures of life, the lungs become stronger. Deep breathing (filling the chest to the 12th thoracic vertebra, feeling the depths of the lungs) and mindfulness meditation deliver a person into the present moment—therefore bolstering the lungs. Conserve and protect the lungs by managing energy output wisely, speaking with integrity, reducing unnecessary talking, and avoiding polluted environments. A lifestyle honoring discipline and order helps the lungs regulate qi in the body. Emotional trauma disrupts this flow. However, when the lungs are strong, they can quickly harmonize the qi circulation, endure future trauma, and avoid emotional reactivity.

## Upholding Integrity

Ethical behavior transforms grief (Bridges 2012, p.204) and prevents it from lodging in the lung and large intestine channels. Adopting positive ideals and empowering belief systems (and letting go of those beliefs which deplete the energy) builds self-esteem and promotes a healthy metal element. Encourage patients to strike a balance between striving for ideals and letting go of the drive to achieve perfection. Ideals can serve as a compass for guiding a patient to successful living. Embodying self-forgiveness and self-acceptance safeguards the patient from clutching to perfectionism. Conducting life in this way, while establishing healthy boundaries, galvanizes the Po to confront future trauma with grace, confidence, and tenacity.

**NUTRITIONAL RECOMMENDATIONS TO SUPPORT THE METAL ELEMENT**

| General Recommendations | Recommended Foods | Foods to Avoid |
|---|---|---|
| • Increase consumption of soups, liquids with cooking, fish oil, protein, and steamed vegetables. | • *To nourish fluids:* yogurt, pears, apples, bananas, millet, almonds, peanuts, eggs, tofu, and pork.<br>• *If phlegm/damp accumulates:* radish, daikon, onion, turnip, and mustard greens.<br>• "Super Blood and Qi" and "The Determined Leader" soups. | • *Drying foods:* crackers, chips, breads.<br>• *Heat-generating foods:* spicy foods, sugar, chocolate, alcohol. |

# The Golden Path and Utilizing Given Talents

Successfully enduring the dark night of the soul shatters illusions and illuminates one's true calling. Chinese medicine has methods to guide a patient into this awareness. Facial diagnosis offers great insight into the talents and abilities a person possesses—these are the foundation of manifesting their destiny or "Golden Path" (a term used by Lillian Bridges in her teachings; see Lotus Institute 2017).

## Using the Face to Determine the Patient's Golden Path

Facial features, markings, and other aspects of the face—when viewed collectively—display the individual talents a person brings to the human family. The process of a practitioner pointing out and communicating the meaning of the patient's unique facial markers assists with the realization of their destiny. A person with flared nostrils, vertical lines in front of the ears, and horizontal lines above the eyebrows has a knack for "sussing out" truth and might be well suited for a profession in the critical examination of details and information. Every person possesses talents. If they are not being used, access to Jing is compromised and the person's energy is not operating at full potential. Thus, emotional trauma is likely to cause chronic issues.

## Reflex of Purpose

Dr. Van der Kolk describes Pavlov's theory of "Reflex of Purpose" in his book *The Body Keeps the Score*, and elucidates, "All creatures need a purpose—they need to organize themselves to make their way in the world… One of the most devastating effects of trauma is that it often damages that Reflex of Purpose…[and] invites us to focus on emotions and movements, not only as problems to be managed, but also as assets that need to be organized to enhance one's sense of purpose" (Van der Kolk 2014, p.78). This idea is the keystone to Golden Path work. Helping a patient discover their purpose shifts their energy and deflates the intensity of the trauma memory. The patient can move forward in the present and plan. When the patient walks their Golden Path, the physiological balance is reset, the body is functioning harmoniously, and a patient can live life to the fullest. As Joseph Campbell explains, "The privilege of a lifetime is being who you are" (Moyers 1988).

## Singing to Resolve Trauma

Many examples are rich with people transforming their lives through embodying their individual talents. The musical *Alive!* in New York City features singers who are 55 or older who use song to share their stories and heal their past traumas. Their expression shifts the trauma from being a hindrance to being a catalyst. The performers realize their purpose and transform the emotional traumas into gifts for themselves and for the audience.

## Guides to Realize Purpose

Life coaches, shamans, astrologers, and other similar professionals can be a great resource for patients. Ultimately, using the resolution of trauma as a catalyst to determine a patient's calling in life can shift the perception of being a victim of trauma to one who is empowered with change. Martin Luther King Jr. exclaimed, "We shall overcome!" This call to action was beautifully exemplified by Theodore Roosevelt Jr., who conquered his fear of never being healthy (he suffered from childhood asthma and frequent illness), endured the loss of his beloved father, and braved the ending of his relationship with his childhood sweetheart Edith Carow. President Roosevelt built up his fragile body through various exercise routines and embraced his love of nature. He overcame his strong childhood fears, rose to power, and protected the natural beauty of America by establishing several national parks. (He eventually did re-unite with Carow after several years apart.) President Roosevelt helped people realize that anything is possible. Having found his path, he transformed early traumas into gifts, and inspired a nation.

## Summary of Prevention of Emotional Trauma

The human family is connected and inter-woven. Feeling part of the bigger picture shifts perception and gives a person the ability to see their path as connected to all humanity. They can sense themselves as a vessel containing heavenly and earthly energies. Each experience, when navigated with grace and determination, can further unlock the flow of energy between the sky and earth.

### Tuning into the Changes Within

Storing and protecting the various energies of the organ systems prevent future emotional traumas from lodging in the body. Keith Richards, a man who has experienced multiple events—and substances—is in his seventies and still traveling and performing in front of thousands of people. When discussing his various life experiences and ability to continue rocking, he explains, in his autobiography *Life*, "I read my body very well" (Richards 2010). This aptitude to understand and feel the body is essential in preventing a stressful event from becoming trapped in the body.

To know one's body is to connect with one's heart. When connected, and the heart pool is stilled, a person's purpose is realized; they embody love and their perceptions are clear. Thoughts can provoke emotions through memories, fears, "what-ifs," and so on. When the mind races, the heart is muddled. As Tripitaka, a character in the epic tale *The Journey to the West*, explains, "When the mind is active all kinds of mara [negative energy] come into existence; when the mind is extinguished, all kinds of mara will be extinguished" (Yu 2006, p.204).

### Gracefully Navigate the Winds of Change

Recognizing and transforming old belief systems reduces the triggering of emotions and the unsettling of the mind. Events inevitably stir the winds of emotion. Having strong Jing, Qi, and Shen increases resilience to emotional reactivity, lets the winds of emotions move through, and allows the body to quickly re-establish balance. In so many cases, pathogens can only take root where deficiency is found. Finding joy in small things ensures a healthy spirit and keeps the body buoyant, regardless of the changes in life. Patients see the world as a place for growth and expansion, which encourages a great metamorphosis—they ultimately untangle patterns and fly freely, sailing on the winds of change.

**References**

Almli, L.M., Fani, N., Smith, A.K., and Ressler, K.J. (2014) "Genetic approaches to understanding post-traumatic stress disorder." *Int. J. Neuropsychopharmacol. 17*, 2, 355–370.

Bridges, L. (2012) *Face Reading in Chinese Medicine* (Second Edition). London: Churchill Livingstone Elsevier.

Brinol, P., Petty, R.E., and Wagner, B. (2009) "Body posture effects on self-evaluation: a self-validation approach." *European Journal of Social Psychology 39*, 1053–1064.

Centers for Disease Control and Prevention (1997) *The CDC-Kaiser ACE Study*. Available at www.cdc.gov/violenceprevention/acestudy/about.html, accessed on 31 May 2017.

Chen, K., and Zheng, S. (1996) *Opening the Dragon Gate*. Trans. T. Cleary. North Clarendon, VT: Tuttle.

Cleary, T. (trans.) (1989) *Immortal Sisters: Secret Teachings of Taoist Women*. Berkeley, CA: North Atlantic Books.

Eagleson, C., Hayes, S., Mathews, A., Perman, G., and Hirsch, C.R. (2016) "The power of positive thinking: pathological worry is reduced by thought replacement in Generalized Anxiety Disorder." *Behavior Research and Therapy 78*, 13–18.

Farrell, Y.R. (2016) *Psycho-Emotional Pain and the Eight Extraordinary Vessels*. London: Singing Dragon.

Fischer, J., Fischer, P., Englich, B., Aydin, N., and Frey, D. (2011) "Empower my decisions: the effects of power gestures on confirmatory information processing." *Journal of Experimental Social Psychology 47*, 1146–1154.

Fox, G.R., Kaplan, J., Damasio, H., and Damasio, A. (2015) "Neural correlates of gratitude." *Front. Psychol. 6*, 1491.

Galdino, G., Romero, T., Silva, J.F., Aguiar, D., *et al.* (2014) "Acute resistance exercise induces antinociception by activation of the endocannabinoid system in rats." *Anesth. Analg. 119*, 3, 702–715.

Grape, C., Sandgren, M., Hansson, L.O., Ericson, M., and Theorell, T. (2003) "Does singing promote well-being? An empirical study of professional and amateur singers during a singing lesson." *Integr. Physiol. Behav. Sci. 38*, 1, 65–74.

Hendrichs, M., Baumgartner, T., Kirschbaum, C., and Ehlert, U. (2003) "Social support and oxytocin interact to suppress cortisol and subjective responses to psychosocial stress." *Biological Psychiatry 54*, 12, 1389–1398.

Houri-Ze'evi, L., and Rechavi, O. (2016) "Plastic germline reprogramming of heritable small RNAs enables maintenance or erasure of epigenetic memories." *RNA Biol. 13*, 12, 1212–1217.

Hyniewska, S., and Sato, W. (2015) "Facial feedback affects valence judgments of dynamic and static emotional expressions." *Front. Psychol. 6*, 291.

Infurna, F.J., and Luthar, S.S. (2016) "Resilience to major life stressors is not as common as thought." *Journal of the Association of Psychological Science, Perspectives on Psychological Science 11*, 2, 175–194.

Kellermann, N.P. (2013) "Epigenetic transmission of Holocaust trauma: can nightmares be inherited?" *Isr. J. Psychiatry Relat. Sci. 50*, 1, 33–39.

Kirste, I., Nicola, Z., Kronenberg, G., Walker, T.L., Liu, R.C., and Kempermann, G. (2015) "Is silence golden? Effects of auditory stimuli and their absence on adult hippocampal neurogenesis." *Brain Struct. Funct. 220*, 2, 1221–1228.

Korb, A. (2015) *The Upward Spiral*. Oakland, CA: New Harbinger.

Lambert D'raven, L.T., Moliver, N., and Thompson, D. (2015) "Happiness intervention decreases pain and depression, boosts happiness among primary care patients." *Prim. Health Care Res. Dev. 16*, 2, 114–126.

Light, K.C., Grewen, K.M., and Amico, J.A. (2005) "More frequent partner hugs and higher oxytocin levels are linked to lower blood pressure and heart rate in premenopausal women." *Biological Psychology 69*, 1, 5–21.

Lipton, B.H. (n.d.) *Maternal Emotions and Human Development*. Available at www.allthingshealing.com/Family-Parenting/Maternal-Emotions-and-Human-Development-/10347#.V7jdnI-cGDs, accessed on 1 June 2017.

Lotus Institute (2017) *Golden Path Workshop*. Available at https://lotusinstitute.com/pages/golden-path-program, accessed on 1 June 2017.

Maclean, W., and Lyttleton, J. (2002) *Clinical Handbook of Internal Medicine, Vol. 2*. Sydney: University of Western Sydney.

Maclean, W., and Lyttleton, J. (2010) *Clinical Handbook of Internal Medicine, Vol. 3*. Sydney: University of Western Sydney.

Moazzami, Z., Dehdari, T., Taghdisi, M.H., and Soltanian, A. (2015) "Effect of an ergonomics-based educational intervention based on transtheoretical model in adopting correct body posture among operating room nurses." *Glob. J. Health Sci. 8*, 7, 52804.

Moyers, B. (1988) *Ep. 3: Joseph Campbell and the Power of Myth—"The First Storytellers."* Available at http:// billmoyers.com/content/ep-3-joseph-campbell-and-the-power-of-myth-the-first-storytellers-audio, accessed on 31 May 2017.

Nabkasorn, C., Miyai, N., Sootmongkol, A., Junprasert, S., *et al.* (2006) "Effects of physical exercise on depression, neuroendocrine stress hormones and physiological fitness in adolescent females with depressive symptoms." *Eur. J. Public Health 16*, 2, 179–184.

Nauert, R. (2016) *Is Resiliency Inherited?* Available at http://psychcentral.com/news/2006/12/01/is-resiliency-inherited/447.html, accessed on 1 June 2017.

Richards, K. (2010) *Life.* New York: Little, Brown.

Riskind, J.H., and Gotay, C.C. (1982) "Physical posture: could it have regulatory or feedback effects on motivation and emotion?" *Motivation and Emotion 6*, 3, 273–298.

Romney, L., Larson, M.J., Clark, T., Tucker, L.A., Bailey, B.W., and LeCheminant, J.D. (2016) "Reduced sleep acutely influences sedentary behavior and mood but not total energy intake in normal-weight and obese women." *Behav. Sleep Med. 14*, 5, 528–538.

Rosenbaum, S., Vancampfort, D., Steel, Z., Newby, J., Ward, P.B., and Stubbs, B. (2015) "Physical activity in the treatment of post-traumatic stress disorder: a systematic review and meta-analysis." *Psychiatry Res. 230*, 2, 130–136.

Sharma, M., and Majumdar, P.K. (2009) "Occupational lifestyle diseases: an emerging issue." *Indian J. Occup. Environ. Med. 13*, 3, 109–112.

Singer, M. (2007) *The Untethered Soul.* Oakland, CA: New Harbinger.

Take Charge Counseling (n.d.) *So What Exactly is a Belief System?* Available at www.takechargecounseling.org/ yahoo_site_admin/assets/docs/Article_2_-_What_Is_A_Belief_System.326110726.htm, accessed on 31 May 2017.

Tye, S.K., Kandavello, G., and Gan, K.L. (2017) "Types of social supports predicting health-related quality of life among adult patients with CHD in the Institut Jantung Negara (National Heart Institute), Malaysia." *Cardiol. Young 27*, 1, 46–54.

Ursell, L.K., Metcalf, J.L., Parfrey, L.W., and Knight, R. (2012) "Defining the human microbiome." *Nutr. Rev. 70*, Suppl. 1, S38–S44.

Van der Kolk, B. (2014) *The Body Keeps the Score.* London and New York: Penguin.

Wang, J.-Y., and Robertson, J. (2008) *Applied Channel Theory in Chinese Medicine.* Seattle: Eastland Press.

Wiseman, N., and Feng, Y. (1998) *A Practical Dictionary of Chinese Medicine* (Second Edition). Brookline, MA: Paradigm.

Wolynn, M. (2016) *It Didn't Start with You.* New York: Viking.

Yehuda, R., Daskalakis, N.P., Bierer, L.M., Bader, H.N., *et al.* (2016) "Holocaust exposure induced intergenerational effects on FKBP5 methylation." *Biol. Psychiatry 80*, 5, 372–380.

Yehuda, R., Hoge, C.W., McFarlane, A.C., Vermetten, E. *et al.* (2015) "Post-traumatic stress disorder." *Nat. Rev. Dis. Primers 1*, 15057.

Yu, A.C. (2006) *The Monkey and the Monk: An Abridgement of The Journey to the West.* Chicago and London: University of Chicago Press.

Zahn, R., Moll, J., Paiva, M., Garrido, G., *et al.* (2009) "The neural basis of human social values: evidence from functional MRI." *Cerebral Cortex 19*, 2, 276–283.

CHAPTER 6

# Western Medicine and Chinese Medicine Joining Hands

Brain research conducted in the 1990s revealed a greater understanding of the bio-mechanism of PTSD and trauma (Van der Kolk 2014, p.21). Positron emission tomography (PET) and functional magnetic resonance imaging (fMRI) allowed scientists to observe brains processing memories, which led to discoveries of how the brain responds to trauma. Researchers found that trauma affects the communication between three major areas of the brain: the brainstem, the limbic system, and the pre-frontal cortex. Learning how the different parts of the brain communicated— or did not—contributed to a comprehensive awareness of how trauma stresses the body systems. Harmonized communication in the brain is required for a healthy body. Emotional trauma and its memory disrupt the communication between the three areas of the brain, causing stress on the body and chronic health conditions.

## The Trauma Brain Triad

The brainstem is formed in the womb, the limbic system when a person is born, and the neocortex (including the pre-frontal cortex) between ages one and seven (Figure 6.1). These three aspects of the brain are involved in emotional trauma. Dr. Van der Kolk refers to these as "The Triune Brain" (Van der Kolk 2014, p.59). The brainstem and limbic system can be thought of as the "emotional brain" (a term coined by David Servan-Schreiber in his book *The Instinct to Heal*), while the pre-frontal cortex is the "rational brain." Communication between the emotional brain and the rational brain is essential when dealing with trauma (Van der Kolk 2014, pp.55–57).

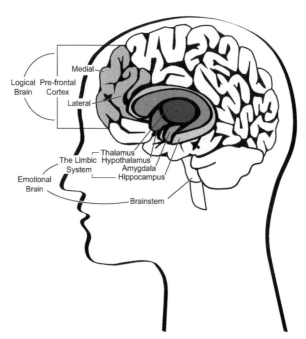

*Figure 6.1 The Aspects of the Brain Involved in Emotional Trauma*
*Source:* Kirsteen Wright

### The Emotional Brain

The brainstem maintains homeostasis and controls the heart, lungs, and immune and endocrine systems. It receives signals from the limbic system and responds by regulating these aspects of the body. The limbic system consists of brain structures that control the basic emotions (anger, fear, pleasure) and drives of the body (sex, hunger, care of offspring); the structures include the amygdala, hippocampus, thalamus, and hypothalamus, and sit on top of the brainstem. These areas of the brain are involved in creating/controlling/initiating several of the impulses of the body, especially those having to do with survival, such as monitoring for danger and preparing people to cope with living in groups. The brainstem and limbic system are the core of the nervous system. When these areas of the brain react to danger, the amygdala sends nerve impulses to the body to protect itself, triggering the release of stress hormones.

The amygdala stores memories and houses neurons related to fear conditioning (an associative behavior pattern developed from a stimulus that elicits fear). The amygdala is involved in activation of the fight-or-flight response and serves the body effectively when one is faced with a real, harmful situation. However, when a person hears or sees something that reminds them of an old trauma, the emotional brain responds as if there is a real current danger. It is up to the pre-frontal cortex (the logical brain) to regulate these reactions.

## *Miscommunication between the Logical Brain and Emotional Brain*

The pre-frontal cortex is responsible for decision making, personality expression, and moderating social behavior. It determines which stimulus is real and when to terminate the fight-or-flight feedback loop. Brain imaging has shown that this area shuts down when patients are faced with trauma or when the trauma memory is triggered. The limbic system takes over and the body is caught in the past; communication between lobes is interrupted. This is likened to a false alarm being triggered and the body reacting as if the experience is real. PTSD scrambles the communication by affecting both the emotional brain and the rational brain, resulting in hypervigilance, overreactions, and shutting down. The intensity of the emotional trauma directly correlates to the level of miscommunication between the different areas of the brain (Frick *et al.* 2016). It is the job of the pre-frontal cortex, along with the hippocampus, to mentally process the trauma.

## *The Hippocampus*

The hippocampus forms, processes, and stores long-term memories/experiences and connects them to new input (Van der Kolk 2014, p.60). When a person is faced with a trauma or its memory, the hippocampus determines the context and meaning of the situation. The brain's ability to coordinate proper reactions to situations is compromised when there is a miscommunication between the hippocampus and the amygdala; that is, the hippocampus becomes less active when faced with an image of trauma, whereas the amygdala becomes overactive (Bisby *et al.* 2016). Thus, the amygdala can cause an inaccurate response to a stimulus, resulting in a fight-or-flight reaction. Individuals suffering from PTSD and emotional trauma have a chronic, constant dysfunction of the amygdala and the hippocampus circuitry even in a resting state (without exposure to the trauma trigger) (Marin *et al.* 2016).

ADDITIONAL AREAS OF THE BRAIN AFFECTED WHEN
RELIVING THE EMOTIONAL TRAUMA

| Brain Area | Function | Reaction to the Trauma Memory |
|---|---|---|
| Left Hemisphere | In charge of making plans and maintaining logical thought processes. | Shuts down (Van der Kolk 2014, p.45)—patients live in the past. |
| Right Hemisphere | Responsible for emotions, spatial connections, intuition, and tactile sensations. | Takes over (Van der Kolk 2014, p.45)—patients feel as if trauma is occurring again. |
| Broca's Area | In charge of speech. | Decreases in function (Van der Kolk 2014, p.45)—patients commonly shut down and are unable to express themselves. |

| Brain Area | Function | Reaction to the Trauma Memory |
|---|---|---|
| Broadman's Area | Responsible for registering images. | Increases in function (Van der Kolk 2014, p.44)—patients will see the images of a past trauma again. |
| Anterior Cingulate Cortex (ACC) | Regulates autonomic and endocrine functions, processes fear, "involved in conditioned emotional learning, vocalizations associated with expressing internal states…assigning emotional valence to internal and external stimuli…" (Devinsky, Morrell, and Vogt 1995). | Shuts down and fails to control the response of the amygdala (Shin *et al.* 2001)—body's physiology is falsely triggered. |

### The Body Physiology Reacting to a False Survival Situation

The emotional brain triggers the nervous system when faced with danger, and the vagus nerve responds. This is the body's safety mechanism, protecting the person from harm in a real survival situation. It activates the ventral vagal complex, signaling a fight-or-flight response (Van der Kolk 2014, pp.82–83). This stays active for as long as the person believes they are experiencing a traumatic event. Therefore, reliving a trauma memory causes a stressed state in the body (elevated blood pressure, breath rate, and heart rate) (Van der Kolk 2014, p.77). If the memory remains active, in time a person believes there is no way out of the situation. The dorsal vagal complex is initiated, and the body shuts down, reducing heart rate and slowing digestion. Essentially, the body freezes and the person withdraws (Van der Kolk 2014, p.86). The patient can shift this response by becoming cognizant of the present moment and their surroundings. This realization is a result of their pre-frontal cortex functioning properly. Managing reactions to situations is learned from mirroring.

### Mirroring and the Formation of a Healthy Pre-Frontal Cortex

Mirroring is a large part of brain development. The mirror neurons fire when a person carries out the same behavior as another person. These neurons enable a person to respond to others' feelings. Therefore, if a person is exposed to someone in a heightened emotional state, they can take on their reactions. Moreover, a person suffering from emotional trauma can be strongly affected by other people's emotions (Van der Kolk 2014, pp.58–59).

The pre-frontal cortex allows a person to react appropriately and manage desires and emotions. Experiencing an emotional trauma, especially at a young age, can alter the development of the pre-frontal cortex. As the intensity of the trauma increases, so does the level of difficulty of the pre-frontal cortex function to curb the emotional brain (Van der Kolk 2014, p.60). When a person experiences trauma or its memory, the thalamus is activated, sending signals to both the amygdala and the pre-frontal cortex. (The pre-frontal cortex receives the signals microseconds after the amygdala.) If the pre-frontal cortex is disabled, the amygdala takes over and the person loses control over their thoughts, feelings, emotions, and reactions (Van der Kolk 2014, pp.60–62). Patients "re-experience the visceral sensations felt during the original event," frequently resulting in hypersensitivity or numbness (Van der Kolk 2014, p.97).

### *Chronic Pain due to Reliving the Trauma Memory*

The pre-frontal cortex coordinates with the insula (responsible for body awareness and pain sensations) to send messages to the viscera. When the insula is activated (e.g., the trauma memory is triggered), the pain threshold is lowered and the patient's ability to feel sensations increases. Patients who continually relive a memory are likely to develop hypersensitivity and pains throughout their bodies (Korb 2015, p.26). Treatment benefiting the pre-frontal cortex is crucial to improve proper communication between the different lobes and halt the cascade of reactions.

The pre-frontal cortex has plasticity, meaning it changes over time based on trauma and input. Successful treatments rely on the ability of the pre-frontal cortex to morph and send appropriate signals to other areas of the brain, which allow the person to live in the moment. This has positive implications for the benefit of behavior-based therapy to change the functioning of a misfiring pre-frontal cortex (McEwen and Morrison 2013). In addition to addressing the pre-frontal cortex, there are methods to reset the limbic system and brainstem to stop the reliving of a past trauma.

## Conventional Western Medical Treatment Approaches

Western medicine treats emotional trauma by working on both the rational brain and the emotional brain. Re-establishing harmonious communication between the two allows patients to gain control of their emotions/impulses and restores homeostasis in the body.

**CONVENTIONAL WESTERN MEDICAL TREATMENT**

| | |
|---|---|
| *Psychotherapy* | Cognitive therapy and behavior therapy. |
| *Pharmaceutical Medication* | Antidepressants, antipsychotics, selective serotonin reuptake inhibitors (SSRIs), anti-anxiety medications, sedatives/hypnotics, and Prazosin. |

### *Psychotherapy*

Psychotherapy, both cognitive and behavioral therapy, focuses on retraining the patient's reaction to past trauma. In cognitive therapy, patients are given the opportunity to express the trauma, which leads to the identification of the faulty belief systems contributing to the patient being stuck in the trauma memory. Therapists help patients process fear, and other attached emotions, to remove them from their consciousness.

Behavior therapy is frequently incorporated into treatment, which exposes the patient to triggers reminding them of their past trauma. Utilizing Pavlov's theory, the more they are shown these reminders, the less intense the triggers become. Over time, patients can see they are safe and in tune with the present moment. Advancements in technology have assisted this approach, re-establishing the equilibrium of homeostasis and restoring the nervous system.

### *Incorporating Virtual Reality with Psychotherapy*

Clinical psychologist Skip Rizzo, at the University of Southern California Institute of Creative Technologies, designed a virtual reality program (a form of exposure therapy) that takes combat veterans through 14 different "worlds"—simulating combat scenarios—in the treatment of PTSD (Quart 2016). This method helps them process their trauma and clear the intensity of its memory. The use of virtual reality has the potential to be used for those not suffering from combat trauma. Specific individual trauma scenarios could be simulated to process their trauma.

### *Retraining the Brain Using Auditory and Visual Signals*

New techniques are emerging to retrain the amygdala using brain imaging. A study published in *Biological Psychiatry* utilized neurofeedback to have patients alter their own emotional responses to stressful events. Amygdala activity was measured by a low-cost electroencephalography (EEG) imaging tool and the subjects were taught how to implement the device with neurofeedback, thus reducing their amygdala activity (Medical Express 2016). In a secondary study, patients used the device to reduce the activity of the amygdala. Research concluded that patients could "modify both the neural processes and behavioral manifestations of their emotions" (Medical Express 2016).

The success of this low-cost bedside imaging tool has wide implications for the use of neurofeedback techniques to retrain the brain and alter its response to stressful events. Patients utilizing the device can practice breathing exercises and other techniques and monitor the response of their brain. This ultimately aids in healthy brain communication and can reset the brain's reaction to old trauma and, possibly, to future traumatic events.

### *Pharmaceutical Medication*

Medication treatment does work on some symptoms of emotional trauma. However, researchers reviewed several studies regarding PTSD treatment effectiveness and concluded that medication is not recommended as the first-line treatment of the disorder (Greenberg, Brooks, and Dunn 2015).

**SHORTCOMINGS OF USING PHARMACEUTICAL MEDICATION FOR TREATING EMOTIONAL TRAUMA/PTSD**

| Medication(s) | Benefit | Downside |
|---|---|---|
| SSRIs, anti-anxiety medications | Soothe the intensity of the trauma and aid the pre-frontal cortex. | Potentially divert attention from dealing with the underlying issues. |
| Sedative/hypnotic (i.e., benzodiazepines, Ativan) | Reduces anxiety associated with trauma. | Habit forming and only used short term. |
| Prazosin | Clinically used to stop nightmares. | Not approved by the FDA for PTSD treatment. |
| Antipsychotic medications (i.e., Abilify, Zyprexa, and Seroquel) | Reduces and blocks the sensations of the trauma. | Have serious negative side effects. |

*Source:* Adapted from Van der Kolk 2014, pp.36–37

## Alternative Treatments Utilized in Western Medical Settings

Patients suffering from PTSD are often unable to see a positive outcome and remain stuck in a trauma memory. When a patient is stuck in the trauma, their nervous system reacts to the world differently and they live with internal chaos. They struggle to suppress the memory. Dr. Van der Kolk states, "These attempts to maintain control over unbearable physiological reactions can result in a whole range of physical symptoms, including fibromyalgia, chronic fatigue, and other autoimmune diseases. This explains why it is critical for trauma treatment to engage the entire organism, body, mind, and brain" (Van der Kolk 2014, p.53).

### Role-Playing to Process Trauma

Peter Levine, in his book *Waking the Tiger*, tells a story of three cheetah cubs processing a trauma, learning from it, and using it to their advantage. One day, the cubs were left on their own while their mother went out to hunt. Subsequently, a lion approached and tried to eat them. The cubs ran from the predator for some distance before finding safety in a tree. The lion, discouraged by waiting, left the cubs. After the coast was clear, the cubs came down from the tree and re-enacted the event. Each played the predator and the prey and went over the chase again and again. When the mother cheetah returned, the cubs proudly acted out the scene for her. Through processing the trauma and learning a new skill, the cubs turned a near tragedy into a gift of education (Levine 1997, p.174).

Dr. Van der Kolk uses treatments that focus on both the rational brain (pre-frontal cortex) and the emotional brain (limbic system and brainstem). He refers to this as treating the brain from the top down or from the bottom up—the "top" being the rational brain, and the "bottom" being the emotional brain. The rational brain responds to mindfulness, meditation, and yoga; the emotional brain to breathing, movements (such as qigong and yoga), and touch (Van der Kolk 2014, pp.63–64 and 268). The goal is for a patient to fully process the trauma, move forward, and see solutions. Thus, the body and mind can live in the present, no longer caught in the memory.

*Alternative Treatments Utilized in Some Western Medical Settings*

- Eye Movement Desensitization and Reprocessing (EMDR)
- Meditation/Mindfulness/Affirmations
- Qigong/Yoga/Movement/Touch
- Dance, Drumming, and Singing Therapy.

## Resetting the Brain with EMDR

EMDR (comprised of eye movement therapy) is one of the newly implemented and integrated treatments being used in Western medical treatment to resolve trauma memories and restore proper brain function. EMDR acts to reset how a patient responds to the trauma and allows them to react differently to the memory. Therapy is conducted to clear the belief systems established during a trauma and provides a new perspective. When undergoing EMDR, it is important that the patient works with a therapist who is well trained in dealing with trauma, since memories surface and the patient can be triggered into a crisis state. Patients will frequently feel scattered during a series of EMDR sessions, and acupuncture assists in stabilizing them.

**STUDIES SHOWING THE EFFECTIVENESS OF EMDR**

| Medical Journal/Book (Date) | Research Finding |
| --- | --- |
| *Frontiers in Human Neuroscience* (2015) | EMDR helps the ACC regain control over the limbic system (Boccia *et al.* 2015). |
| *Psychological Trauma* (2016) | Patients undergoing EMDR require less conventional therapy sessions and have greater gains compared with those simply treated with conventional therapy alone (McLay *et al.* 2016). |
| *The Body Keeps the Score* (2014) | Patients undergoing EMDR experienced significantly better results in resolving trauma than those patients taking Prozac (Van der Kolk 2014, p.256). |

## *Reducing PTSD with Meditation and Yoga*

Patients who practice mindfulness and yoga improve the function of their pre-frontal cortex. This allows clear communication between the rational brain and the emotional brain (Tomasino and Fabbro 2016); thus the patient is no longer stuck in a trauma memory. A study published in *Military Medicine* measured two groups of military service members diagnosed with PTSD being treated with psychotropic drugs. One group practiced meditation regularly and the other did not. After one month, those in the meditation group had significantly reduced or ceased taking medication compared with the non-meditating group. A six-month follow-up yielded the same results and found that the severity of PTSD symptoms in the non-meditating group actually increased (Barnes *et al.* 2016).

TREATING EMOTIONAL TRAUMA WITH YOGA

| Medical Journal (Date) | Research Finding |
| --- | --- |
| *Journal of Alternative and Complementary Medicine* (2016) | A study of adult women showed that yoga reduced the mental and physical symptoms of PTSD (Rhodes, Spinazzola, and Van der Kolk 2016). |
| *International Journal of Yoga* (2015) | A study measured 100 ex-combatants from illegal armed groups suffering from PTSD. Half the group practiced yoga and the other half went through the regular demobilization program. The yoga group scored over 18 percent better on the Post Traumatic Checklist (Quiñones *et al.* 2015). |
| *Journal of Alternative and Complementary Medicine* (2015) | Orphans in Haiti (between the ages of seven and 17) practiced yoga, breathing exercises, and mindfulness meditation and successfully reduced trauma-related issues (Culver *et al.* 2015). |

## *Dancing, Drumming, and Singing Away Distress*

The emotional brain responds to activities such as breath work, dance, drumming, bouncing on a yoga ball, tossing a beach ball back and forth, and EFT (Emotional Freedom Technique). These exercises help the person live in the present and shift the memory. People feel safe and they begin to trust their environment; with each success, a new way to process reality is revealed. Their emotional brain no longer takes over when they feel sensations related to their trauma memories.

| Modality | Finding of Study |
|----------|------------------|
| Dancing | Dance Movement Therapy (DMT) reduced "anxiety, depression, intrusive recollection, elevated arousal, and aggression" for African adolescent torture survivors (Harris 2007). Several studies confirm the effectiveness of dance to treat trauma-related distress (Levine and Land 2016). |
| Drumming | Drumming improved the brain's coordination/communication and released emotional trauma (Winkelman 2003). |
| Singing | Singing alleviated anxiety, lifted depression, and improved patients' energy to endure cancer treatment by Western medicine (Hamilton *et al.* 2016). |

## Parallels of Trauma Pathophysiology

Understanding correlations between Western medicine and Chinese medicine is helpful. It is important to not make direct connections between the two paradigms since they are profoundly different; however, comparing the Chinese medicine understanding of trauma pathophysiology to the recent brain research in Western medicine uncovers interesting parallels. Yin and yang are akin to the right and left hemispheres.

**APPROXIMATE COMPARISON OF THE RIGHT AND LEFT HEMISPHERES AND YIN AND YANG**

| Right Hemisphere | Left Hemisphere |
|------------------|-----------------|
| Related to intuition, emotions, and tactile, spatial, and visual sensations. | Oversees verbalizing and organizing experiences. |
| Yin (associated with feeling, emotions, and feminine). | Yang (associated with structure, planning, logic, and masculine). |

The two halves of the brain operating in harmony enable a person to process feelings, and express them—remaining in the present moment. When a trauma is relived, the left hemisphere shuts down and the right takes over, sending the patient into a flood of emotions that goes unchecked as they spiral into the trauma memory. Yin is associated with water, deep with feeling. This mystery of emotion overwhelms and causes a sense of drowning. Bringing yang brightness will guide a patient to the present moment and empower them to swim free from the undercurrent of emotions. However, too much yang (logic/structure) can lead to operating like a robot (the opposite of being emotional—e.g., Mr. Spock from *Star Trek*) and going to the other extreme; balance is essential.

Another similarity is found comparing the three aspects of the brain involved in emotional trauma and the three Dantians of Chinese medicine, as shown in the table below and Figure 6.2.

**APPROXIMATE CORRESPONDENCE BETWEEN THE
BRAIN TRIAD AND THE THREE DANTIANS**

| | |
|---|---|
| Pre-Frontal Cortex | Upper Dantian |
| Limbic System | Middle Dantian |
| Brainstem | Lower Dantian |

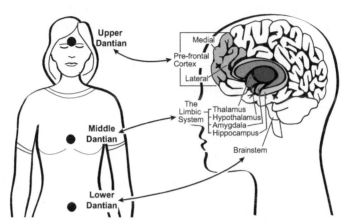

*Figure 6.2 Comparison of the Brain Triad and the Three Dantians Here*
*Source:* Kirsteen Wright

## The Pre-Frontal Cortex and the Upper Dantian

The pre-frontal cortex is responsible for empathy and appropriate responses to stimuli, akin to the upper Dantian governing a person's intent and thoughts. Both provide perspective on experiences, providing a person with a clear understanding of their current situation. The person relates to their environment in a global context (free from personal drama) and is liberated from the triggering of the trauma memory. Therefore, the pre-frontal cortex notes the absence of any actual trauma and the amygdala does not send fight-or-flight signals or shut down the body—similar to the upper Dantian providing clarity and presence.

Several acupuncture points can be stimulated to open the upper Dantian. Yin Tang, DU-20, DU-24, and DU-19 activate the upper Dantian to help improve the function of the pre-frontal cortex. The area on the face relating to the third eye is associated with the liver. Therefore, utilizing points such as LV-2, LV-3, LV-4, and LV-5 opens the upper Dantian and helps the pre-frontal cortex's ability to bring a patient into the present moment and out of the trauma memory.

## The Limbic System and the Middle Dantian

The limbic system is the middle aspect of the brain and is the emotional center. When emotions are excited, the amygdala sends signals to the body, and the organ systems are put into fight-or-flight mode—or shut down. The middle Dantian relates to the heart, and in Chinese medicine the heart stores the spirit. The heart is considered the emperor of the body, and when peaceful, rules with grace and harmony. If the emperor is disturbed by emotion (the stirring of the heart mirror), the body suffers from the disruption. The limbic system and the heart in Chinese medicine rely on clear perception to effectively govern the body. Thus, both share a connection to the emotional aspect of the body and when disturbed cause physiological responses.

Settling the mind can be accomplished by stimulating points that affect the heart and, as a result, calm the limbic system. Activating points on the pericardium, heart, and gallbladder channels, along with DU-11, R-17, and auricular acupuncture points (Anxiety, Shen Men, and Heart), achieves stillness in the heart pool and thus stabilizes the limbic system.

### The Brainstem and the Lower Dantian

In some ways, the brainstem is like the lower Dantian as it is the first part of the brain to develop and links people to their reptilian ancestry. The lower Dantian relates to the root and connects to the ancestors. The Du and Ren vessels originate in the lower Dantian and are the first channels to form in the body. The brainstem governs the basic physiological functions, which roughly compares to the Jing. Jing is held in the kidneys and resides in the lower Dantian.

Benefiting the Jing via the kidneys can be achieved by activating points on the kidney and san jiao channels. Specifically, KD-3, KD-6, KD-7, and SJ-4 prove clinically helpful in the re-ordering of the physiologic functions, akin to brainstem regulation. Using local points is also helpful, such as R-4, R-6, DU-4, and KD-16.

The kidneys can influence how the brainstem sends signals to the body. One researcher discussed the connection between fear-induced kidney deficiency and the amygdala–hippocampus–pre-frontal cortex nervous pathway. His article proved that fear depleting the kidneys (the material foundation of the central nervous system) created miscommunication in the brain, which in turn triggered a response in the body's physiological functions (Liu *et al.* 2010). Qigong practitioners emphasize rooting one's energy in the lower Dantian to stabilize and harmonize the body, akin to a correctly functioning brainstem sending appropriate signals to maintain balance in the body.

## Similarities in Treatment Approaches

Both Western medicine and Chinese medicine address trauma by constructing treatment approaches based on the various aspects of trauma pathophysiology described above. Dr. Van der Kolk utilizes two approaches—the bottom-up method (focusing on the emotional brain) and the top-down method (targeting the rational brain) (Van der Kolk 2014, p.63). These can be roughly compared to the Chinese medicine acupuncture protocols "Gathering the Qi" (mothering the body) and "Soothing the Trauma Memory" (fathering the body).

### SIMILARITIES IN MODERN WESTERN MEDICAL APPROACHES AND ACUPUNCTURE PROTOCOLS

| Van der Kolk's Approach | Acupuncture Protocol |
|---|---|
| *Bottom Up—Treats the Emotional Brain* | *"Gathering the Qi"—Yin (Mothering)* |
| 1. Concentrates on the limbic system and the brainstem to maintain internal stability. | 1. Connects the three Dantians to ground the patient and stabilize the organ systems. |
| 2. Utilizes body-centered modalities (breathing, movement, and touch). | 2. Supplies blood to the organs and spaces in the body to coordinate body functions. |
| 3. Harmonizes body functions and emotions to maintain internal stability. | 3. Calms the spirit to settle emotions. |
| | 4. Supports the earth element to restore a harmonious rhythmic function in the body. |
| *Top Down—Treats the Rational Brain* | *"Soothing the Trauma Memory"—Yang (Fathering)* |
| 1. Focuses on the pre-frontal cortex function to reduce and eliminate the triggers causing disruption in homeostasis. | 1. Brings cosmic water down to the mind to clear the heat and wind of the trauma memory, which improves the coordination of the organ systems. |
| 2. Uses thought-based treatments (mindfulness, meditation, and yoga). | 2. Activates the medial pre-fontal cortex (view of self) and the dorsolateral pre-frontal cortex (view of environment). Therefore, the patient is prevented from being transported to the time of trauma. |

## *Differentiation Beginning in Western Medical Treatment of Trauma*

To fully clear a trauma, treatments must be individualized, focusing on the specific imbalances in each patient. Chinese medicine places a strong emphasis on differential diagnosis and individualized treatments. Western medicine now is beginning to offer customized treatment approaches for emotional trauma. EMDR, cognitive behavior therapies, and, in some cases, individualized medications seek to tailor treatment to each patient's specific issues (Ponteva *et al.* 2015).

## Chinese Medicine and Western Medicine Working in Harmony

> *Coming together is a beginning. Keeping together is progress. Working together is success.*
>
> *Henry Ford*

Many medical facilities across the globe integrate Chinese medicine into the treatment of mental health issues. Programs that utilize acupuncture, herbal medicine, qigong, shamanic drumming, and EFT—along with counseling and medication—prove effective (Aung, Fay, and Hobbs 2013). Auricular acupuncture is utilized at several U.S. military facilities as a complement or alternative to traditional treatments. Its use increased after various clinics treating veterans for PTSD found it effective in reducing trauma symptoms (King, Moore, and Spence 2016). An additional study of 55 service members showed that acupuncture decreased PTSD symptoms (including depression and pain) and improved physical and mental health function (Engel *et al.* 2014).

WESTERN MEDICAL RESEARCH OF CHINESE MEDICINE
(ACUPUNCTURE AND HERBAL MEDICINE)

| Chinese Medicine | Western Research Findings |
|---|---|
| Bleeding jing-well points | Slowed the interstitial fluid flow in the thalamus (Fu *et al.* 2016), suggesting that this technique can affect the hypothalamus stress hormone response to emotional trauma. |
| Needling ST-36 versus sham acupuncture | ST-36 produced different EEG and fMRI patterns than sham acupuncture (Wong 2016). |
| True acupuncture versus sham | True acupuncture positively affected communication in the brain to reduce pain (Egorova, Gollub, and Kong 2015). |
| Electro-acupuncture on DU-20 and DU-24 (with support points Sishencong (M-HN-1) and Fengchi GB-20) | "Electro-acupuncture has certain improving effects on PTSD symptoms, which is likely to be related with enhancing the connectivity between parietal lobe and hippocampus…leading to an indirect influence on [the] limbic system" (Zheng *et al.* 2015). |
| Sailuotong (SLT)—consists of Xi Yang Shen, Bai Guo, and Hong Hua (Panax ginseng, Ginkgo biloba, and Crocus sativus) | Improved memory and cognitive function (Steiner *et al.* 2016), thus showing that certain herbs increase brain communication and demonstrate their potential in treating emotional trauma. |
| Review of over 1500 papers discussing Chinese herbs to treat anxiety | Several herbs successfully treat anxiety (Sarris, McIntyre, and Camfield 2013). |

## *Processing Trauma with the Help of Both Chinese Medicine and Western Medicine*

Therapies such as acupuncture offer patients body awareness to shift them out of the trauma memory state and reformulate ways of interpreting trauma. The patients become present in their bodies as the trauma is processed on a physical level, enabling them to clear old emotions. Utilizing these body-oriented modalities with cognitive therapy provides patients a means with which to express their feelings, as blockages in the channels and organs are released. This synergistic approach increases the transformation of the trauma and its memory.

Promising research and an increased openness to Chinese medicine by the Western medical community gives hope that integrated treatments will continue to be developed and utilized to treat the complicated issue of emotional trauma. Isaac Newton declared, "We build too many walls and not enough bridges." May innovations in the treatment of emotional trauma perpetually turn this phrase around and bring a bounty of effective multi-disciplinary treatments.

## Summary of Western Medicine and Chinese Medicine Joining Hands

Practitioners of both Western medicine and Chinese medicine both seek advancement in treating emotional trauma. This budding field blooms as practitioners consistently strive for increasingly effective treatments and new studies provide more information and insight to expand the knowledge of trauma. Joining hands and working together will prove to be the best way to transform trauma, thus stopping it from being passed down to future generations. Resetting patients' nervous systems and harmonizing their organ systems allows them to live to their full potential.

Many practitioners recognize the power of the healer's intention in the success of treatment. The clearer the practitioner is about the mechanism of disease and how they want to treat it, the better the result. This clarity relates to the stilling of their heart pool, since the heart of the healer plays a significant role in caring for patients. One study proved how the subtle heart energy does connect with patients. The author demonstrated that those patients who sat at a three- to four-foot range from the practitioner, compared with patients who sat at a 15- to 18-foot range, produced substantial heart-rate synchronization. The patients closest to the providers experienced less stress and an improvement in mood (Bair 2008). Practitioners of Western medicine and Chinese medicine working with a combined intention—as their hearts sync up—will bring wonders to the field of treating emotional trauma.

### References

Aung, S.K., Fay, H., and Hobbs, R.F. (2013) "Traditional Chinese medicine as a basis for treating psychiatric disorders: a review of theory with illustrative cases." *Med. Acupunct. 25*, 6, 398–406.

Bair, C.C. (2008) "The heart field effect: synchronization of healer–subject heart rates in energy therapy." *Adv. Mind Body Med. 23*, 4, 10–19.

Barnes, V.A., Monto, A., Williams, J.J., and Rigg, J.L. (2016) "Impact of transcendental meditation on psychotropic medication use among active duty military service members with anxiety and PTSD." *Mil. Med. 181*, 1, 56–63.

Bisby, J.A., Horner, A.J., Hørlyck, L.D., and Burgess, N. (2016) "Opposing effects of negative emotion on amygdalar and hippocampal memory for items and associations." *Soc. Cogn. Affect. Neurosci. 11*, 6, 981–990.

Boccia, M., Piccardi, L., Cordellieri, P., Guariglia, C., and Giannini, A.M. (2015) "EMDR therapy for PTSD after motor vehicle accidents: meta-analytic evidence for specific treatment." *Front. Hum. Neurosci. 9*, 213.

Culver, K.A., Whetten, K., Boyd, D.L., and O'Donnell, K. (2015) "Yoga to reduce trauma-related distress and emotional and behavioral difficulties among children living in orphanages in Haiti: a pilot study." *J. Altern. Complement. Med. 21*, 9, 539–545.

Devinsky, O., Morrell, M.J., and Vogt, B.A. (1995) "Contributions of anterior cingulate cortex to behaviour." *Brain 118*, Pt 1, 279–306.

Egorova, N., Gollub, R.L., and Kong, J. (2015) "Repeated verum but not placebo acupuncture normalizes connectivity in brain regions dysregulated in chronic pain." *Neuroimage Clin. 9*, 430–435.

Engel, C.C., Cordova, E.H., Benedek, D.M., Liu, X., *et al.* (2014) "Randomized effectiveness trial of a brief course of acupuncture for posttraumatic stress disorder." *Med. Care 52*, 12, Suppl. 5, S57–S64.

Frick, A., Åhs, F., Palmquist, Å.M., Pissiota, A., *et al.* (2016) "Overlapping expression of serotonin transporters and neurokinin-1 receptors in posttraumatic stress disorder: a multi-tracer PET study." *Mol. Psychiatry 21*, 1400–1407.

Fu, Y., Li, Y., Guo, J., Liu, B., *et al.* (2016) "Bloodletting at jing-well points decreases interstitial fluid flow in the thalamus of rats." *J. Tradit. Chin. Med. 36*, 1, 107–112.

Greenberg, N., Brooks, S., and Dunn, R. (2015) "Latest developments in post-traumatic stress disorder: diagnosis and treatment." *Br. Med. Bull. 114*, 1, 147–155.

Hamilton, J.B., Worthy, V.C., Kurtz, M.J., Cudjoe, J., and Johnstone, P.A. (2016) "Using religious songs as an integrative and complementary therapy for the management of psychological symptoms among African American cancer survivors." *Cancer Nurs. 39*, 6, 488–494.

Harris, D.A. (2007) "Dance/movement therapy approaches to fostering resilience and recovery among African adolescent torture survivors." *Torture 17*, 2, 134–155.

King, C.H., Moore, L.C., and Spence, C.D. (2016) "Exploring self-reported benefits of auricular acupuncture among veterans with posttraumatic stress disorder." *J. Holist. Nurs. 34*, 3, 291–299.

Korb, A. (2015) *The Upward Spiral.* Oakland, CA: New Harbinger.

Levine, B., and Land, H.M. (2016) "A meta-synthesis of qualitative findings about dance/movement therapy for individuals with trauma." *Qual. Health Res. 26*, 3, 330–344.

Levine, P. (1997) *Waking the Tiger.* Berkeley, CA: North Atlantic Books.

Liu, S.K., Yan, C., Wu, L.L., and Pan, Y. (2010) "Study strategies for neurobiology mechanism of 'kidney storing will and responding to fear.'" [In Chinese.] *Zhong Xi Yi Jie He Xue Bao 8*, 2, 106–110.

Marin, M.F., Song, H., Van Elzakker, M.B., Staples-Bradley, L.K., *et al.* (2016) "Association of resting metabolism in the fear neural network with extinction recall activations and clinical measures in trauma-exposed individuals." *Am. J. Psychiatry 173*, 9, 930–938.

McEwen, B.S., and Morrison, J.H. (2013) "The brain on stress: vulnerability and plasticity of the prefrontal cortex over the life course." *Neuron. 79*, 1, 16–29.

McLay, R.N., Webb-Murphy, J.A., Fesperman, S.F., Delaney, E.M., *et al.* (2016) "Outcomes from eye movement desensitization and reprocessing in active-duty service members with posttraumatic stress disorder." *Psychol. Trauma 8*, 6, 702–770.

Medical Express (2016) *When Output Becomes Part of Input.* Available at http://medicalxpress.com/news/2016-09-amygdala-emotions.html, accessed on 1 June 2017.

Ponteva, M., Henriksson, M., Isoaho, R., Laukkala, T., Punamäki, L., and Wahlbeck, K.; Päivitystiivistelmä (2015) "Update on current care guidelines: post-traumatic stress disorder." [In Finnish.] *Duodecim 131*, 6, 558–559.

Quart, J. (2016) *Treating PTSD with Virtual Reality Therapy: A Way to Heal Trauma.* Available at http://abcnews. go.com/Technology/treating-ptsd-virtual-reality-therapy-heal-trauma/story?id=38742665, accessed on 1 June 2017.

Quiñones, N., Maquet, Y.G., Vélez, D.M., and López, M.A. (2015) "Efficacy of a Satyananda yoga intervention for reintegrating adults diagnosed with posttraumatic stress disorder." *Int. J. Yoga Therap. 25*, 1, 89–99.

Rhodes, A., Spinazzola, J., and Van der Kolk, B. (2016) "Yoga for adult women with chronic PTSD: a long-term follow-up study." *J. Altern. Complement. Med. 22*, 3, 189–196.

Sarris, J., McIntyre, E., and Camfield, D.A. (2013) "Plant-based medicines for anxiety disorders, part 2: a review of clinical studies with supporting preclinical evidence." *CNS Drugs 27*, 4, 301–319.

Shin, L.M., Whalen, P.J., Pitman, R.K., Bush, G., *et al.* (2001) "An fMRI study of anterior cingulate function in post-traumatic stress disorder." *Biol. Psychiatry 50*, 12, 932–942.

Steiner, G.Z., Yeung, A., Liu, J.X., Camfield, D.A., *et al.* (2016) "The effect of Sailuotong (SLT) on neurocognitive and cardiovascular function in healthy adults: a randomised, double-blind, placebo controlled crossover pilot trial." *BMC Complement. Altern. Med. 16*, 1, 15.

Tomasino, B., and Fabbro, F. (2016) "Increases in the right dorsolateral prefrontal cortex and decreases the rostral prefrontal cortex activation after 8 weeks of focused attention based mindfulness meditation." *Brain Cogn. 102*, 46–54.

Van der Kolk, B. (2014) *The Body Keeps the Score.* London and New York: Penguin.

Winkelman, M. (2003) "Complementary therapy for addiction: 'drumming out drugs.'" *Am. J. Public Health 93*, 4, 647–651.

Wong, Y.M. (2016) "Commentary: differential cerebral response to somatosensory stimulation of an acupuncture point vs. two non-acupuncture points measured with EEG and fMRI." *Front. Hum. Neurosci. 10*, 63. Available at http://journal.frontiersin.org/article/10.3389/fnhum.2016.00063/full, accessed on 2 June 2017.

Zheng, C., Tan, L., Zhou, T., and Zhang, H. (2015) "Effects of electroacupuncture on resting-state encephalic functional connectivity network in patients with PTSD." [In Chinese.] *Zhongguo Zhen Jiu 35*, 5, 469–473.

CHAPTER 7

# Case Studies

The body, mind, and spirit of countless people have benefited from the effectiveness of Chinese medicine for millennia. The theories and treatment methods posed in this text are expanded upon in the following case studies to display their validity in clinical practice and, more importantly, in the resolution of emotional trauma. The collection of cases exhibits the diverse spectrum of emotional trauma and the various diagnostic and treatment methods in action. Both detailed and abbreviated case studies demonstrate the flow of first "Gathering the Qi" and then "Soothing the Trauma Memory," followed by addressing specific channel and organ systems. They are presented in the highest spirit of appreciation for the people who agreed to share their stories and outcomes. Without their generosity, the text would merely be a book filled with hypotheses and lack real support.

## Case 1: 58-Year-Old Female Transcended Feeling Unsafe in the World

(Also see Holman 2016.)

### *Initial Visit*

*Background*

A 58-year-old woman, "Grace," reported strong right hip and left low back pain after experiencing a traumatic event. While on vacation with her partner, she woke in the middle of the night to distressing noises. She discovered that her partner was having a grand mal seizure. Grace alerted the friends they were staying with and called 911. Her partner was treated and soon recovered.

Although this experience was disturbing in its own right, it triggered a trauma memory from Grace's childhood. When she was nine years old her father had a medical emergency in the middle of the night. Grace found him and went for help, but when she returned to his room, he was dead.

Feelings of vulnerability and insecurity had haunted her ever since her father's death, and resurfaced intensely following her partner's trauma. She felt alone, often crying and feeling anxious. In the clinic, she appeared small and unsure, as if she had reverted to her nine-year-old self. Grace had recently retired and said she was feeling a lack of purpose. She had just survived a life-threatening illness which contributed to her feeling of uncertainty.

Physically, she had intense local pain in her right hip that increased with activity and radiated down her leg. The pain varied from 3 to 7 on a scale from 1 to 10, and was achy and sometimes burning. She also experienced constant deep, aching left low back pain that wrapped around to her hip. Grace used heat, stretching, and tiger balm to alleviate the pain, but it remained intense. She also reported an increase of phlegm in her sinuses. She had begun seeing a counselor to address the anxiety and crying episodes.

*See Figure 7.1.*

## Diagnosis

Scattered Qi, Ungrounded Shen, Kidney Deficiency with Heat, and Local Qi and Blood Stagnation in the Shao Yang Channel and Dai Vessel.

**DIAGNOSTIC SIGNS**

| Diagnostic Method | Finding | Meaning |
| --- | --- | --- |
| *Face* Jing Markers | Lost love lines. | Lost some part of herself. |
| | Emotional lines—grief, impatience, stress, and bitterness. | Feeling sad, irritated, stressed, and had a sense things didn't work out as she had hoped respectively. |
| *Face* Qi Markers | Dimpled, wobbly, and lined chin. | A strong feeling of fear. |
| | Redness on her entire nose and around her mouth. | Heat in the lungs and digestive system respectively. |
| | Lines and paleness at the bridge of her nose. | Spleen deficiency and blood sugar instability. |
| | Tears in her eyes. | Raw presence of the emotional trauma. |
| | Indentation in her forehead. | Deep despair. |
| *Face* Shen Markers | Dark and muddy Shen. | Qi and blood stagnation and confusion. |
| | Sad, lost, timid look and powerless demeanor. | Feeling alone, scared, and lacking a sense of purpose and clarity. |

| Diagnostic Method | Finding | Meaning |
|---|---|---|
| *Channel Palpation* | A general tightness in the pericardium channel and nodules at PC-6. | Impaired blood circulation to the organs due to tightness in the pericardium. |
| *Pulse* | Thin and choppy. | Blood deficiency and stagnation. |
| *Tongue* | Entire tongue body was dusky red. | Blood stagnation with heat. |
| | A thick white coat that was dry on the surface. | Phlegm misting the heart, along with an accumulation of dampness generating heat and drying the fluids. |
| *Physical Symptom Energetics* | Pain wrapping around her waist to her hip. | Involvement of the Dai vessel—where her childhood trauma had been repressed. |
| *Spirit Perception* | Powerlessness. | Weak Zhi. |

## Treatment Principle

Gather the Qi, Soothe the Trauma Memory, Calm and Ground the Shen, Clear Heat, Tonify the Kidneys, Move Qi and Blood, and Transform Phlegm.

**TREATMENT**

| Modality | Explanation |
|---|---|
| • "Gathering the Qi" protocol with the addition of the Master Tung point Xia Bai 22.07.<br>• *Infrared heat on her abdomen.*<br>• *EFT.*<br>• *Counseled on doing minimal physical exercise for one to two weeks.* | The "Gathering the Qi" protocol was used to center and ground the patient. After 15 minutes, 22.07 was incorporated to address the right-side hip pain associated with the kidney deficiency. The heat and EFT were used to settle her spirit. |

## Second Visit
**CHANGES AFTER TREATMENT**

| *Subjective Changes* | She felt calm and settled and reported realizing how her insecurity encompassed her life and was triggered frequently. Her low back pain was reduced, although her right-side hip pain was intense and still radiated down her leg. She also still had phlegm. |
|---|---|
| *Objective Changes* | Her face had shifted from having the look of a scared little girl to an adult processing her emotional history (the darkness under her eyes reflected the use of her kidneys to work through the old trauma). The indentation on her forehead was filling in—displaying a new-found hope. The nodules at PC-6 reduced and softened, showing an improved circulation of blood. Her tongue was less red and dusky, indicating reduced heat and blood stagnation. |

*See Figure 7.2.*

**TREATMENT**

| Modality | Explanation |
|---|---|
| *Acupuncture*<br>• Baihui DU-20<br>• Shenting DU-24<br>• "Gathering the Qi" protocol<br>• Huangshu KD-16<br>• Xia Bai 22.07 on the left<br>• Zulinqi GB-41 on the right | The "Soothing the Trauma Memory" and the "Gathering the Qi" protocols were combined to help her process the trauma and stay in the present moment. Only part of the "Soothing the Trauma Memory" protocol was used in order to limit the number of needles and avoid overstimulation. KD-16 was added to tonify her kidneys since she was processing old fear and trauma. Because the point is on the abdomen, it helped to center her qi. 22.07 was combined with GB-41 (the opening point on the Dai vessel) to treat her hip pain. |
| • *Infrared heat on her abdomen.*<br>• *A gentle hip exercise to open the joint was taught to her.* | Heat was directed to her abdomen to center her energy. The exercise facilitated the opening of the Dai vessel. |

## Third Visit

**CHANGES AFTER TREATMENT**

| Subjective Changes | Grace said she felt much better overall. She felt relaxed and less anxious. The triggers of feeling unsafe and small were minimal. She felt more in her body. Her hip pain was lessened but she still ached with some workouts. The pain was focused in her right low back. |
|---|---|
| Objective Changes | Grace looked taller and more powerful. She is a strong woman and her strength was showing. Her Shen was light and present. Her face literally became soft and round. The redness on her nose and chin reduced. The lines and dimpling on her chin had softened. Her eyes were lighter and she didn't have tears when talking about the old trauma. |

*See Figure 7.3.*

## Analysis

Grace shifted from being caught in the trauma to being present as an adult. She was grounded, settled, and full of energy. The "Soothing the Trauma Memory" protocol enabled her higher self to communicate with her earthly self and step into a place of strength and composure. The addition of GB-41 reduced the hip pain, and KD-16 helped her to process her fear and stand tall. Her emotional trauma was no longer overbearing, allowing detailed work on her kidneys and blockage in the gallbladder channel.

**TREATMENT**

| Modality | Explanation |
|---|---|
| *Acupuncture* <br> • Baihui DU-20 <br> • Shenting DU-24 <br> • Yinxi HT-6 <br> • Huangshu KD-16 <br> • Taixi KD-3 <br> • Zulinqi GB-41 <br> • Juliao GB-29 and Fengshi GB-31 with electric stimulation, both on the right | Grace stabilized from the trauma, which allowed for more specific treatment of the affected channels and organ systems. Her third treatment occurred in mid-December—the heavenly stem was Gui (the kidney organ), the earthly branch was Zi (shao yin weather), and the open channel was gallbladder. Since her pain was located on the gallbladder channel, local point GB-29 was paired with GB-31. Electric stimulation (with gentle intensity and frequency) was used to promote qi and blood flow in the channel. KD-3 was used to tonify the kidneys. In hindsight, KD-7 might have been a better choice to nourish the fluids depleted by the heat, created by the trauma. HT-6 was selected to clear heat and calm the spirit. Activation of GB-41 and KD-16 was repeated. |
| • *Infrared heat on her right hip.* | Heat was directed to her hip to open the gallbladder channel and Dai vessel. |

## *Summary*

*See Figure 7.4.*

Fifteen days after her third treatment, Grace reported feeling emotionally stable, with only one occurrence of mild anxiety. Her hip and low back pain were less intense. Her Shen glowed through her skin and her eyes were clear. Grace appeared strong, present, and confident. Her face underwent a significant transformation from oval to round and lifted, and the indentation in her forehead filled in. The tightness in the pericardium channel relaxed. Her choppy pulse resolved and her white tongue coating reduced, which showed her blood was now moving more smoothly and the fluid accumulation was transforming.

Grace had experienced an intense traumatic event which triggered an old trauma memory, from which she had created a faulty belief system of being unsafe in the world. The recent trauma acted as a gateway to the old trauma, which is common. Also, frequently after retirement or a life-threatening illness, a person's ability to ground and feel safe is affected, giving rise to old trauma memories. Grace had experienced both and was intensely shaken by her partner's seizure.

The initial treatment focused first on stabilizing her body and mind and re-establishing homeostasis. If the primary focus at the first visit was to address only the hip and low back pain, this would likely mean her qi flow would continue to be disrupted. After the first treatment, she felt grounded and could begin to process her emotions. Incorporating the "Soothing the Trauma Memory" protocol into the second treatment was essential to help her feel present in the moment and stop reliving the old trauma.

This case demonstrates the importance of grounding a patient after a trauma and helping them process old trauma to break the cycle. Grace gained a new perspective on her old trauma. She could now move forward without going back into the nine-year-old state of mind. Continued treatment on soothing the trauma and benefiting the kidneys would be necessary to fully clear her issues.

Looking at this case from a Western perspective, there was miscommunication between Grace's rational brain and emotional brain. When her trauma was triggered, her pre-frontal cortex appeared to not be registering the present moment surroundings and her limbic system had taken over control. Her emotional brain continued to send fight-or-flight signals to her nervous system each time the trauma was triggered, being transported in time back to her nine-year-old self. The "Gathering the Qi" protocol grounded her and helped her body regain a peaceful homeostatic state so that she could clearly see her present situation. The "Soothing the Trauma Memory" protocol benefited her pre-frontal cortex and limbic system communication. The treatments helped her to step into the world and move forward on her path with confidence. Grace could then shine, present and illuminated.

## Case 2: 57-Year-Old Female Released from the Trauma Memory of Late Husband's Suicide

### Initial Visit

#### Background

"Vivian" was in a car accident and suffered neck, shoulder, and hip pain. The accident triggered grief about her late husband's suicide two years prior and she was as distraught and shaken as when she found him in January 2014. (He had taken his life with a gunshot to the head.) Vivian had high levels of anxiety, poor sleep, and migraines. Her right-side neck and shoulder pains were rated at a level of 8 (on a scale of 1–10), and her left hip pain was at a 7. Due to the intensity of her emotional state, documenting her case with pictures started with the third treatment.

*See Figure 7.5.*

#### Diagnosis

Scattered Qi, Qi and Blood Stagnation in the Shao Yang Channel, Heart/Spleen Qi and Blood Deficiency, Heart Blood Stagnation, and Kidney Yin Deficient Heat.

**DIAGNOSTIC SIGNS**

| Diagnostic Method | Finding | Meaning |
| --- | --- | --- |
| *Face* Jing Markers | Faint line encircling her mouth. | Fear of abandonment, starvation, and not having enough money to survive. |
| | Vertical line on both her nose tip and in her philtrum. | Gives of herself to others (especially those close to her) to the point of creating blood deficiency and limiting her creativity. |
| | Several emotional lines. | Grief, irritation, over-nurturing, stress, and disempowerment. |
| *Face* Qi Markers | Dusky nose (especially on the right), indented (as if pushed in), and wobbly or unstable. | Symbolizes the spine and how a person is in the world—the accident and the trauma memory were limiting her ability to move forward. |
| | Swelling in lower lip. | Difficulty letting go. |
| | Dimpled red chin. | Heat in the kidneys and fear. |
| *Face* Shen Markers | Dusky skin tone, reflecting stagnation. | Stagnation. |
| | Cloudy eyes. | Muddled spirit. |
| *Channel Palpation* | Small nodules in the pericardium channel. | Tightness/blockage in her heart. |
| *Pulse* | Thin, tight, smooth vibration, and choppy. | Qi stagnation, instability, and blood stagnation. |
| *Tongue* | Slightly dusky, indentation on the tip. | Stagnation and heart blood deficiency. |
| *Physical Symptom Energetics* | Her hip suffered from the impact of the car accident—mobilized her Dai vessel. | Repressed trauma can be stored in the Dai vessel—the accident dislodged the embedded trauma of her late husband's suicide. |
| *Spirit Perception* | Felt frozen and disorientated. | Fear of being alone; scattered Shen from the shock of the trauma memory affecting her heart and kidneys. |

## Treatment Principle

Gather Qi, Stabilize the Shen, Tonify the Zhi, Soothe the Trauma Memory, Regulate Shao Yang, Tonify Heart and Spleen, Clear Heat, and Nourish Yin.

## TREATMENT

| Modality | Explanation |
|---|---|
| • "Gathering the Qi" protocol. | The "Gathering the Qi" protocol was used to |
| • *Infrared heat on her abdomen.* | center her, help her let go of the past, gain a new |
| • *Shamanic Journey Drumbeat.* | perspective, secure her spirit, and help build self- |
| • *She was taught gentle qigong exercises for her shoulder.* | love. The Shamanic Journey Drumbeat was played to ground her spirit and support her heart. |

## *Second Visit*

Vivian reported feeling grounded and calm. She complained of fatigue (a common phenomenon after settling the qi) but was feeling less nervous energy.

## TREATMENT

| Modality | Explanation |
|---|---|
| *Acupuncture* | San Cha San and Biyi were substituted for PC-6 |
| • Yin Tang (M-HN-3) | to support her energy. The earthly branch at the |
| • San Cha San (similar to Yemen SJ-2) | time of treatment was Hai (pig); thus San Cha San, |
| • Zhongwan R-12 | on the shao yang channel, was selected. |
| • Sanyinjiao SP-6 | |
| • Biyi 1010.22 | |
| • *Encouraged to follow a structured routine of eating, sleeping, and gentle exercise.* | To stabilize her Shen. |

## *Third Visit*
### CHANGES AFTER TREATMENT

| Subjective Changes | Increased energy but still feeling the sad loss of her husband and having bouts of restless sleep. Shoulder and hip pain had lessened to a 5 out of 10. Neck pain was the most aggravating—rated at a 7. |
|---|---|
| Objective Changes | Shadowing on her nose reduced. Vertical line on her nose tip faded, but the other lines (disempowerment, irritation, grief, stress, abandonment, and over-nurturing) remained the same. Chin was less red and dimpled, indicating a reduction of fear and heat. Her eyes started to sparkle. The skin Shen was beginning to lighten. |

**TREATMENT**

| Modality | Explanation |
|---|---|
| *Acupuncture*<br>• "Soothing the Trauma Memory" protocol<br>• Shenmen HT-7<br>• Sanyinjiao SP-6<br>• Yangfu GB-38 on the left<br>• Xuanzhong GB-39 on the left | The "Soothing the Trauma Memory" protocol was used (since her qi was grounded) in combination with HT-7 and SP-6 to calm spirit and build blood. The heavenly stem at the time of this treatment (and the treatments subsequently listed) was Gui, relating to the kidney organ. The earthly branch was Zi (rat), associated with the shao yin weather pattern and the gallbladder channel. Therefore, points were selected from the shao yin and gallbladder channels to calm the spirit, build blood, clear heat, and stop pain. (The gallbladder points benefited her heart due to the same movement pivot channel pairing.) |
| • *Infrared heat on her feet.*<br>• *Affirmation: "I am safe, healthy, and strong."* | Heat was directed to her feet to ground her energy. An affirmation was given to empower and settle her. |

## Fourth Visit

### CHANGES AFTER TREATMENT

| Subjective Changes | Her sleep and energy improved by 60 percent. She felt grounded, but had episodes of being un-centered and stirred up. Her neck was less tight (a 5 out of 10), and she only had two headaches since the last treatment. |
|---|---|
| Objective Changes | Vivian displayed sparkling Shen that showed her heart was strengthened. Her skin was red, there were small nodules at PC-7, her pulse had the blood heat quality, and her tongue was red. These signs indicated heat. Yet, her skin was glowing and her nose was much less dark. A bouncy liveliness emanated from her energy field. |

*See Figure 7.6.*

**TREATMENT**

| Modality | Explanation |
|---|---|
| *Acupuncture*<br>• Yin Tang (M-HN-3)<br>• Daling PC-7<br>• Zhongwan R-12<br>• Fuliu KD-7<br>• Jianjing GB-21 on the right<br>• Lingdao HT-4 on the left<br>• Yanglingquan GB-34 on the left<br>• Zulinqi GB-41 on the left | The previous treatment had calmed the trauma memory and freed her spirit. Vivian was feeling stronger and processing her past, a positive step in the direction toward resolving her trauma. However, the burst of energy and the processing of the trauma was exciting her heart and creating heat. Her Shen required stabilization and the heat needed to be cleared. An alternative to the "Gathering the Qi" protocol (substituting PC-7 for PC-6) was used to clear heat and nourish yin. The shao yin and gallbladder channels were used to stop neck pain and headaches. Opening the command point (GB-41) on the Dai vessel cleared heat and encouraged the release of her old trauma. |
| • *Taught the Shaking Qigong Form and a gentle qigong hip exercise.* | To trash out old energy and open the Dai vessel. |

## *Fifth Visit*
### CHANGES AFTER TREATMENT

| | |
|---|---|
| *Subjective Changes* | Vivian reported feeling increased joy and reduced pain in her hip (now down to 4 out of 10). Her headaches were fewer, but she now felt pain in her right-side neck and jaw due to teeth clenching. |
| *Objective Changes* | The redness in her tongue cleared (a dusky hue remained) and there were scallops on the sides. |

### TREATMENT

| Modality | Explanation |
|---|---|
| *Acupuncture*<br>• "Soothing the Trauma Memory" protocol<br>• Tinghui GB-2<br>• Sanyinjiao SP-6<br>• Shenmen HT-7 on the right<br>• Shaofu HT-8, Yangfu GB-38, and Xuanzhong GB-39 on the left | Vivian's qi was centered and the "Soothing the Trauma Memory" protocol could be used again. She was clenching her teeth, a sign of stagnation in the wood element due to water deficiency. Processing the trauma required a lot of energy and it created tension. Thus, points on the shao yang channel were selected to resolve her neck and jaw pain. The primary points were HT-8, GB-38, and GB-39, with HT-7 and GB-2 as guide points. |
| • *She was asked to increase rest time laying down.*<br>• *Affirmation: "I embody stillness, I am safe and protected."* | To benefit her Zhi. |

## *Sixth Visit*
### CHANGES AFTER TREATMENT

| | |
|---|---|
| *Subjective Changes* | She had less pain, but was experiencing surges of sadness and stress due to the holidays. She was feeling overwhelmed, reliving the horror of her husband's suicide. |
| *Objective Changes* | The darkness on her nose reduced. However, the line around her mouth was more pronounced, along with the disempowerment lines. She had increased swelling in her lower lip. She also had cloudy Shen in her eyes, pale skin, and increased darkness in her temples and under her eyes. Her chin appeared smaller and darker. Yet, transformation lines appeared and her skin tone was softer and illuminated. |

*See Figure 7.7.*

## Analysis

The patient was processing her husband's suicide. He had killed himself during the holidays, thus making this time of year especially difficult for Vivian. She reported reliving the memory of the trauma and certain facial diagnosis signs were enhanced. The cloudy eyes, pale bluish skin tone, darkness under her eyes, and darkness in her chin showed the tiredness of her kidneys from processing all the emotions. Her shrinking chin, increasing disempowerment lines, and deepening line around her mouth reflected her working through feeling powerless and abandoned. The darkness in her temples revealed stagnation of the liver as she wrestled with her feelings of depression. However, there was clarity in her Shen, as reflected in the illuminated skin tone, and an inner strength present (indicated by her stronger nose, i.e., her stronger spine/backbone). Although she was feeling extreme emotions, there was lucidity present. The transformation lines (diagonal lines on the forehead) indicated that her third eye had opened and she was advancing on her path, breaking free from the trauma memory.

### TREATMENT

| Modality | Explanation |
| --- | --- |
| *Acupuncture* <br> • "Gathering the Qi" protocol | The "Gathering the Qi" protocol was needed to center her and support her sense of strength. Revisiting this protocol helped her maneuver through the dark night. |
| • *Shamanic Journey Drumbeat.* <br> • *Infrared heat on her feet.* <br> • *Cupping on her upper back.* | Drumming and heat were utilized to ground her energy. Cupping was applied to stop pain in her shoulders and clear the old toxin of the trauma memory from her body. This assisted with her processing. |

## Seventh Visit

Vivian felt secure and was ready to start letting go of her husband's belongings. She had started to boost her physical activity and reorganize her house, which moderately aggravated her neck, hip, and back pain.

**TREATMENT**

| Modality | Explanation |
|---|---|
| *Acupuncture*<br>• Baihui DU-20<br>• Shenting DU-24<br>• Yinxi HT-6<br>• Zhongwan R-12<br>• Fuliu KD-7 | The patient was grounded and beginning to move forward. Half of the "Soothing the Trauma Memory" protocol was used to help continue to clear the charge of her trauma memory. She was processing several emotions which generated heat and depleted fluids; thus, HT-6 and KD-7 were selected to nourish her fluids and calm her spirit. |
| • *Affirmation: "I am calm and settled, moving forward with grace."* | To assist with processing the trauma memory. |

## After the Rounds of Treatments

**CHANGES AFTER TREATMENT**

| *Subjective Changes* | Vivian had removed more of her late husband's belongings from her house and was feeling less triggered by memories of him. She felt grounded. She was able to work again, finish school, and apply for her massage license. Her energy was improved and she was sleeping soundly. All pains reduced to 4 out of 10. |
|---|---|
| *Objective Changes* | Her face was rosy, glowing, and clear. Joy and clarity were in her eyes. Her philtrum had lightened and the line down the center was reduced. Disempowerment, grief, irritation, wei qi, and over-nurturing lines lessened. Her chin was stable and less red. The swelling under her lip diminished. Her nose appeared stronger and its darkness had faded. |

*See Figure 7.8.*

## Summary

*See Figure 7.9.*

Vivian was frozen in the past, with memories of her late husband taking his life. It had left her disoriented and stuck, powerless to step forward on her path. The car accident served as a blessing in disguise to unlock the trapped trauma. Chinese medicine stabilized her Shen and strengthened her Zhi so that she could process her trauma and continue on with her life. The pictures taken throughout her treatments document her metamorphosis. She was mired in the trauma, then opened to growth, then deeply processed the stored trauma, and finally emerged from being trapped in her past. Acupuncture, shamanic drum healing, affirmations, lifestyle modifications, and dietary recommendations provided her with the means to navigate through the dark night and appear on the other side, grounded and clear. Vivian stood strong and found her passion as a massage therapist and an avid gardener. She embodied the universal spirit with beauty.

# Case 3: 60-Year-Old Female Conquered Her Fear

## *Initial Visit*

### *Background*

"Lulu" was crossing the street when she was hit by a car and knocked to the ground. Her left knee, right elbow, and rib area were bruised. Lulu came to the clinic 26 days after being hit, feeling shaken and fearful. She had swelling on her knee and was unable to flex it. Her right elbow area and rib were tender to the touch. Every time she thought about the trauma, she experienced indigestion and waves of powerlessness and fatigue.

*See Figure 7.10.*

### *Diagnosis*

Scattered Qi with Liver Qi and Blood Stagnation, Heat, and Kidney Qi Deficiency.

**SUPPORTING SIGNS OF LULU'S DIAGNOSIS**

| Diagnosis | Signs |
|---|---|
| Scattered Qi | • Dusky Shen and clouded/red third eye.<br>• Scattered pulse and an overall smooth vibration quality. |
| Liver Qi and Blood Stagnation | • Significant irritation lines, deep lines coming down from the corners of her mouth, darkness in her temples, dusky Shen, and anger in her eyes.<br>• Tightness in the pericardium channel. |
| Heat in the Blood | • Redness in her third eye and red chin.<br>• Small, firm nodules around HT-6 to HT-7 and tightness in the pericardium channel.<br>• Slippery pulse.<br>• Dry tongue coat and a deep center crack. |
| Kidney Qi Deficiency with Stagnation | • Darkness under her eyes, a bumpy quality to her chin, and a dusky, marbled look to her whole face (especially on her forehead).<br>• Stick-like change at KD-3.<br>• Soft pulse.<br>• Pale tongue. |

TREATMENTS (FIRST AND SECOND VISITS)

| Modality | Explanation |
|---|---|
| *Acupuncture*<br>• "Gathering the Qi" protocol<br>• Yingu KD-10 on the right | The first two treatments consisted of the "Gathering the Qi" protocol. KD-10 on the right side was added to regulate and tonify the kidneys, clear damp accumulation, and reduce her knee and elbow pain. |
| • *Infrared heat on her abdomen.*<br>• *Shamanic Journey Drumbeat.*<br>• *Affirmation: "I am safe and protected."* | The Shamanic Journey Drumbeat and infrared heat were used to center her energy. The affirmation was given to instill courage. |

Lulu felt grounded and less fearful after these treatments. Her face was softer, and the intense anger had diminished. Over the span of nine days, her pains were reduced, especially in the elbow. On the way to the clinic for her third treatment Lulu was almost hit by a car when she was crossing the street. This incident triggered her fear and the trauma memory.

## Third Visit

TREATMENTS (THIRD AND FOURTH VISITS)

| Modality | Explanation |
|---|---|
| *Acupuncture*<br>• "Soothing the Trauma Memory" protocol<br>• Neiguan PC-6<br>• Taixi KD-3<br>• Yingu KD-10 on the right<br>• Shaohai HT-3 on the right<br>• Rangu KD-2 on the left | The "Soothing the Trauma Memory" protocol was applied since she was centered. PC-6 was used to calm her spirit and stop the knee pain. The treatment was in December; the earthly branch is Zi (shao yin weather pattern) and heavenly stem is Gui (kidney organ). Thus, KD-3 was substituted for SP-6 to address her kidney deficiency. HT-3 was used to stop elbow pain and stabilize her spirit. KD-2 (the ying-spring point) was activated to reduce inflammation in the kidney channel. |

See Figure 7.11.

## After Four Treatments

See Figure 7.12.

Lulu reported a reduction in fear and was feeling calmer. The triggering of the old trauma was less intense and she had begun walking to work again, reporting flexibility and reduced pain in her knee. Her rib pain resolved and her elbow pain was minimal.

Several diagnostic signs changed over the 15-day period: less redness in her third eye, softening of both the irritation lines and of the lines coming down from the corners of her mouth, lightening in her temples and Shen, and a lessening of the anger in her eyes. The darkness under her eyes faded, her chin was less red/bumpy, and the stick-like change found at KD-3 was significantly reduced—reflecting the reduction of inflammation and strengthening of her kidneys. Her Shen softened and brightened, and her face became round and full—revealing her grounded spirit. Her pulse was stronger and its scattered quality resolved, indicating stabilized Shen and increased energy.

### Summary

*See Figure 7.13.*

One of the most remarkable transformations for Lulu was the transformation of fear. After the four treatments, the shock and frozen aspect of her Shen resolved (her Zhi was stabilized). The change in the shape of her face demonstrated a significant increase in her earth energy and grounding. She resumed her routine of walking to work, felt secure, and wanted to be more engaged with life (the unfreezing of water freed her Hun). Lulu continued Chinese medicine treatment and was encouraged to dance—something she had always enjoyed. She also started seeing a professional for EMDR to assist with resolving old trauma. The "Gathering the Qi" and "Soothing the Trauma Memory" protocols were used, as needed, while she processed old trauma uncovered by the EMDR.

## Case 4: 36-Year-Old Female Restored Her Motivation

### Initial Visit

#### Background

"Tasha" had recently divorced and become the sole guardian of her six-year-old son. She had endured several subsequent relationships/breakups and said it was like she kept "starting over" every few years. Tasha, feeling discouraged, stressed, fearful, and lonely, encountered a resurgence of past trauma. When she was two years old, her mom died and she had grown up feeling abandoned. The stress was causing shoulder pain, neck tension, fatigue, and food cravings. Tasha was seeing a counselor and was hoping to get additional relief from Chinese medicine.

*See Figure 7.14.*

#### Diagnosis

Scattered Qi, Heat in the Blood, Blood Stagnation, Damp Accumulation, Tai Yin Deficiency, and an Underlying Kidney Deficiency.

## SUPPORTING SIGNS OF TASHA'S DIAGNOSIS

| Diagnosis | Signs |
|---|---|
| Scattered Qi | • Muddy, clouded Shen and a cloudy third eye.<br>• Overall smooth vibration pulse quality. |
| Heat in the Blood | • Red face (especially redness on the upper lip, red swollen nose, and a red, dimpled chin).<br>• Red tongue. |
| Blood Stagnation | • Nodules at PC-6 and LI-6 to LI-9. |
| Damp Accumulation | • Personal grief lines.<br>• Puffiness in her legs (especially along the spleen channel).<br>• Slippery pulse.<br>• Greasy tongue coat. |
| Tai Yin Deficiency | • Pale nose bridge and disempowerment lines. |
| Underlying Kidney Deficiency | • Faint line around her mouth, darkness under her eyes, dark Shen, and a dimpled chin. |

## FIRST TREATMENT AND OUTCOME

| Treatment | Result |
|---|---|
| • "Gathering the Qi" protocol.<br>• *Shamanic Journey Drumbeat.*<br>• *Counseled on a heat-reducing diet.* | Eight days after the first visit, she reported a significant decrease in fear but felt worried. Her shoulder and neck tension was reduced and she was recovering from the stomach flu. The redness and swelling in her face lessened and her Shen was brighter. |

## *Second Visit*
### TREATMENT

| Modality | Explanation |
|---|---|
| *Acupuncture*<br>• Shenting DU-24<br>• Zhongwan R-12<br>• Sanyinjiao SP-6<br>• Shaofu HT-8<br>• Auricular points: Shen Men, Stomach, and Anxiety | Tasha was grounded; thus a point from the "Soothing the Trauma Memory" protocol was combined with aspects of the "Gathering the Qi" protocol. HT-8 was substituted for PC-6 to clear heat. The auricular points were added to assist with calming and counter food cravings. |

## Third Visit

TREATMENT

| Modality | Explanation |
|---|---|
| *Acupuncture*<br>• Baihui DU-20<br>• Shenting DU-24<br>• Yinxi HT-6<br>• Gongsun SP-4<br>• Auricular points: Shen Men, Stomach, and Anxiety | Tasha was improved—the heat had significantly cleared, as seen in the reduction of redness in her face and tongue. The third treatment incorporated the "Soothing the Trauma Memory" protocol and continued to address the heat in the blood. HT-6 was used to regulate the heart blood and clear heat. SP-6 was replaced with SP-4 to open the Chong vessel and clear the trauma revolving around her mom's death. |
| • *Cupping on her upper back.* | Cupping was applied to reduce her pain and lift the trauma memory from her energy field. |

*See Figure 7.15.*

## Fourth Visit

TREATMENT

| Modality | Explanation |
|---|---|
| *Acupuncture*<br>• "Soothing the Trauma Memory" protocol<br>• Chize LU-5<br>• Yinlingquan SP-9<br>• Auricular points: Shen Men, Stomach, and Anxiety | She was grounded and her heat had cleared; thus the fourth treatment engaged the whole protocol of "Soothing the Trauma Memory." The he-sea points on the tai yin channel were included to regulate the qi. |

*See Figure 7.16.*

Tasha reported minimal fear and worry and was less triggered by her trauma memories. She felt motivated and subsequently registered to take the licensed clinical social worker exam that she had put off for months. Her energy improved and she felt the courage to take her son on a road trip. The food cravings Tasha had struggled with resolved and she had the impetus to begin exercising.

Tasha's face changed significantly after the series of treatments. Her skin tone and eyes were vibrant and sparkling, the redness, bloating, and greasiness of her skin cleared, and she had less darkness under her eyes. Her third eye opened, the strength in her chin improved, and the personal grief and disempowerment lines softened. The puffiness in her legs and the nodules in the pericardium and large intestine channels were reduced. The smooth vibration pulse quality abated, and the thick tongue coating disappeared.

## Summary

*See Figure 7.17.*

Tasha's case demonstrated a smooth transition from the "Gathering the Qi" to "Soothing the Trauma Memory" protocols. It also exemplified the regimen of first centering her energy, then clearing excess, followed by addressing the underlying trauma, and finally regulating the qi to process the shock of her mom's death.

A few months after the series of treatments, Tasha reported a strong fear of flying. Using a combination of the "Gathering the Qi" and "Soothing the Trauma Memory" protocols, she confidently flew to California with minimal issues. A few weeks later, Tasha passed her licensing exam and took a position managing a counseling program at a pediatric clinic. All these accomplishments reflected her empowerment and confidence to move forward on her life path.

## Case 5: 59-Year-Old Male Realized His Self-Assurance

### Initial Visit

*Background*

"Stuart" was physically assaulted by a female co-worker and put on a temporary leave of absence. The event was emasculating. Although he was innocent of any wrongdoing, he was ostracized from his workplace, which created emotional trauma and triggered an old pattern of being bullied. It also brought up his feelings of not having faith in authority and not being supported. He felt incredibly anxious, defeated, and unable to cope with his situation; he sought help with Chinese medicine. Stuart's diagnosis was scattered qi with heart qi and blood deficiency. He underwent treatments to center his energy, soothe the trauma memory, and improve his feeling of self-worth. He took the Chinese herbal formula modification of Gan Mai Da Zao Tang (Licorice, Wheat, and Jujube Decoction with Bai He (Bulbus Lilii), Long Gu (Os Draconis), Hu Po (Succinum), and Yuan Zhi (Radix Polygalae)) and did affirmations.

Two months later, Stuart felt secure and returned to the workplace. It took some adjustment, but in time he was again interacting with his co-workers and felt like things were getting back to normal. One morning an inappropriate drawing was taped to his computer monitor and it sent him into a negative spiral. The "Gathering the Qi" protocol was used and his self-worth was recovered.

Stuart felt settled and reported the inappropriate drawing to the human resources department, which launched an investigation. The drawing had triggered the memory of the assault and caused bouts of anxiety. During this time, he was rear-ended and suffered low back and neck pain. He returned to the clinic for help. Stuart had a

meeting scheduled the next day with several department heads to discuss the drawing and he felt especially distressed about the outcome of the meeting.
*See Figure 7.18.*

## Diagnosis

Destabilized Po, Liver Qi Stagnation, and Ungrounded Shen.

**SUPPORTING SIGNS OF STUART'S DIAGNOSIS**

| Diagnosis | Signs |
|---|---|
| Destabilized Po | • Deep grief lines, sad eyes, and lines in the wei qi area.<br>• His energy field was perceived as weak and fragile. |
| Liver qi stagnation, ungrounded Shen, and an inability to grasp the bigger picture | • Red, cloudy third eye.<br>• Tense pulse. |

**TREATMENT**

| Modality | Explanation |
|---|---|
| *Acupuncture*<br>• "Soothing the Trauma Memory" protocol<br>• Neiguan PC-6<br>• Zhongwan R-12<br>• Sanyinjiao SP-6<br>• Shenmai UB-62 on the right<br>• Da Bai 22.04 and Ling Gu 22.05 on the left | Stuart needed a combination of gathering and soothing to build self-love, open his third eye, establish healthy boundaries, and stabilize his spirit. Points were added to relieve his right-side, low back pain. |
| • *EFT homework.*<br>• *Affirmation: "I am strong and I stand up for myself."* | To stabilize his Po and Shen. |

## Second Visit

Stuart returned seven days later and said he felt strong and had held his ground in the meeting (his back pain had also reduced). His face shifted from having a look of defeat to a person engaged in dealing with the trauma. Stuart was processing, and his grief lines, sad eyes, and lines in the wei qi area resolved. Stuart's tense pulse reduced and his Shen was present.

Stuart felt closure with the traumatic situation, akin to successfully passing a test. His third eye had remarkably opened, reflecting his realization that the initial assault had been a catalyst for him to finally claim his energy. A feeling of security and calm was detected in his energy field that had not been present before.
*See Figure 7.19.*

A similar treatment was applied to reduce the charge of the trauma memory and to ground Stuart. SI-3, the command point of the Du vessel, was substituted for PC-6 to bolster his courage and to reduce the pain throughout his spine from the car accident (literally and figuratively to strengthen his backbone). R-6 was added to build his qi and fortify his yang.

**TREATMENT**

| Modality |
| --- |
| *Acupuncture* |
| • "Soothing the Trauma Memory" protocol |
| • Houxi SI-3 |
| • Zhongwan R-12 |
| • Qihai R-6 |
| • Sanyinjiao SP-6 |
| • *Infrared heat on his feet.* |
| • *Refilled Gan Mai Da Zao Tang Modified Formula.* |

*See Figure 7.20.*

## Summary

*See Figure 7.21.*

Stuart had initially regained his confidence to return to the workplace after the initial series of treatments, but was still trapped in a cycle of reliving the trauma memory. The two treatments chronicled in this case demonstrate the freeing of a pattern. Stuart achieved clarity of his situation and processed the old trauma. Having cleared a pattern of victimization, he reclaimed a sense of self-assurance and advanced on his life path.

# Case 6: 78-Year-Old Female Returned to the Source

## Initial visit

### Background

"Marilyn" received devastating news from her Western medical doctor. The medication she was taking to treat her atrial fibrillations (A-Fibs) was too strong for her heart and he said her heart was too weak to undergo pacemaker surgery. He told her to discontinue all heart medication, "think positive," and then he released her from care.

Frustrated and scared, she decided to try Chinese medicine. Marilyn was having intense A-Fibs (during which her heart rate went up to 235 bpm) and strong sensations of heat. She was also experiencing extreme fatigue, anxiety, and low back and leg pains.

Marilyn was traumatized by having been released from Western medical treatment and was hoping anything would help.

*See Figure 7.22.*

## Diagnosis

Scattered Qi, Damp Accumulation, Blood Stagnation, and Heart Yin Deficiency with Heat.

### SUPPORTING SIGNS OF MARILYN'S DIAGNOSIS

| Diagnosis | Signs |
|---|---|
| Scattered Qi | Disoriented and vacant Shen.<br>Energy field felt muddy. |
| Damp Accumulation | Moist face and thick upper eyelids.<br>Puffy/swollen sensation detected on palpation of the spleen channel.<br>Enlarged, scalloped tongue.<br>Energy field was perceived as heavy. |
| Blood Stagnation | Dusky nose tip and tongue.<br>Choppy pulse. |
| Heart Yin Deficiency with Heat | Multiple lines on her nose tip (also some red-colored areas), three-sided eyes, flushed cheeks, and red lower eyelids.<br>Feeble absent quality pulse in her heart position.<br>Overall thin pulse.<br>Red, dry tongue.<br>Nodules on the san jiao channel. |

### INITIAL TREATMENT

| Modality | Explanation |
|---|---|
| *Acupuncture*<br>• Yin Tang (M-HN-3)<br>• Chize LU-5<br>• Yinlingquan SP-9<br>• Diji SP-8<br>• Yanglingquan GB-34 | Marilyn needed hope and grounding to move forward after hearing the news from her Western medical doctor. Her earth element was weak and congested, causing dampness. The accumulation of fluids and blood strained her heart and kidneys and produced intense A-Fibs. A modification of the "Gathering the Qi" protocol was used. (The time of treatment was in July.) Thus, points on the tai yin channel were active. The heavenly branch is Ji, relating to spleen, and the earthly branch is Wei, associated with the tai yin weather pattern. LU-5 and SP-9 were substituted for PC-6 and SP-6, to regulate qi, liberate the Yi, and regulate the fluids. The xi-cleft point, SP-8, was added to regulate the blood. GB-34, a he-sea point, was selected to address her heart and regulate the blood. It was also selected to regulate overaction of wood on earth since Marilyn was frustrated and angry that Western medicine could not help her. |

## *Treatment Series*

FOLLOW-UP TREATMENT SERIES

| Modality | Explanation |
|---|---|
| *Acupuncture*<br>• Shenting DU-24<br>• Baihui DU-20<br>• Laogong PC-8 or Neihuan PC-6<br>• Shaofu HT-8 or Shenmen HT-7<br>• Yinlingquan SP-9<br>• Zusanli ST-36 | After the initial treatment, Marilyn responded well and the A-Fibs reduced. She underwent several acupuncture treatments that focused on benefiting earth, clearing heat, tonifying the heart, and calming the spirit. These varied between points on the heart or pericardium channels and incorporated both the "Gathering the Qi" and "Soothing the Trauma Memory" protocols. When there was strong heat present, the ying-spring points, PC-8 and HT-8, were needled. Other points with similar functions were substituted depending on the month of treatment. |

## *After the Treatment Series*

Over several months of treatment, Marilyn underwent a great transformation. She felt calmer, experienced minimal A-Fibs, and her heat abated. Marilyn was happy and had the energy to engage with neighbors and do activities. She went to see her Western medical doctor and he determined she was strong enough to have pacemaker surgery and to resume taking Western medication.

Marilyn continued Chinese medicine treatments one to two times per month. Her energy improved and she found a healthy balance between activity and resting. Her nose tip (representing the heart) transformed dramatically over the months of treatment.

*See Figure 7.23.*

## *Summary*

*See Figure 7.24.*

TRANSFORMATION OF MARILYN'S DIAGNOSTIC SIGNS

| Initial Diagnosis | Transformation of Signs |
|---|---|
| Scattered Qi | • Energy field felt light, sparkly, and harmonized. |
| Damp Accumulation | • Greasy sheen to Marilyn's skin cleared.<br>• Spleen channel was less puffy.<br>• Enlarged tongue reduced. |
| Blood Stagnation | • Nose tip changed to pink.<br>• Choppy pulse and dusky tongue cleared up. |
| Heart Yin Deficiency with Heat | • Red and lined areas on nose cleared.<br>• Three-sided eyes disappeared.<br>• Flushed cheeks cleared.<br>• Redness in lower eyelids reduced.<br>• Reduction of nodules in the san jiao channel. |

*See Figure 7.25.*

Emotional trauma can stem from being given a medical diagnosis or, in this case, a release from Western medical treatment. Marilyn was traumatized, but had the will to seek another solution. Chinese medicine alleviated her symptoms and, more importantly, strengthened her to have heart surgery and resume taking medication. Ultimately, Chinese medicine and Western medicine worked together and offered the best care to Marilyn.

### *Returning to the Source*

*See Figure 7.26.*

Ancient Chinese wisdom traditions emphasize returning to the source by embodying a child-like innocence, while retaining the accumulated wisdom of a lifetime. As people age, it is common for the proportions of the five elements to shift. The goal is for the person to return to their original elemental makeup. Marilyn's progression, from a baby (earth-fire), to a teen (fire-metal), to a grown woman (wood-water), to that in her recent picture (earth-fire), exhibits the shift back to her earthy, fiery nature. Chinese medicine—along with her phenomenal spirit—assisted Marilyn with reclaiming a grounded, jovial spirit.

## Summary of Case Studies

Emotional trauma can stem from a variety of conditions—from childhood and physical trauma to fear of mortality. Chinese medicine stabilizes a person, enabling them to process past trauma. Establishing harmony between the organ systems and channels allows a patient to move forward on their path, resilient to endure future traumas, and to share their talents. Patience on the part of the practitioner helps the person untangle ingrained beliefs and blockages. Staging the treatments from a global outlook to a more detailed approach ultimately brings quick trauma resolution and frees the patient from reliving the memory and "being stuck." The ancestors of Chinese medicine and shamanism bestowed great gifts to the modern-day practitioner. May the human family continue discovering gems to enlarge the treasure trove of this time-honored medicine.

**Reference**

Holman, C.T. (2016) "The treatment of emotional trauma and PTSD with Chinese medicine." *Journal of Chinese Medicine 112*, 35–51.

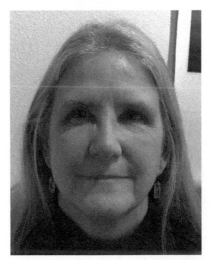

*Figure 7.1 Grace at initial visit*

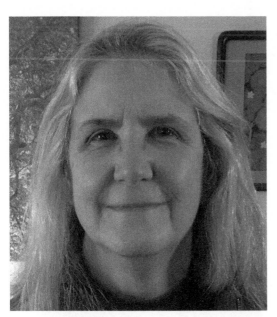

*Figure 7.2 Grace at second visit*

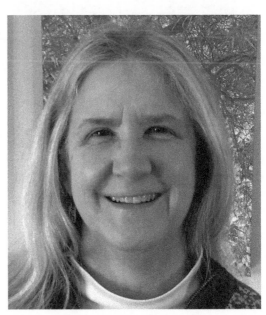

*Figure 7.3 Grace after treatments*

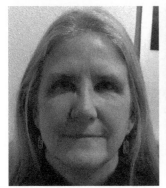
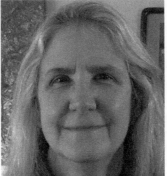
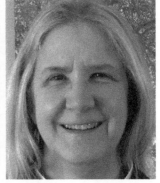

*Figure 7.4 Grace's transformation*

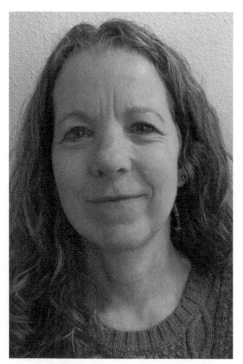

*Figure 7.5 Vivian at third visit, the beginning of documenting her case*

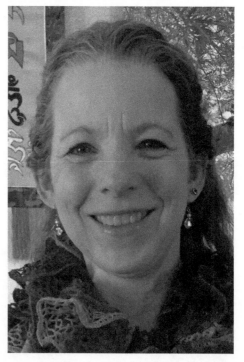

*Figure 7.6 Vivian at fourth visit*

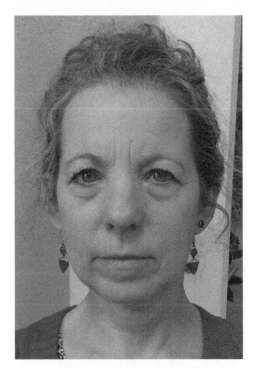

*Figure 7.7 Vivian at sixth visit*

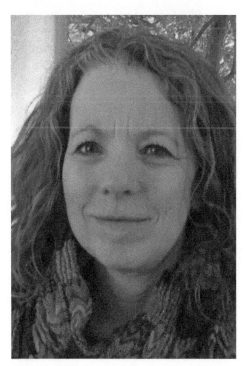

*Figure 7.8 Vivian after treatments*

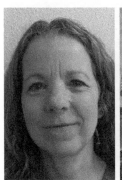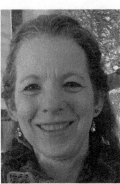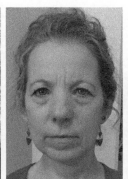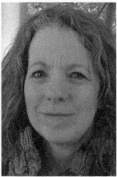

*Figure 7.9 Vivian's transformation*

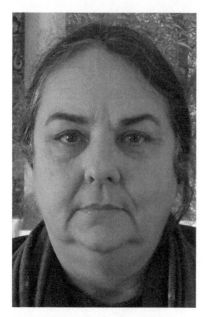

*Figure 7.10 Lulu at initial visit*

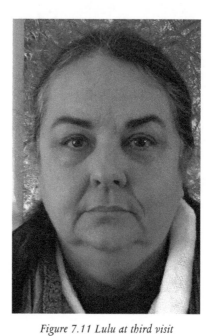

*Figure 7.11 Lulu at third visit*

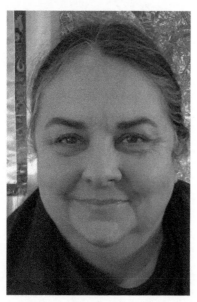

*Figure 7.12 Lulu after treatments*

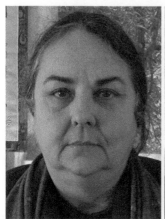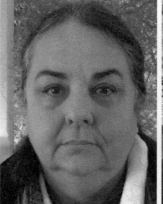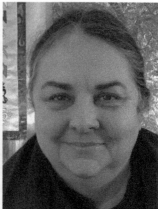

*Figure 7.13 Lulu's transformation*

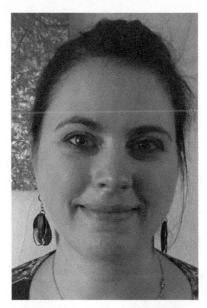

*Figure 7.14 Tasha at initial visit*

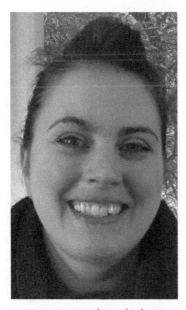

*Figure 7.15 Tasha at third visit*

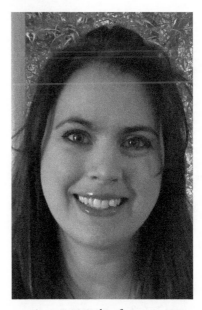

*Figure 7.16 Tasha after treatments*

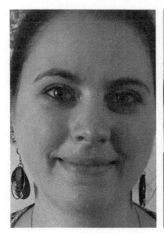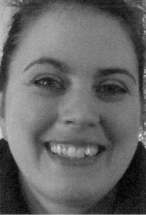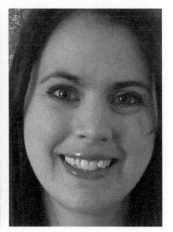

*Figure 7.17 Tasha's transformation*

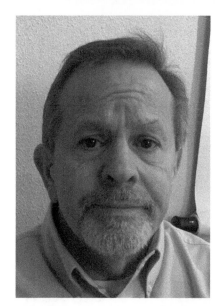

*Figure 7.18 Stuart at initial visit*

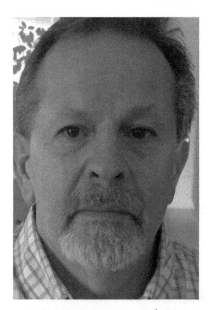

*Figure 7.19 Stuart at second visit*

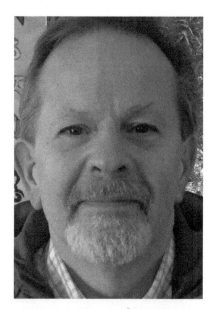

*Figure 7.20 Stuart after treatments*

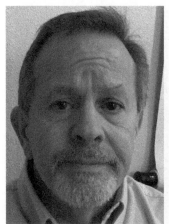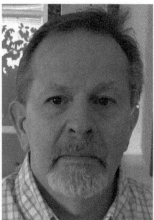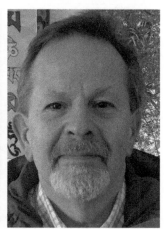

*Figure 7.21 Stuart's transformation*

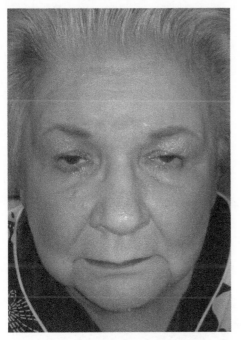

*Figure 7.22 Marilyn at initial visit*

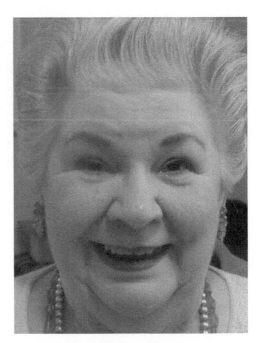

*Figure 7.23 Marilyn after treatments*

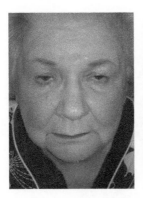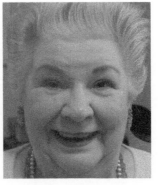

*Figure 7.24 Marilyn's transformation*

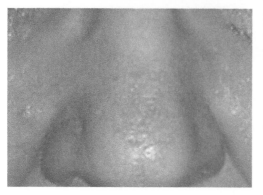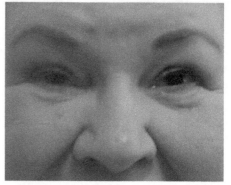

*Figure 7.25 Marilyn's nose before and after the treatment series*

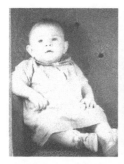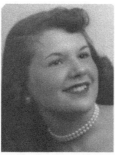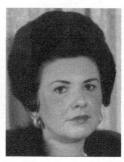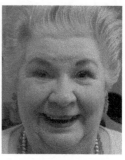

*Figure 7.26 Progression through Marilyn's lifetime demonstrating the five elemental proportional changes*

# Eight Limbs of Chinese Medicine

The eight limbs of Chinese medicine[1] are akin to rungs on a ladder. People are encouraged to utilize and rely primarily on those modalities ("rungs") at the top of the ladder. The bottom rung represents the most invasive treatment, and the top rung represents the least invasive, that is, the patient is solely in charge of their healing. However, there are times when invasive measures are needed based on the severity of the pathogen. Some of the rungs are paired because of their interdependent nature. The goal of Chinese medicine is to instill confidence in patients and increase their practice of the upper rung modalities. Modern society typically wants immediate results, but the upper rungs require increased time and effort. With repetition and experience, patients actualize their self-healing power that in many ways outshines intervention methods. However, there are conditions that require medical attention in addition to the upper-rung modalities.

The limbs or rungs are as follows (from top to bottom):

1. **Mind:** Meditation, qigong, prayer, affirmations, visualizations—anything that changes the psychological state. The patient is fully in charge of the healing process.

2. **Diet:** Food and fluids. Proper nutritional choices are essential for healthy organ systems. The patient oversees these choices. Diet, paired with exercise, is the yin aspect.

3. **Exercise:** Exercise (the yang of the diet and exercise pair) keeps the body moving and the channels open. The adage "the door hinge that keeps moving does not rust" encapsulates the importance of exercise. Exercise is paired with diet because without proper nutrition the body would not have the energy for physical activity.

---

1    Personal training with Nam Singh.

4. **Geomancy or Feng Shui:** This is the science of placement. Where a person lives, the design of their home, the arrangement of the contents in their home or business, and so on all affect health. It is at this rung when intervention is needed by an expert to provide accurate advice. This rung is paired with Astrology.

5. **Astrology:** The science of timing is applied to many aspects of life, including for example marriage, health, and business. The patient is less in control of their health and an expert is needed.

6. **Massage/Tui Na:** At this rung, someone is placing their hands on the patient.

7. **Acupuncture:** An expert inserts needles into the patient.

8. **Herbal Medicine:** This is the most invasive treatment. Chinese herbal medicine, which includes plants/minerals/animal products, ends up in the patient's bloodstream.

# Clear Broth Soups

Clear broth soups are foundational to Chinese medicine dietetics. One cup a day is recommended as an efficient means to assimilate nutrients, infuse strength into the organs, and restore the earth element after trauma. Emotional trauma scatters energy and weakens the earth element, creating spleen and stomach deficiency, making it difficult to digest foods. These clear, long-cooked soups deliver a variety of nutrients to benefit digestion. Given busy lives, concocting soup is viewed as a time-consuming and daunting task. However, soups are one of the easiest dishes to prepare, made simply by chopping up vegetables and roots and putting them—along with animal organs—into a pot of water. The broth can be added easily as a side dish to any meal. Breakfast is a meal that frequently lacks protein, and soup is a wonderful addition.

## Animal Organ Soups

Classically, in Chinese culture, if a person has a problem with some part of their body, then they eat that same part of an animal. For example, a person with tendonitis would eat animal tendons, or someone with cardiovascular issues would eat animal heart. The organ meats also benefit the emotional body. For instance, a patient lacking courage would benefit from eating animal liver. This elementary yet powerful approach enhances the other modalities used when treating emotional trauma.

There are many animal organ soup combinations possible. Those listed below all have the same base ingredients of roots and vegetables. Organic roots, vegetables, and organs are recommended. Many grocery stores and markets can specially order organs if they are not already stocked. The variety of roots and vegetables in the soup stock mask the organ taste. However, for those who do not wish to use organ meats, simply use the roots and vegetables to nourish the body and support the digestive system. The vegetable/root stock is the same for each of the five organ soups and can be modified based on the time of the year when the vegetables are in season.

## THE FIVE ANIMAL ORGAN SOUPS

| Soup | Animal Organs Used | Action |
|---|---|---|
| **The Great Communicator** | • Heart<br>• Tongue<br>• Kidney | • Harmonizes the heart and kidney<br>• Nourishes yin<br>• Clears heat<br>• Stabilizes the Shen<br>• Tonifies the Zhi |
| **Determined Leader** | • Liver<br>• Kidney (can substitute with oxtail) | • Nourishes yin and blood<br>• Stabilizes the Hun<br>• Strengthens the Zhi |
| **The Root of Inspiration** | • Heart<br>• Oxtail | • Nourishes the heart and kidney yin<br>• Settles the heart mirror<br>• Harmonizes the heart and kidney |
| **Fortify the Will** | • Kidney<br>• Oxtail | • Nourishes the water element<br>• Strengthens the Zhi<br>• Consolidates the Jing |
| **Super Qi and Blood** | • Liver<br>• Heart<br>• Spleen | • Builds blood and qi<br>• Supports the Hun, Shen, and Yi<br>• Calms the spirit<br>• Benefits digestion |

## VEGETABLES AND ROOTS FOR THE BASE SOUP STOCK

| | |
|---|---|
| Beets | Two medium-sized bunches |
| Carrots | Eight or nine large |
| Celery | One bunch |
| Turnips | One bunch |
| Daikon | One large |
| Sweet Potatoes | Two or three large |
| Celery Root | One large |
| Rutabaga | One or two medium |
| Ginger Root (optional) | One half |

## *Cooking Directions*

Chop the ingredients into one-inch pieces and place them, along with the organs, in approximately six to eight liters of filtered water with two tablespoons of vinegar and one teaspoon of sea salt. Bring to a boil and simmer for four to five hours. Some chefs will allow the soup to cook for 24 hours in a crock pot to extract more energy from the ingredients. However, four to five hours is sufficient.

# Suggested Resources

## Books

*Fourth Uncle in the Mountain* by Quang van Nguyen and Marjorie Pivar

*Opening the Dragon Gate* by Chen Kaiguo and Zheng Shunchao

*Face Reading in Chinese Medicine, Second Edition* by Lillian Pearl Bridges

*Tian Gan Di Zhi, Heavenly Stems and Earthly Branches* by Master Zhongxian Wu

*Seeking the Spirit of the Book of Change* by Master Zhongxian Wu

*Vital Breath of the Dao* by Master Zhongxian Wu

*Applied Channel Theory in Chinese Medicine* by Wang Ju-Yi and Jason Robertson

*Lectures on Tung Acupuncture System: Points Study* by Wei-Chieh Young

*Lectures on Tung Acupuncture System: Therapeutic System* by Wei-Chieh Young

*The Five Transport Points* by Wei-Chieh Young

*Chinese Pulse Diagnosis: A Contemporary Approach* by Leon Hammer

*Clinical Handbook of Internal Medicine, Volumes 1–3* by Will Maclean and Jane Lyttleton

*Five Spirits: Alchemical Acupuncture for Psychological and Spiritual Healing* by Lorie Dechar

*Psycho-Emotional Pain and the Eight Extraordinary Vessels* by Yvonne R. Farrell

*Atlas of Tongue Diagnosis, Volume 2* by Barbara Kirschbaum

*The Body Keeps the Score: Brain, Mind, and Body in the Healing of Trauma* by Bessel Van der Kolk

*It Didn't Start with You: How Inherited Family Trauma Shapes Who We Are and How to End the Cycle* by Mark Wolynn

*The Upward Spiral: Using Neuroscience to Reverse the Course Depression, One Small Change at a Time* by Alex Korb

*Peace is Every Step* by Thich Nhat Hanh

*Road to Heaven: Encounters with Chinese Hermits* by Bill Porter

*Monkey and the Monk: An Abridgement to The Journey to the West* translated by Anthony C. Yu

*Waking the Tiger: Healing Trauma* by Peter Levine and Ann Frederick

*You Can Heal Your Life* by Louise Hay

*The Key to Self-Liberation* by Christiane Beerlandt

## Films

*Red Beard* directed by Akira Kurosawa

*Amongst White Clouds* directed by Edward A. Burger

*Happy* directed by Roko Belic

## Websites and Seminars

Lillian Pearl Bridges: https://lotusinstitute.com

Master Zhongxian Wu: www.masterwu.net

Dr. Wang Ju-Yi: http://channelpalpation.org

Jason Robertson: http://kentuckyginseng.com

Dr. Wei-Chieh Young (Master Tung Style Acupuncture): www.drweichiehyoung.com

Susan Johnson: http://tungspoints.com/seminars

Shen/Hammer Pulse Diagnostic System: www.dragonrises.org

Nam Singh/Academy of Cooking with Herbs of China: +1(415) 334-0616

Shamanic Drumming/Toby Christensen: www.healingdrummer.com

C.T. Holman: www.redwoodspring.com

# Subject Index

# Author Index

**CT Holman** practices Chinese medicine in Salem, Oregon. His full-time clinic was founded in 2001. CT teaches courses internationally, operates a mentorship program, and is the Director of Development for the Lotus Institute. He studied in China (1999, 2001, and 2003) and has extensive post-graduate education with several leading teachers in the field. CT helped edit and contribute to the textbook, *Applied Channel Theory in Chinese Medicine* and has been published in the *Journal of Chinese Medicine*. He trains masters and doctoral students as an off-site supervisor of the Oregon College of Oriental Medicine. *www.redwoodspring.com*